THE Mulligan Concept
OF Manual Therapy, 2e

THE Mulligan Concept

OF Manual Therapy, 2e

textbook of techniques

Wayne Hing, PhD, MSc (Hons), ADP(OMT), Dip MT, Dip Phys, FNZCP
Toby Hall, PhD, MSc, Post Grad Dip Manip Ther, FACP
Brian Mulligan, Dip MT, FNZSP (Hon)

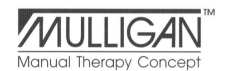

ELSEVIER

Elsevier Australia. ACN 001 002 357
(a division of Reed International Books Australia Pty Ltd)
Tower 1, 475 Victoria Avenue, Chatswood, NSW 2067

ISBN: 978-0-7295-4282-1

National Library of Australia Cataloguing-in-Publication Data

A catalogue record for this book is available from the National Library of Australia

NATIONAL LIBRARY OF AUSTRALIA

Senior Content Strategist: Melinda McEvoy
Content Project Manager: Fariha Nadeem
Edited by Christine Wyard
Proofread by Matt Davies
Cover by Lisa Petroff
Index by Innodata Indexing
Typeset by Toppan Best-set Premedia Limited
Printed in China by RR Donnelley

Last digit is the print number: 9 8 7 6 5 4 3 2

Contents

Foreword

I thank Elsevier for pressuring, in a nice way, Professor Wayne Hing and Dr Toby Hall to write a second edition of this textbook on my concepts. In this edition are technique improvements that needed to be shared as well as new essential techniques. I must again acknowledge and thank my teaching colleagues Mark Oliver and Frank Gargano for the new techniques and material they have contributed.

I believe the contents of this book, in its second edition, are priceless. All who deal with musculoskeletal conditions and practise manual therapy should have a copy.

As I stated in the first edition, what makes our concepts so special is that when indicated they are immediately effective. The Mobilisation With Movement techniques described within this book are only to be used when they produce no pain when indicated and, of course, are immediately effective. I know of no other manual therapy concepts for the entire body that follow these guidelines. What is really special about them is that it only takes about two minutes to decide whether they are indicated. Not to be able to use our concepts may be denying patients their best treatment option. I now have many hours of video showing the efficacy of our concepts, from personally treating patients on stage in many cities in America before my peers. The hundreds who have witnessed these occasions are left in no doubt as to the efficacy of these techniques because of the regular positive and instant pain-free outcomes. I should add that when I lecture on our concepts I always treat patients on stage to show what we can do – it is much better than telling people what we can do.

Forgive the repetition, but our concepts have come a long way from 1985 when, by chance, I had an unexpected instant pain-free success with a traumatised finger using what are now known as 'Mobilisations With Movement'. The patient, who was a young woman in her early twenties, presented with a swollen interphalangeal joint that was painful and would not flex. I applied traction to the joint several times, which accomplished nothing. I then applied joint (glide) translations in the recommended biomechanically appropriate direction for flexion. Like the tractions, these glides were also ineffective and painful. I then tried a medial translation accessory movement, which was unacceptable to the patient because of

pain. Without much enthusiasm I then gently tried a lateral translation, which prompted the patient to say 'it does not hurt'. Something prompted me to sustain this translation and ask her if she could flex her finger. To my astonishment and her delight the finger flexed without pain! She then said something like 'You have fixed me'. 'Of course!' I replied. She still had a small loss of flexion range owing to some residual swelling but she departed my rooms with a smile.

The young woman returned two days later and her finger had completely recovered. Why, I asked myself? The only explanation I could come up with for my chance success was that as a result of her trauma there was a minute positional fault of the joint that prevented flexion movement. When this positional fault was corrected it enabled a full recovery to take place. It was a simple hypothesis and because of this I began to look differently at all joints that I treated and experimented to see whether I could achieve similar results by repositioning other joint surfaces. I began having unbelievable successes in the clinic. A 'miracle a day' I called them. Louis Pasteur once said that chance only favours the prepared mind. When I, by chance, had my first 'miracle' with the young woman and her painfully limited interphalangeal joint, I did indeed have a prepared mind.

Today the concepts that have grown from this chance finding have come a long way and guidelines are now in place for their successful clinical use; these are fully described within this textbook. To optimally succeed with our concepts, you need advanced clinical reasoning and excellent handling skills. The detailed descriptions in this book will help you immensely in both these aspects. Ideally, of course, the reader should attend the courses that are available around the world by accredited Mulligan Concept teachers. Teachers and courses are listed at www.bmulligan.com.

While on the topic of teachers, I always acknowledge and thank my mentor Freddy Kaltenborn. Freddy came many times from Europe to teach in faraway New Zealand. He taught me how to manipulate every joint in the spine and to mobilise the extremity joints. His able teachings gave me excellent handling skills. He also increased my knowledge and the importance he placed on the clinical significance of treatment planes led me to successfully develop Mobilisation With Movement. If you do not know each joint's treatment plane you will never be able to successfully manipulate or effectively apply the Mulligan concepts.

I must stress that the techniques contained within this book are not set in stone. They are all based on repositioning joint surfaces, or muscles and their tendons, to see whether one can achieve pain-free resolution of a musculoskeletal problem. The techniques described in the book are those we, in the Mulligan Concept Teachers Association, have clinically found to be effective. If any clinicians applying them, who have the requisite knowledge and handling skills, can improve upon these techniques then this would be most welcome. It is hoped these clinicians would share their significant worthwhile improvements with other clinicians and teachers.

I feel very humble to have the support of such scholars as Wayne and Toby, and thank them and Elsevier sincerely for this wonderful publication.

Brian Mulligan

Preface

This second edition of the textbook entitled *The Mulligan Concept of Manual Therapy: Textbook of Techniques* presents new techniques in addition to the original ones covered in the first edition. More than 250 Mulligan Concept techniques are shown and these include therapist techniques as well as home exercises and taping techniques. The pictures illustrating this book have been re-taken for improved clarity, with the number of images greatly increased to enable the reader to better conceptualise the execution of each technique. The text has also been updated throughout each chapter, with new references to inform the reader about the current evidence base for the Mulligan Concept.

The book is aimed at being a comprehensive and easy-to-follow resource for the novice and the experienced clinician as well as researchers. It has been written for the clinician, teacher and student interested in furthering their familiarity with the wide array of techniques under the Mulligan Concept umbrella. Mulligan Concept techniques are effective and safe when applied in accordance with easy-to-follow guidelines and clearly identified underlying principles.

When Brian Mulligan first described Mobilisation with Movement (MWM) in 1984 he shared his techniques through his original book entitled *Mulligan's Manual Therapy: NAGs, SNAGs and MWMs*, of which there have been seven editions over the past 30 years. This book has been written to expand on and fully describe in a standardised format all the techniques mentioned in Brian Mulligan's aforementioned original texts, as well as including new techniques that were not contained in those earlier landmark editions. This book is also intended as an accompaniment to our first book entitled *Mobilisation with Movement: the Art and the Science*, which was published in 2011.

Our first book presented the science underpinning MWM and also described aspects of 'the art' inherent in its successful implementation. In that book the basic principles of MWMs were outlined, potential mechanisms underpinning the successful application of MWMs were canvassed, and in-depth aspects of its clinical application were critiqued including guidelines on dosage and troubleshooting. Over half of the first text presented the application of MWM in a series of case reports. These case studies focused on the clinical reasoning underlying the application of the Mulligan Concept, including consideration of the evidence base. The case studies followed the application of the Mulligan Concept from the first session to discharge, showing how the techniques were selected, applied and progressed over the treatment programme. However, the purpose of that first book was not to provide a detailed description of all the techniques under the Mulligan Concept umbrella, which is the scope of the first and second edition of the current book as it continues the work of the preceding landmark book *Mulligan's Manual Therapy: NAGs, SNAGs and MWMs*.

There was a real need for a comprehensive presentation of the wide array of techniques under the umbrella of the 'Mulligan Concept'. These techniques include MWM and other Mulligan techniques such as pain release phenomenon (PRP). Each technique has been described in a consistent and logical format fully explaining the indications, application and modifications for each technique. In addition, we have detailed the current available evidence for each technique in each chapter.

The book is divided into 14 regional chapters, covering the whole body and encompassing the whole range of musculoskeletal disorders that present to clinical practice, including apparent non-joint disorders such as lateral epicondylalgia. The first chapters focus on MWM, home exercise and taping techniques for the upper quadrant, which includes the cervical spine through to the thorax. These chapters include cervicogenic headache and cervicogenic dizziness, the temporomandibular joint, shoulder complex, elbow, forearm, wrist and hand. The subsequent chapters cover the lower quadrant, including the lumbar spine, sacroiliac joint, hip, knee, ankle and foot. The final chapter covers commonly used PRPs, which are distinct to MWM but can be very helpful in the right clinical presentation, usually after the condition being treated has proved resistant to other Mulligan Concept techniques.

The techniques in this text are drawn from those presented on the Mulligan Concept courses taught worldwide and as such form the curriculum of the different levels of those Mulligan Concept courses. Also presented is a dictionary of annotations for the techniques described, along with an explanation of the rationale underlying the system of annotations.

Professor Wayne Hing
Brisbane, Australia, 2019
Adjunct Associate Professor Toby Hall
Perth, Australia, 2019
Brian Mulligan
Wellington, New Zealand, 2019

Authors

Wayne Hing, PhD, MSc (Hons), ADP(OMT), Dip MT, Dip Phys, FNZCP
Professor in Physiotherapy and Head of Program, Bond University, QLD, Australia

Toby Hall, PhD, MSc, Post Grad Dip Manip Ther, FACP
Adjunct Associate Professor, School of Physiotherapy and Exercise Science, Curtin University, Perth, WA, Australia;
Director of Manual Concepts;
Fellow of the Australian College of Physiotherapists

Brian Mulligan, Dip MT, FNZSP (Hon)
Lecturer, Author, President MCTA, New Zealand

Contributors

Elisa F D Canetti, PhD, MSc (High Perform Sci), BPhty
Assistant Professor, Bond University, QLD, Australia

Daniel Harvie, PhD, MMusc & Sports Physio, BPhysio (Hons)
NHMRC Early Career Research Fellow, The Hopkins Centre, Menzies Health Institute Queensland, Griffith University

Jill McDowell, Dip Phys, Reg Physio Acup, Post Grad Cert Sports Med, Dip MT, Cred MDT, Cred Mulligan Concept, MNZCP (Acup), MNZCP (Manip), MPhty, MNZSP, MCTA

Mark Oliver, MAppSc (Curtin), Grad Dip Manip Ther (Curtin), Dip Manip Ther (NZMPA), Dip Physio (AIT), MNZSP, MCTA
Musculoskeletal Physiotherapist

Acknowledgments

Wayne Hing

The completion of the second edition of this Mulligan Concept book on techniques is now complete. A huge thank you to my good friend Toby Hall for his commitment and expertise to complete this goal.

Brian, this is once again a tribute to you for your gift to the physiotherapy profession! You taught me a philosophy of manual therapy that is practical and functional. To my kids, Matthew and Philippa, who make my life meaningful, thank you.

Toby Hall

To the many people who have supported me: foremost are my family, Liz, Sam and Amy, and parents, Christine and Douglas. You give the meaning to my life. I am also privileged to have worked and learnt from esteemed colleagues, Kim Robinson, Bob Elvey and Brian Mulligan, among many others. Of course, a huge shout-out to my friend and colleague, Wayne Hing, without whom this book would not exist. Thanks to all of you.

Brian Mulligan

Like I say below, this second edition, like the first, will be welcomed by all those involved in the field of musculoskeletal medicine. This edition will also be a first-class addition to the literature on manual therapy. It is superbly authored by Drs Wayne Hing and Toby Hall.

It brings the reader up to date with new techniques and with all the recent journal articles supporting our concepts. There are format changes that the reader will appreciate. What is really unique is that, with all the techniques dealt with, the authors give the levels of evidence that support them.

I am indebted to both Wayne and Toby for this textbook.

Special acknowledgment

Special acknowledgment goes to Daniel Harvie, Mark Oliver, Jillian McDowell and Elisa Canetti for their contribution to this edition: Daniel's specific contribution to the introduction, Mark's to the sacroiliac and temporomandibular chapters, Jillian's to the overall nomenclature and annotations throughout the book and finally Elisa Canetti for her specific assistance in updating all chapter introductions to the literature and levels of evidence.

Lastly, a huge thank you to Brian Mulligan for giving the authors the opportunity to write this book; also for his vision, support and guidance through the journey of planning and then writing of the book.

Finally, to the Mulligan Concept Teachers Association (MCTA), thank you all for contributing to the first and second editions of this book, *The Mulligan Concept of Manual Therapy; Textbook of techniques*. Without all your support and contribution this would not have been possible. For details of the current members please refer to the website at https://www.bmulligan.com/teachers.

TABLE 1 Abbreviations for use in Mulligan Concept annotations

Start position	Side	Joints/anatomy	Glides (text)	Mulligan technique	Movement	Repetitions/time/sets
pr ly=prone lying s ly=side lying sit=sitting st=standing sup ly=supine lying WB=weight-bearing	L=left R=right	ACJ=acromioclavicular joint Ank=ankle Calc=calcaneum CV=costovertebral joint Cx=cervical spine C3=cervical spine 3rd vertebra Elb=elbow Fib=fibula Fra=forearm Gastroc=gastrocnemius GH=glenohumeral Inn=innominate Kn=knee L5=lumbar spine 5th vertebra MC=metacarpal MCP=metacarpophalangeal joint MT=metatarsal MTP=metatarsophalangeal joint PFJ=patellofemoral joint PIP=proximal interphalangeal joint PS=pubic symphysis RUJ=radioulnar joint SCJ=sternoclavicular joint Sh=shoulder SIJ=sacroiliac joint Sx=sacrum Tib=tibia TMJ=temperomandibular joint Tx=thoracic spine T4=thoracic spine 4th vertebra Wr=wrist	Ant=anterior AP=anteroposterior# Comp=compression(φ) Dist=distraction gl=glide Inf=inferior Lat=lateral(φ) Med=medial(φ) PA=posteroanterior* Post=posterior Prox=proximal Sup=superior/separates multiple individual glides – indicates combined glides **Glides (symbol)(φ)** ↑=anteroposterior# ←=lateral glide left →=lateral glide right ↔=longitudinal ⌐=posterior glide left ¬=posterior glide right ↓=posteroanterior*	BLR=bent leg raise HA SNAG=headache sustained natural apophyseal glide MWM=Mobilisation with Movement NAG=natural apophyseal glide Rev HA SNAG=reverse headache sustained natural apophyseal glide Rev NAG=reverse natural apophyseal glide SMWAM=spinal mobilisation with arm movement SMWLM=spinal mobilisation with leg movement SNAG=sustained natural apophyseal glide Tr SLR=traction straight leg raise Trans SNAG=transverse sustained natural apophyseal glide **Movement direction (symbol)(φ)** ↺=lateral rotation ↻=medial rotation ↰=side flexion left ↱=side flexion right	Ab=abduction(φ) Ad=adduction(φ) Approx=approximation Depr=depression Dev=deviation DF=dorsiflexion(φ) DFIS=dorsiflexion in standing Downw=downward E=extension(φ) EiL=extension in lying ❖ El=elevation(φ) ER=external rotation Ev=eversion(φ) F=flexion(φ) HBB=hand behind back HE=horizontal extension(φ) HF=horizontal flexion(φ) Inv=inversion(φ) IR=internal rotation LF=lateral flexion Occl=occlusion Opp=opposition PF=plantarflexion(φ) PKB=prone knee bend Pron=pronation Rot=rotation SKB=small knee bend Supin=supination	min=minutes sec=seconds ×=times ()=sets **Other** +A=with assistant +2A=with 2 assistants Bilat=bilateral OP=overpressure Res=resistance Unilat=unilateral

#Acceptable interchangeable terms for anteroposterior include dorsal and posterior.
*Acceptable interchangeable terms for posteroanterior include anterior and ventral.
(φ)Denotes established Maitland abbreviations and symbols; although supination is recorded as 'Sup' in Maitland's abbreviations it has been altered here to avoid confusion with superior glide 'sup gl', which is more commonly used than cephalad (ceph) and caudad (caud) in Mulligan Concept terminology.
❖ Denotes established McKenzie acronym.

Mulligan Concept annotations

The Mulligan Concept of Manual Therapy uses the annotational framework established by McDowell and colleagues (McDowell et al., 2014).

'Annotation' refers to the specific formula used to record a manual therapy technique within patients' records. They may be likened to a specific shorthand, using abbreviations to allow the efficient and accurate recording of treatment in sufficient detail to allow reproduction by another practitioner.

Accurate recording of Mulligan Concept techniques has specific challenges for practitioners as they must encompass additional treatment parameters above those required of other manual therapy approaches.

Mulligan Concept annotations should include the following details preferably in sequential framework order:

- start position
- side
- joint(s)
- method of application (belt, self)
- glide(s) applied
- terminology (e.g. MWM, SNAG, NAG)
- movement or function performed by the patient
- assisted (indicates a second or third therapist required)
- over-pressure (and by whom)
- repetitions or time
- sets.

So, for example, a simple cervical SNAG is sitting with ipsilateral contact on C2 and patient-generated over-pressure, performed with three sets of six repetitions, which may be recorded as follows using common abbreviations (see Table 1):

sit L C2 SNAG Rot L +OP×6(3)

(start position / side / joint / technique / movement direction / over-pressure / repetitions / sets)

encompassing 8 of a possible 11 framework parameters. A more comprehensive description is required for a scapulothoracic MWM where an assistant applies the posterior glide to the humerus and the therapist alters four positional faults with a combination of corrective glides:

sit R scapulothoracic Inf gl / Downward rot / Med gl / ER + Post gl GH MWM F +A×6(3)

(start position / side / joint / glides applied to scapula and glenohumeral joints / technique / movement direction / assisted by second therapist / repetitions / sets)

The following operational rules for the annotational framework have been established by McDowell and colleagues (McDowell et al., 2014).

- NAGs and SNAGs – the therapist's contact points are central on the spine unless notated otherwise. Documentation must stipulate whether the therapist's contact position is on the right or left of the spinal segment as a SNAG may be ipsilateral or contralateral to the active movement.
- Transverse SNAGs (formerly called positional SNAGs), SMWAM and SMWLM – if the annotation states 'L T1' this notates the therapist contact point; that is, the therapist applies pressure to the left of the T1 spinous process and applies a transverse glide towards the right.
- If over-pressure is applied then it should be recorded. Special notation should occur if it is performed by a third party or has a special application; for example, the patient's partner administers the over-pressure during a self-cervical rotation SNAG. Otherwise all over-pressure should be considered patient generated.
- If a technique has both a manual and a treatment belt method of application then the use of a belt should always be recorded. When 'belt' is missing from the annotation the practitioner will assume it is a manual technique.
- If more than one corrective glide is applied (e.g. to the scapula for a scapulothoracic MWM) then the glides should be listed in the order of emphasis or magnitude of force. If more inferior glide is needed than external rotation, medial glide and downward rotation then it should be listed as 'Inf gl / ER / Med gl / downward rotation'. Forward slash lines separate multiple glides (in keeping with Maitland's combined movements (Maitland, 1978) and dashes indicate combined glides (e.g. in the 'Post-sup gl' of the inferior tibiofibular joint).
- The clinical reasoning underpinning the Mulligan Concept recommends that only three repetitions of a technique be performed if a patient's condition is highly acute or irritable (Vicenzino et al., 2011). Accordingly, the number of repetitions should be recorded as '×3'. Once a condition is sub-acute or chronic then six to ten repetitions may be used in three to five sets. The annotation '×6(3)' would indicate six repetitions were performed three times with a rest between each set.

- As a pain release phenomenon (PRP) is a sustained technique it is best recorded by duration but the technique also may have sets applied; for example '×20 sec(3)' indicating that three 20 second contractions, stretches or compressions were performed with a rest between each set.
- NAGs are applied at the rate of three per second and here each second should be considered a set. Typically, three to four seconds are performed per segment before retesting (personal communication, Brian Mulligan). If 'sit L C5 NAG×4sec' is recorded this should be interpreted as 12 glides to the C5 segment.
- Rib MWM with a single point of contact over the posterior chest wall should be recorded using 'costovertebral' (CV) in the annotation. This abbreviation allows differentiation from the double hand rib MWM where the rib is lifted anteriorly and posteriorly and recorded using 'rib' in the annotation.
- Self-treatments may be performed with a handgrip, fist, towel or treatment belt with the method of application also included when recording home exercise prescriptions.
- Mulligan Concept annotations use 'elevation' (El) when an arm movement is in the plane of scaption, 'flexion' (F) when in the sagittal plane and 'abduction' (Ab) when in the frontal plane.

(reproduced with permission)

References

McDowell, J.M., Johnson, G.M., Hetherington, B., 2014. Mulligan Concept manual therapy: standardising annotation. Man. Ther. 19 (5), 365–508.

Maitland, G., 1978. Musculo-Skeletal Examination and Recording Guide. Lauderdale Press, Adelaide.

Vicenzino, B., Hing, W.A., Rivett, D., Hall, T., 2011. Mobilisation With Movement: The Art and the Science. Elsevier, Sydney.

Introduction

In the history of manual therapy, specific individuals have been influential in contributing innovative and original insight and developing novel manual therapeutic approaches and techniques. These include the likes of Maitland, McKenzie, Kaltenborn, Elvey and, last but not least, Mulligan. As quoted in the first *Mobilisation with Movement* (MWM) book (Vicenzino et al., 2011a):

> These aforementioned utilised their skills in clinical observation, palpation and reasoning to open new fields in manual therapy which effectively shifted practice paradigms and transcended professional boundaries. Indeed, their names have over time become synonymous with manual therapy itself. Almost without exception, these outliers of manual therapy exhibited self-deprecation and a continual drive to share their ideas, techniques and experiences with other practitioners.

Mulligan's unique MWM concept has significantly impacted on manual therapy practice worldwide over the last two decades. The history of MWM is well documented in our first book (Vicenzino et al., 2011a). Mulligan began his career as a physiotherapist graduating from the Otago School of Physiotherapy in Dunedin in 1954. In the late 1950s, after attending seminars based on Dr James Cyriax's approach to orthopaedic medicine, which included spinal manipulation (high-velocity thrust) and passive joint mobilisation techniques, he quickly developed his keen appreciation and interest for manual therapy. Mulligan, Paris and McKenzie's interest in manual therapy led Paris and McKenzie to visit Kaltenborn in Europe. They then returned to New Zealand and shared their knowledge with Mulligan and other physiotherapists.

In those early times the physiotherapy schools did not include this form of manual therapy training, with the key components consisting of exercise therapy and massage, as well as electrotherapy modalities.

Mulligan eventually expanded his knowledge in manual therapy by travelling to Helsinki to attend a Kaltenborn peripheral joint mobilisation course. Upon returning to New Zealand he employed the techniques in his clinic, found them very useful and so then began to teach these new skills to local private practitioners. He went on to run his first weekend course on Kaltenborn mobilisation techniques in 1970 and then taught similar courses in Australia.

It was in 1985 that Mulligan had his first MWM success, which ultimately changed his whole approach to manual therapy. After applying a series of contemporary treatment techniques of passive joint mobilisation and ultrasound to a swollen and painful second proximal interphalangeal joint with little improvement, out of frustration Mulligan trialled a sustained pain-free lateral glide with active flexion. The technique was immediately successful and restored a full range of pain-free movement with complete return to function and resolution in swelling following this single application of treatment. The concept of applying a sustained glide to a joint and maintaining this during active movement was born and applied in other clinical situations. All MWMs that have since been developed arose from this single observation of a recalcitrant clinical problem.

Mulligan had developed the concept of MWM and went on to apply the same idea to all his patients with finger joint problems, and then to other joints. Medial and lateral glides and rotations with movement were developed first in the fingers, then shortly after in the wrist. Sustained natural apophyseal glides (SNAGs) soon followed in the spine. Mulligan then started to teach these new techniques along with other concepts on courses throughout New Zealand through the manual therapy special interest group of the New Zealand Society of Physiotherapists known as the New Zealand Manipulative Therapists Association.

Mulligan's first Mulligan Concept course was held in 1986 and his text entitled *Manual Therapy: NAGs, SNAGs, MWMs Etc.*, which this current book replaces, is now in its 7th edition, which is due to be released soon (Mulligan, 2019 in press) and has sold more than 80 000 copies worldwide. The interest in Mulligan's courses eventually led to the establishing of the international Mulligan Concept Teachers Association (MCTA), which had its inaugural meeting in Stevenage, United Kingdom (UK) in 1998. This teaching group was set up to standardise the teaching of the Mulligan Concept around the world. There are currently 54 members of MCTA providing courses for physiotherapists all over the world (www.bmulligan.com). The impact that the Mulligan Concept has had on clinical practice was highlighted when Mulligan was named one of 'The Seven Most Influential Persons in Orthopaedic Manual Therapy' as the result of a poll of members of the American Physical Therapy Association.

Our first book, entitled *Mobilisation with Movement: the Art and the Science*, was published in 2011. The text defines and operationally describes the MWM concept in terms of its parameters and how these may be manipulated in order to achieve clinically beneficial outcomes. It is important that the therapist is familiar with the principles behind the MWM concept before attempting to use the techniques described in the current textbook of techniques. While the concept is quite simple in its approach, failure to follow the following guidelines will at best most likely lead to treatment failure, and at worse could exacerbate the patient's condition.

Within the book the importance of therapist knowledge and skill, patient–therapist collaboration and patient cooperation are highlighted in the acronym **CROCKS**, which is favoured by Mulligan (personal communication, 2009) in his teaching and is summarised in Table 1.

Contraindications. Manually induced forces applied to a patient by a therapist ought to be considered in light of the state of the underlying tissues, as well as any underlying pathology both locally (e.g. infection, inflammation) and generally (e.g. sero-positive arthropathy, rheumatoid, cancer). For example, bone quality (e.g. osteoporosis, fractures), joint structure integrity (e.g. unstable joint), blood vessel patency (e.g. vertebral artery, aortic aneurism), and skin integrity (e.g. frail skin in diabetes or peripheral vascular disease), which could likely be compromised in patients presenting with painful conditions, need to be considered. Novice manual therapists, including novices to MWM, should make themselves familiar with conditions that are contraindications to manual therapy and those in which caution is required (Gay & Nelson, 2003). Notwithstanding this, MWM techniques have a built-in safety mechanism because they are to be applied without symptoms (e.g. pain, giving way, pins and needles) and with the least amount of force to achieve an improvement in the patient's movement impairment. The technical and conceptual aspects required to apply safe MWMs are presented within this text, which is an updated edition of *The Mulligan Concept of Manual Therapy: Textbook of Techniques* (Hing et al., 2015) as well as our previous one *Mobilisation with Movement: the Art and the Science* (Vicenzino et al., 2011a).

Repetitions. The number of repetitions per set and the number of sets per session vary between techniques as well as the stages of the intervention. It is generally advisable that fewer repetitions should be used when treating the spine compared with peripheral joints, particularly on initial application and in more recently injured joints

TABLE 1 Summary of acronym CROCKS	
C	Contraindications
R	Repetitions
O	Over-pressure
C	Communication and cooperation
K	Knowledge
S	Sustain, skill, sensibility and subtle

or in injuries with severe pain presentation (or neural or joint instability symptoms). More repetitions are used in more-longstanding cases (often those recalcitrant to previous treatments) and as a progression when the patient's condition improves. Table 2 presents a guide to the numbers of repetitions.

Over-pressure. All joints have an active and passive available range of movement (ROM), with slightly more passive range available than active. The maximum passive range is achieved by therapist-applied firm over-pressure at the end of the joint's active range. If pain-free over-pressure can be achieved at the symptomatic joint as a consequence of a MWM technique, then this is believed to ensure optimal recovery. Failure to test over-pressure for pain responses may hinder the recovery of the specific joint being treated.

Communication and cooperation. These are essential features of safe and effective MWM application. Practitioners must inform patients of expected effects and patients must communicate with practitioners the presence of any symptoms, discomfort or pain during each treatment session.

Knowledge. Practitioners must have knowledge of musculoskeletal medicine, pathology, biomechanics and anatomy. This will enable the safe, efficient and accurate application of techniques.

Sustain. MWM techniques incorporate accessory glide with active movement. Ensure the glide is maintained during the entire duration of the movement, even on return to the start position. **S** also stands for skill, sensibility and subtle, as described below.

Skill in the manual handling of the physical application of the technique. MWM is a skill like any form of manual therapy. The more the therapist perfects their technique, the better the technique will be performed.

Sensibility. Again, with practice, the therapist will gain greater sense and feeling through their hands. This will enable awareness of joint gliding, physiological movement, and subtle changes in muscle tone associated with pain and guarding.

Subtle changes in glide direction, which are often required when a technique does not achieve the desired aims. For example, a patient may feel movement is improved by the application of MWM, but may still feel some pain with movement (i.e. they are not completely better). Subtle changes in the direction of the glide may eliminate the pain completely.

Finally **S** also stands for **common Sense**. Most of all, therapists ought to bring a reasoned approach (common sense) to rationalising indications, contraindication, communication, cooperation, knowledge, evidence and skill in individualising the MWM to the patient they are treating.

Another of Mulligan's acronyms that he uses in his teaching is **PILL**, which is defined in Table 3. This is related to the desired response from the technique's application.

Pain-free application refers to the glide / mobilisation and movement components. This is the most important principle that must always be adhered to. If pain (or other presenting symptoms) cannot be eliminated during a technique then this requires the therapist to make changes to the technique. If pain is reduced during the application of a technique but not eliminated then subtle changes in glide direction and glide force should be attempted to eliminate pain completely. If pain is increased during the initial application of the glide, then this often indicates that the correct glide would be in the reverse direction. If pain with movement is unchanged by the application of a glide, then this usually indicates that a glide in a different plane is required.

TABLE 2 Repetitions: an approximate guide

Location		Repetitions	Sets
Spine	First session	3	1
	Subsequent	6–10	3–5
Peripheral joints	First session	6	3
	Subsequent	6–10	3–5

TABLE 3 Summary of acronym PILL

P	Pain-free
I	Instant effect
L	Long
L	Lasting

Instant means that the effect must be immediate at the time of application. This means an immediate improvement in pain-free ROM or an immediate improvement in the functional activity the patient is having issues with.

Long and **Lasting** refer to the results that should be obtained beyond the technique's application. If the effects of treatment are only short lived, then this indicates that the practitioner must make significant changes during subsequent treatment sessions. This might include an increased number of sets or repetitions, the addition of over-pressure, home exercise, or the addition of sports taping where applicable.

The practitioner can help facilitate **patient compliance** with treatment, in particular the self-management aspect, by showing the patient that the application of MWM can produce an immediate pain-free change (the 'P' and 'I' of PILL) in their most provocative or restricted movement or functional activity. Such a response may potentially have the power to change negative beliefs or expectations that the patient may have brought with them to the clinical session.

MOBILISATION WITH MOVEMENT

An MWM can be defined as the application of a **sustained passive accessory force / glide** to a joint while the patient actively performs a task that was previously identified as being problematic.

A critical aspect of the MWM is the identification of a task that the patient has difficulty completing, usually due to pain or joint stiffness. This task is most frequently a movement or a muscle contraction performed to the onset of pain, or to the end of available ROM or maximum muscle contraction. This task is referred to as the **Client Specific Impairment Measure (CSIM)** (refer to Chapter 2 in Vicenzino et al., 2011a).

The passive accessory force usually exerts a translatory or rotatory glide at the joint and as such must be applied close to the joint line to avoid undesirable movements. It may be applied manually with the therapist's / patient's hands, or via a treatment belt, or even with sports tape applied on the skin. The direction of the accessory movement that is used is the one that effects the greatest improvement in the CSIM. It is somewhat surprising that a lateral glide is the most commonly cited successful technique used in peripheral joints (Vicenzino et al., 2011a).

An iterative approach might be required to find the right direction of the glide. The glide should be applied parallel to the treatment plane (Fig. 1) (Vicenzino et al., 2011a), which is a line drawn across the concave joint surface. For example, at the tibiofemoral joint the tibial plateau forms the treatment plane. The treatment plane will vary from person to person, and may change as a result of bone remodelling following trauma or disease such as osteoarthritis. The treatment plane will also vary according to the patient's start position. For example, in the extended knee the treatment plane is horizontal in standing but almost vertical in supine. Particular to SNAGs or MWM in the spine, the gliding direction is always in the plane of the facet joint. The orientation of the spinal facets varies from level to level, and needs to be understood before attempting a SNAG. A full review of the evidence and explanation of application, repetitions and progression is found in Chapter 2 of our first book (Vicenzino et al., 2011a).

MWM can be easily integrated into the standard manual therapy physical examination to evaluate its potential as an intervention. A seamless integration can be undertaken after examining the appropriate active / functional movements, static muscles tests and passive accessory movements. They can also be readily trialled and implemented in the first treatment session. Reassessment is generally just a matter of the practitioner taking their hands off the patient and asking them to move (without having to change position) and assessing the effect of the MWM. Usually the treatment and its reassessment is applied in weight-bearing positions for lower limb and spine problems, as the majority of CSIM are in functional weight-bearing positions. There is also a notion that treatment in weight-bearing usually brings about greater improvement in the patient's condition.

The indications for MWM both in the physical examination and for treatment are essentially the same as for other manual therapy approaches, as are the contraindications. This was discussed more comprehensively in our first book (Vicenzino et al., 2011a). Generally, mobilisation techniques, including MWM, have been conceptualised as being indicated for mechanically induced joint pain and joint stiffness limiting ROM. However, MWM has also been proposed by Mulligan to affect what appear to be soft tissue conditions, such as lateral epicondylalgia of the elbow and De Quervain syndrome, and indeed there are a number of randomised controlled trials (RCTs), case series and case studies supporting his assertion (Vicenzino et al., 2011a).

While original in nature, the MWM concept has parallels to other approaches to manual therapy that would facilitate ready adoption by the manual therapist. For example, the consideration of joint mechanics in some MWM techniques is akin to the approach advocated by Kaltenborn (1980), and the strong emphasis on

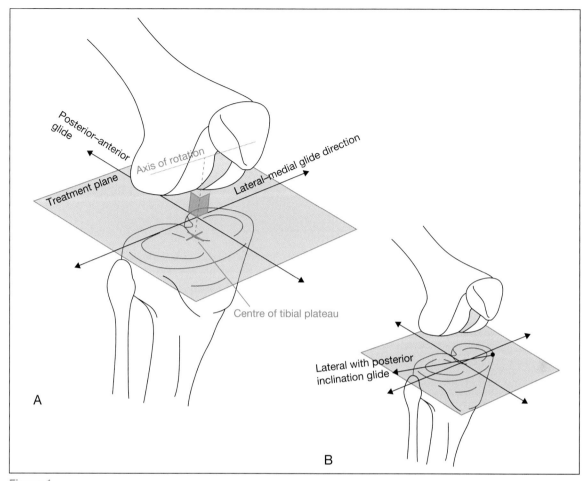

Figure 1
Treatment plane. (A) The treatment plane defined with reference to an example at the tibiofemoral joint. The treatment plane is perpendicular to a line drawn from the centre of rotation of the femoral condyles (convex member) to the centre of the tibial plateau (concave member). Glides and rotations that occur in this plane are thought to be the most mechanically effective. (B) Demonstrates fine-tuning of a lateral glide with a slight posterior inclination with the filled in circle representing the contact point and the arrow the direction. Note how the contact point and application will be modified when fine-tuning the direction (refer to Fig. 2.4, p. 16 in Vicenzino et al. (2011a)).

self-management using repeated movements would be familiar to McKenzie practitioners (McKenzie & May, 2003). This is not surprising given that Mulligan was mentored and influenced early in his career by both these practitioners. In common with both the Maitland (2005) and the McKenzie approaches a change in pain response is used as an indication that the correct technique is being applied, although rather than provoking or localising pain the aim of MWM is its immediate and total elimination.

In contrast to the Maitland and Kaltenborn approaches, there is no system of grading the force and amount of movement in MWM. Rather, when applying MWM the practitioner will apply as much force in the mobilisation as is required to improve the CSIM without causing pain. Sometimes pain may be provoked by the application of too much glide force, or too strong a grade of mobilisation. Gentle force is often all that is required to achieve an improvement in pain-free function. If improvement in function is not achieved with gentle force, then the force (and therefore grade) would be increased until it is effective or shown to be inappropriate and dismissed. In addition to these differences between the MWM concept and other manual therapy approaches, MWM uniquely combines both passive and active elements. This is in contrast to just focusing on one aspect (e.g. passive joint movement as per Kaltenborn). In regard to the latter, there is some similarity to the combined movement approach described by Edwards (1999), in which pain-free joint positioning is used to enable end-range passive mobilisation.

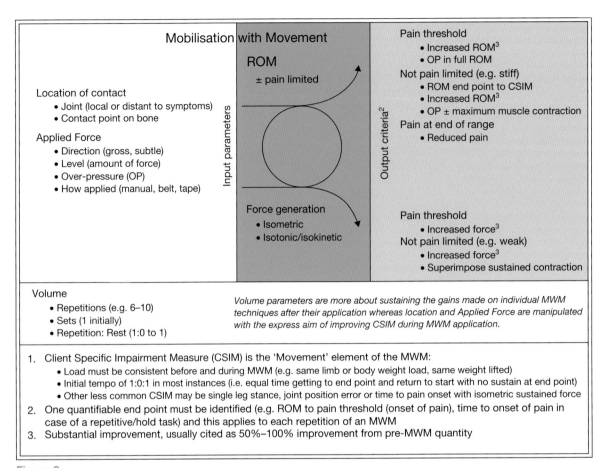

Figure 2
The mobilisation element of MWM. The input parameters of the 'mobilisation' element of MWM are listed in the left column. Pain threshold refers to measuring some quantity of the task other than pain, such as ROM or force generated when the patient first feels the onset of pain. That is, pain is not the variable, but rather the ROM or force generation are the key output criteria. Where pain is not the main limiting feature of the patient's problem then measures of pain, ROM and force generated become the possible output criteria. From these criteria, decisions can be made to modulate the input parameters (location and force in the left column, and volume in the middle row above footnotes) of the mobilisation (first 'M' in **M**WM). Implicit in this flow chart is the iterative nature of MWM applications (refer to Fig. 2.2, p. 14 in Vicenzino et al. (2011a)).

MWM was defined as the application of a specific vector of force to a joint (mobilisation or the first 'M' in **M**WM), which is sustained while the patient performs a previously impaired physical task. The key to successful use of MWM is the skilful and efficient application of this mobilisation force so as to painlessly achieve immediate and long-lasting relief of pain (Vicenzino et al., 2011a).

The mobilisation element of MWM (Fig. 2) is described through the parameters of amount, direction and volume of applied force, as well as the location and mode of application of the force (Vicenzino et al., 2011a). Further, a key feature of an MWM application is the movement or the second 'M' in MW**M**, referred to as the CSIM, as described earlier.

An MWM should be applied only when there is a meaningful clinical measure of a problematic physical task, which is similar to Maitland's comparable sign. That is, the key feature of a CSIM is that it needs to reflect the patient's main concern(s). The measure needs to be patient centred and meaningful to the individual, so consequently we termed it the CSIM. The CSIM assessed in the clinic may be the task itself – for example, placing the hand behind the back to tuck a shirt in for a shoulder problem or walking down a step for a knee problem.

That is, a physical activity or task that is easily **reproducible** in the clinic is likely to be directly incorporated in an MWM, whereas the one that is not readily reproducible in the clinic will need to be approached in a slightly different way. An example of a task reproducible in the clinic but not readily amenable to the application of an

MWM is where a patient may have a pain problem with deep squatting but it may not be desirable to reproduce the deep squat too many times, so alternatively the practitioner can break down these tasks into less stressful and presumably less painful component parts such as a non-weight-bearing (NWB) knee flexion, which would then be the start point for treatment. If this was only mildly painful then four-point kneeling or partial weight-bearing (WB) with a foot up on a chair could be the appropriate start point. In summary, selection of a CSIM, while reflecting the patient's main problem, should also allow a safe MWM to be applied without risk of exacerbating a severe pain problem in fully loaded joints.

Of key importance is that the initial assessment of the patient not only identifies the CSIM / comparable sign or physical task / activity that is problematic (usually painful) to the patient but also establishes the extent to which the physical task interferes with the patient's day-to-day function, as well as the **severity and irritability** of the condition (Vicenzino et al., 2011a). The physical examination will then **quantify the CSIM**. This quantification will be somewhat variable depending on the presenting problem – that is, it will be different for a painful condition versus a stiffness or weakness problem.

In the case of someone presenting with a CSIM in a painful condition, the physical problem is the painful movement (Vicenzino et al., 2011a). The patient would indicate when they first feel pain during the movement and this could be measured with a goniometer, inclinometer, tape measure or some other reference point (e.g. a point on the wall). In the event that a painful muscle contraction is the CSIM, it can be measured with a dynamometer (e.g. grip testing in tennis elbow) (Fig. 3).

In the case where there is pain at end of range or on full-strength contraction upon the application of an MWM the patient reports their perception of pain using a visual analogue scale (VAS) or numerical rating scale (NRS) and the MWM should substantially reduce the pain to no pain or very little pain for it to be of any use in treatment (Table 4).

All these measurements are standard and routine in musculoskeletal healthcare practice. Other examples of the application of MWM to a stiffness or weakness problem, or a combination of these problems, are found in Chapter 2 of the first MWM book.

Another important aspect of MWM is the **application of over-pressure** to the CSIM at the end point of the movement, but only if pain-free. Mulligan (2019 in press) strongly emphasised the necessity of over-pressure in order to optimise the effectiveness of the treatment. Depending on the technique, either the patient or the therapist could apply the over-pressure. Additionally, techniques that already had an over-pressure component (i.e. **active WB**) or included a gravitational effect require no manual application of over-pressure and are often valuable techniques for a patient to perform as a self-MWM.

The second M of MWM (vector force) falls under the separate categories of the direction of force application, the amount of force being applied, the possible interrelationship between direction and amount of force, the locality of the force application, the manner in which the force is applied (e.g. manually, tape, treatment belt) and the overall volume. These aforementioned factors can be considered the input parameters / variables

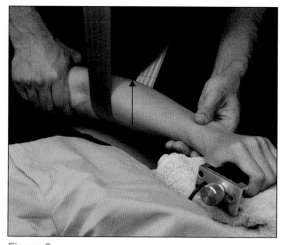

Figure 3
Belt MWM: lateral glide with gripping

TABLE 4 Pain end point, measurement and MWM target

Impairment	End point	Measurement or quantity	MWM target(s)
Pain-limited motion[1]	Pain onset	Degrees of motion[2]	Motion (not pain)
Painful arc	Pain onset and offset[3]	Degrees of motion	Arc of motion and motion at onset (not pain)
Pain at full end of range	End of normal range of motion	Pain (NRS or VAS)[4]	Pain (not range of motion)
Limited range of motion with no pain[5]	Range of motion	Degrees of motion	Motion
Force generation less than normal due to pain	Pain onset	Force output	Force generation[6] not pain
Painful contraction without strength deficit	Normal force output	Pain (NRS or VAS)	Pain not force generation
Weakness without pain	Force output	Force output	Force generation

1. The motion could be of joints, muscle or nerve. This applies for all motion functions in this table.

2. In some instances it may not be degrees, but rather a linear distance achieved (e.g. hand behind back using millimetres along the back, bending forward using linear measurement of reach with fingers to the floor).

3. The pain experienced at pain onset should not increase with further movement so as to prevent further movement.

4. VAS (visual analogue scale). NRS (numerical rating scale).

5. This may also include perceptions of stretch and discomfort that the patient does not describe as being painful per se.

6. In order to have a reproducible measure, the force generation is usually isometric, but this only refers to when pain is involved and when pain is the end point.

(Vicenzino et al., 2011a, Table 2.1, p. 10)

of the mobilisation (or first 'M') part of the MWM (Fig. 2). The figure refers to two reference points for these parameters, the first being the description of the input parameters, such as the amount (*N*) and direction (degrees) of force. The second reference point is the CSIM and in particular how the parameters impact on the CSIM (Fig. 4).

The **direction of force application**/accessory glide that the practitioner applies to a joint varies between a medial, lateral, anterior, posterior and rotational direction. The passively applied glide is sustained and maintained while and after the patient performs their CSIM. The techniques described throughout this text all originated from Mulligan's clinical observations over the course of his practice. They provide novice practitioners with an expert opinion (from the innovator of the techniques) regarding a start point to their applications of MWM, especially as there appear to be no other scientifically based guidelines for the direction of force application in MWM.

The **amount of MWM** that is applied may be conceptualised as a volume, which is defined as the sum total of all MWM applications that a patient experiences. The volume of MWM consists of the MWM that is performed by the practitioner as well as that which the patient does in self-treatment. This is reasonably easy to quantify by multiplying the number of repetitions per set by the number of sets of a specific MWM completed over a period of time. The application of tape is also considered another method of extending the amount/volume of MWM experienced by the patient, but it is relatively less quantifiable and in most cases is worn for a only day or two per application.

An important component of the MWM application is the **self-treatment** element that is required for the majority of patients (i.e. those who are not completely recovered after a session or two with the practitioner) (Fig. 4). The volume of MWM experienced by the patient is likely to be a large driver of the sustainability of the MWM effects and, as such, repetition of the MWM will often require the patient to self-treat (Vicenzino et al., 2011a).

The **application of strapping tape**, applied in a similar direction to the mobilisation, to replicate the manually applied MWM, is another strategy to extend the therapeutic effect of the MWM. Similar to the self-administered MWM, the tape should have some demonstrable effect on the CSIM if it is to be used as part of the treatment plan. With the application of tape the clinician should be familiar with standard safety procedures regarding the use of tape applied to skin, particularly when using rigid tape under tension. These include warnings related to the checking of skin allergies prior to application, warning the patient about potential skin irritation and, of

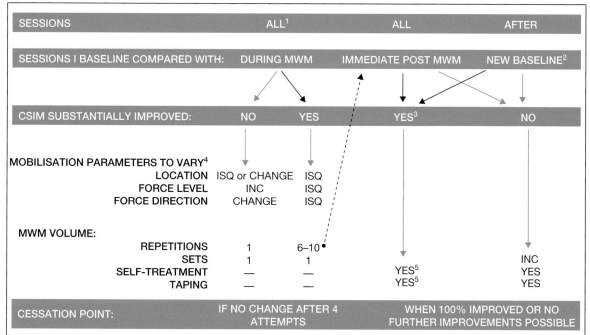

SESSIONS	ALL[1]		ALL	AFTER
SESSIONS I BASELINE COMPARED WITH:	DURING MWM		IMMEDIATE POST MWM	NEW BASELINE[2]
CSIM SUBSTANTIALLY IMPROVED:	NO	YES	YES[3]	NO
MOBILISATION PARAMETERS TO VARY[4]				
LOCATION	ISQ or CHANGE	ISQ		
FORCE LEVEL	INC	ISQ		
FORCE DIRECTION	CHANGE	ISQ		
MWM VOLUME:				
REPETITIONS	1	6–10		
SETS	1	1		INC
SELF-TREATMENT	—	—	YES[5]	YES
TAPING	—	—	YES[5]	YES
CESSATION POINT:	IF NO CHANGE AFTER 4 ATTEMPTS		WHEN 100% IMPROVED OR NO FURTHER IMPROVEMENTS POSSIBLE	

1. After completing a set of MWM repetitions always do a through-range movement with the MWM applied, gradually easing out to the end of range pain free. Failure to do this commonly results in an exacerbation of pain when the patient first moves after the MWM.
2. If patient does not report 100% recovery (to the extent that is possible for their condition) with the application of only one type of MWM technique (usually applied over several sessions) then consideration needs to be given to new MWM techniques being additionally applied, possibly at other locations also (e.g. spine for peripheral problem, or adjacent joint).
3. Care should be exercised at the first session as it is commonly reported that a rebound effect (worsening in ensuing 24–48 hours) may occur if volume is too great.
4. In all MWMs with ROM as an end-point criteria, over-pressure is applied. This over-pressure may be passive as in pain-limited ROM or it may be at maximal contraction in cases of stiff or weakness-limited ROM.
5. This is not always the case following first sessions, but depends on how successful the MWM was, how well the patient can learn the self-treatment and if tape was possible to apply. After the first session, if the patient is very much better (which occurs in some) then self-treatment and tape may not be required.

Figure 4
Proposed decision matrix for MWM. For within-session decisions on application and progression, the clinical-reasoning process largely relies on the response during and immediately post-MWM application compared with that session's preapplication CSIM, whereas for ensuing sessions the preapplication CSIM is compared with the first session's baseline (preapplication) CSIM. Whether or not the CSIM is substantially improved or not will dictate whether changes will be made to the parameters of the MWM and the exact nature of those changes if required. Parameters such as location, level and direction of force are modulated to effect changes during application whereas, as a general guide, a successful MWM session appears to usually involve 1 to 3 sets of 10 repetitions but the exact volume for any individual can be determined with certainty only by using the post-application CSIM response (refer to Fig. 2.3, p. 15 in Vicenzino et al. (2011a)).

extreme importance, the removal of tape if allergies arise (skin itch, burning or other sensations). It is also important that the tape be removed cautiously, even if no reaction has occurred, to prevent skin loss.

CLINICAL REASONING AND THE MULLIGAN CONCEPT

The Mulligan Concept, and in particular MWM, is entirely consistent with autonomous and contemporary manual therapy clinical practice. The effective employment of MWM and other original Mulligan treatment techniques requires the application of skilled clinical reasoning in addition to the hands-on technical skills required to perform the procedures. Indeed, MWM and contemporary, skilled clinical reasoning are critically interdependent if the maximal benefits of the Mulligan approach are to be realised and if the ongoing development of the practitioner's clinical skills is to be sustained. Several key, underpinning principles of skilled clinical reasoning are evident in the application of MWM and these will now each be briefly elucidated.

Patient-centred approach to healthcare

The Mulligan Concept techniques are entirely consistent with patient-centred clinical reasoning and modern healthcare. The concept of evidence-based medicine as promoted by Sackett and colleagues (Sackett et al., 1996, 2000) and the patient-centred model of clinical reasoning in manual therapy proposed by Jones and Rivett (2004) both position the patient as the primary focus of the clinical interaction and the related clinical reasoning process. The patient is unambiguously viewed as a critically important, active collaborator in the process of resolving their problem. Moreover, the patient's clinical presentation and their individual response to management is unique to them and shaped in part by the beliefs, understandings, expectations and experiences they bring to the evolving clinical encounter, as well as their current contextual circumstances (Gifford, 1998). Similarly, central to the Mulligan Concept is that **each patient is an individual** and their clinical presentation is unique, although some features may be in common with others. This means that applying Mulligan's techniques necessitates the use of high-level clinical reasoning skills and that it is not a one-size-fits-all approach.

Consistent with the biopsychosocial approach to healthcare, the application of MWM requires the patient to actively participate in their management and promotes **patient-centred, collaborative clinical reasoning** in several ways.

- The patient must fully comprehend that successful application of the technique is completely without pain / symptoms and that they need to immediately inform the therapist of any pain.
- The patient is usually required to perform an active movement or functional task that is the most painful or limited for them in daily life (the CSIM) as part of the treatment application and also for reassessment purposes. The use of the CSIM in relation to MWM recognises the unique clinical presentation of the individual patient.
- Many MWM and other Mulligan techniques involve the patient applying over-pressure at the end of the movement range in an effort to optimise the clinical response (Mulligan, 2019 in press).
- Finally, as part of the patient's self-management strategies, some MWMs and other procedures can be adapted for prescribed home exercises (e.g. self-MWMs) or by using tape to sustain the accessory movement (or mobilisation) element of the technique.

It is clear that all of the above components of MWM require the patient to understand the basic principles of MWM and be willing to actively contribute to their own management. Accordingly the patient is a core and critical factor in the success of MWM treatment. **Effective communication** is pivotal to the engagement of the patient and thus the effective application of MWM, as well as being critical for meaningful collaborative clinical reasoning. Importantly the patient must immediately communicate the commencement of any pain with either the 'Mobilisation' or the 'Movement' component, or else the technique will not be beneficial. On the other side of the coin, the practitioner must clearly communicate what is expected of the patient at each of the various stages of application of the MWM.

Promotion of knowledge organisation

A well-organised knowledge base will facilitate the application of advanced clinical reasoning skills. The relatively efficient and accurate reasoning process of pattern recognition (in which a cluster of linked clinical cues are readily identified and which is typically employed by experts when dealing with familiar problems) is heavily dependent on a highly organised knowledge base. Specifically, research has shown it to be more accurate in manual therapy diagnosis (Gifford, 1998) than the more linear hypothetico-deductive reasoning process typical of novices. Obviously novice clinicians have gained substantial knowledge from their recent training but it is not just the amount of knowledge that is important in clinical reasoning, but also how these learned understandings and skills are stored and held together in the memory using acquired clinical patterns (Jones & Rivett, 2004). This pattern acquisition requires significant reflective experiences in applying the knowledge to real-world clinical problems.

MWM provides a means by which some of the categories of clinical reasoning hypotheses identified in manual therapy by Jones and Rivett (2004) can be tested and clinical patterns acquired. Clearly hypotheses related to decisions in management and treatment can be immediately confirmed or refuted as any effected clinical changes should be observable instantly (see the PILL acronym earlier in this chapter). It can also be argued that the response to MWM (or other Mulligan procedure) can help the practitioner in implicating the structural source(s) of the patient's symptoms, although caution is needed in this regard owing to pathoanatomical and pathophysiological complexities. Finally, the extent and length of response to MWM can potentially expedite and refine decisions relating to the clinical prognosis.

It can be further argued that the Mulligan Concept **promotes knowledge organisation** by:

- Stimulating research and a growing evidence base of knowledge, which can be used to help guide and inform clinical reasoning (Sackett et al., 1996, 2000). As later chapters indicate, there is an expanding evidence base, both biological and empirical, for MWM and other procedures.
- Identifying and linking key physical examination findings, in particular passive accessory movement findings (the 'Mobilisation') with the CSIM (the 'Movement') in the application of the MWM.
- Facilitating acquisition of clinical patterns (and thus organisation of knowledge) through the immediacy of response to application of the MWM or other procedure. This immediacy of response provides real-time feedback to the practitioner as to the accuracy of the related clinical decision(s) and thus helps to strengthen the association(s) of key clinical findings with correct clinical actions.
- Nurturing the development of metacognitive skills through the requirement to constantly modify the application of the technique on the basis of the patient's initial and varying responses. Metacognitive skills are higher-order thinking skills of self-monitoring and reflective appraisal of one's own reasoning, and are requisite for the acquirement of advanced clinical patterns (Jones & Rivett, 2004).

While the Mulligan Concept, particularly as it relates to MWM, may facilitate the growth of skills in clinical reasoning, there is a risk that the unthinking practitioner may simply and blindly follow treatment recommendations or protocols (Jones & Rivett, 2004). It is not the intention of the authors that this text be used as a recipe book for the treatment of a range of musculoskeletal disorders. Indeed, practitioners should not feel constrained by the techniques covered in this book, but should instead adapt, modify and develop new procedures as required by individual patient presentations, so long as the aforementioned underpinning principles of the Mulligan Concept are followed within a contemporary clinical reasoning framework.

PROPOSED MECHANISMS BY WHICH MWM WORK

When selecting a treatment, clinicians frequently consider not only evidence of efficacy, but also the underlying mechanism of action. That is, it is not only important whether a treatment works, but also how. A holy grail of clinical decision-making in musculoskeletal practice has been the quest to match patients to the most appropriate treatment. Such an aim cannot be fulfilled without understanding both the mechanisms underlying an individual's pain or dysfunction and how various treatments might interact with those mechanisms. Although the potential mechanisms of MWMs have been discussed in the first edition of this book and the accompanying textbook (Vicenzino et al., 2011b, 2011c), it is relevant to revisit this topic as science progresses.

Over recent years our understanding of the mechanisms of pain has greatly expanded. Broadly speaking, pain mechanisms can be divided into contributions from peripheral (input), central (processing) and response (output) system domains (Fig. 5). With respect to **input / peripheral mechanisms**, we consider factors that might contribute to increased nociceptive signalling to the central nervous system (CNS). These factors might be immune / inflammatory, mechanical, neurogenic or a combination thereof. **Central / processing mechanisms** are those that increase synaptic efficacy in pathways relevant to pain and nociceptive processing – broadly termed central sensitisation. Central sensitisation is not one process, but rather an umbrella term for a range of processes, not all of which are well understood. Typically, central sensitisation refers to an increase in the gain at nociceptor-to-nociceptor interfaces. Other centrally acting processes to consider include: (1) bioplastic adaptations often referred to as functional reorganisation (Flor, 2003; Flor et al., 1997; Moseley & Flor, 2012), (2) cognitive and affective variables operating at the level of context, expectations and information processing (Moseley & Arntz, 2007; Tracey, 2010; Wiech et al., 2008) and (3) associative learning mechanisms that are posited to link pain responses to non-nociceptive stimuli (Harvie et al., 2015, 2016, 2018; Madden & Moseley, 2016; Madden et al., 2015). With respect to **output / response systems**, we consider protective nervous system-mediated responses that might initially be adaptive but, if persistent, may contribute to a cycle of pain or movement dysfunction. These potentially maladaptive responses include efferent motor, sympathetic, neuroendocrine and neuroimmune responses (Butler & Moseley, 2013; Mosley & Butler, 2017). Manual therapies such as MWMs – to the extent that they are effective (see reviews of effectiveness by Hing et al., 2009; Vicenzino et al., 2011b, 2011c) – must have

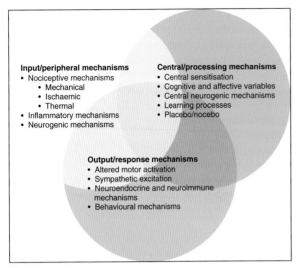

Figure 5
A snapshot of some of the key mechanisms that may underlie a pain state

their effect by interacting with underlying mechanisms of pain and movement dysfunction. After all, they cannot influence pain or movement if they do not influence their underlying biological processes. In the following paragraphs we will discuss possible interactions between MWM and some of the mechanisms underlying pain and movement dysfunction.

MWMs and peripheral mechanisms

Historically, it has been assumed that manual therapies affect pain by altering such factors as alignment, mechanical function, tone or tissue extensibility, and that any change in pain results from alteration of mechanical forces and tissue physiology. In the evolution of MWMs, a number of observations led Brian Mulligan to favour a positional fault hypothesis (PFH) as both the cause of a range of musculoskeletal pain conditions and the explanation for MWM effects. That is, he noticed that many of his patients who presented with peripheral joint problems demonstrated remarkable improvements in pain and ROM following applications of novel manual therapy techniques applied in a way consistent with the PFH (Mulligan, 1989, 1993). More specifically, Mulligan noticed these improvements when applying passive joint mobilisation – typically an accessory glide applied perpendicular to the plane of movement – *during* the (normally) pain-provoking active movement. Importantly, Mulligan found that the direction of glide was critical to the outcome of the technique. It was this direction specificity that led him to speculate that these patients presented with a positional fault at the offending joint, and that the externally applied force of the treatment technique corrected this fault (Mulligan, 1996, 2010). The positional fault could be thought of as a bony incongruence – which may occur as a result of altered soft tissue supports following a sprain, strain or other injury – that resulted in symptoms as a result of interference with normal joint function. Although some evidence has supported suspicions that static bony alignment often deviates from the population mean in some patient groups (Desmeules et al., 2004; Herrington, 2008; Hubbard & Hertel, 2008; Hubbard et al., 2006), there is so far a lack of any evidence that MWMs correct such an alignment, and alternative hypotheses regarding the mechanisms responsible for the effects of MWM have been proposed (Baeske, 2015; Vicenzino et al., 2011b).

Altered mechanoreceptive input during MWM

As with any valid theory, any explanation for the effect of MWM must account for the observed phenomena. These observations include: (1) normally painful and / or restricted motion can be dramatically improved during application of an external force during that motion, (2) a certain degree of force is required to achieve benefit, (3) improvement is generally dependent on the direction of applied force, and (4) the change in movement and pain often persists for at least a short period beyond application. The immediate effects on pain and the direction and force specificity of the effect outlined in points 1–3 can be explained by understanding mechanoreceptor function.

Mechanoreceptors are present throughout the somatosensory system, within afferent nociceptive, tactile and proprioceptive neurons. MWM is applied only where a symptom of pain and / or stiffness coincides with movement, suggesting that mechanoreceptive input is linked to the presenting symptoms. It follows that altering this mechanoreceptive input will then likely alter symptoms, at least for the duration that the input is altered. Animal studies suggest that articular and periarticular mechanoreceptors elicit distinct activation under different loads, and respond to specific directions of strain (Chen et al., 2005, 2006; Pickar & McLain, 1995). The application of an MWM technique may alter the force and / or direction of force exerted to mechanoreceptors in the applied region, which will subsequently alter the suite of mechanoreceptive input to the CNS. Mechanoreceptive input may be nociceptive (pain-facilitating) or tactile / proprioceptive (generally pain-inhibiting (Melzack & Wall, 1965)). Thus, an MWM might reduce symptoms either by reducing nociceptive signalling or increasing non-nociceptive signalling. Of further note, provided that sufficient force is applied to alter mechanoreceptive input, a change in symptoms will likely result, regardless of whether a positional fault is present or corrected. Thus, the positional fault hypothesis is not required to explain the immediate effects of MWM. For an extensive review of the role of mechanoreceptors in MWM see Baeske (2015).

MWMs and central mechanisms

Does pain alleviation by MWM prove peripheral dysfunction?

When pain is predictably provoked by mechanical action and eased by its variation, we quickly implicate a mechanical, or at least peripheral, nociceptive mechanism. Although the logic is attractive, theoretical and established mechanisms exist whereby non-nociceptive mechanical input can come to trigger pain. The most common example of this is allodynia, whereby central sensitisation processes allow non-noxious stimulation to trigger pain (Latremoliere & Woolf, 2009). Although the pathways responsible for non-noxious mechanical information are anatomically distinct from those responsible for noxious (nociceptive) information, potential facilitatory (and inhibitory) connections exist between them, which become activated as part of the sensitisation process – thus allowing tactile and proprioceptive inputs alone to cause pain independently of tissue state or nociception. Further, it has been suggested that associative learning mechanisms – such as the Hebbian learning process characterised by the phrase *neurons that fire together, wire together* – might induce further facilitatory links between non-noxious mechanical / non-mechanical inputs and nociceptive pathways (Moseley & Vlaeyen, 2015), which is further discussed below.

Extinguishing movement–pain associations

The imprecision hypothesis recently proposed an associative learning pathway whereby non-nociceptive information could acquire nociceptive-like effects (i.e. the ability to contribute to or trigger pain) (Moseley & Vlaeyen, 2015). Nociceptors have higher thresholds and slower transmission than tactile and proprioceptive neurons. Therefore, in physiological situations, nociception is always preceded by non-nociceptive input, providing opportunities for associative learning – neurons that fire together, wire together. Utilising the classical (Pavlovian) conditioning framework, the imprecision hypothesis proposes that, after repeated pairing of a non-nociceptive stimulus and a nociceptive stimulus, the non-nociceptive stimulus may come to elicit the response intrinsic to the nociceptive stimulus – thus enabling the normally inert stimulus to contribute to pain as an acquired *conditioned response*. Indeed, pairing a pain-associated cue with nociceptive stimulation seems to facilitate activity in regions responsible for nociceptive processing (Atlas et al., 2010; Diesch & Flor, 2007; Jensen et al., 2014) and a small number of human studies have shown that, after a classical conditioning procedure, a nociceptive stimulus is more painful if it is preceded by a pain-associated cue (Madden et al., 2015). As musculoskeletal pain is frequently associated with movement, kinaesthetic feedback, such as that from mechanoreceptors, might become conditioned stimuli capable of contributing to pain. This provides an intriguing possible explanation for the observations of Mulligan and for the apparent effectiveness of MWMs. That is, if a specific package of normally non-painful mechanosensory input, such as that resulting from a bending movement, comes to contribute to pain because of its prior association with pain, then specific alterations of that mechanosensory input using MWM techniques may help to explain the immediate pain alleviation. Further, repeating the movement in the relatively pain-free manner afforded by application of the MWM may assist to break the association between movement, in this case bending, and pain. Indeed, it has previously been suggested that MWMs might be repeated in order to facilitate relearning of previous pain-free motor memories (Zusman, 2004), and that this might occur through the same physiological and behavioural mechanisms that extinguish aversive memories (Myers & Davis, 2002). That MWM targets the patient's specific physical task associated with pain, and that it does so in a painless manner, lends it to being viewed as a learning strategy (Vicenzino et al., 2011b). In classical conditioning theory, this strategy is known as extinction learning, and is thought to diminish the learned response by weakening the association, in this case between movement and pain, and reinstating implicit pain-free movement memory traces. This theory has historically been applied to fear of movement (Meulders et al., 2011), and has only more recently been seriously considered with direct application to pain (Moseley & Vlaeyen, 2015; Zaman et al., 2015); thus the theory remains to be fully verified, although progress has been made (Harvie et al., 2015, 2016; Madden et al., 2015).

Centrally mediated inhibitory mechanisms

Manual therapy, in general, is known to induce activation of temporarily acting analgesic mechanisms (Bialosky et al., 2009; Malisza et al., 2003; Sterling et al., 2001). Because of their temporary nature, these analgesic mechanisms should rarely be considered useful targets, and perhaps instead practitioners should be cautious that these mechanisms are likely to lead to practitioner and patient bias. Generally speaking, the effects of MWM appear to include analgesic effects similar to those in other manual therapy interventions, including non-opioid-mediated mechanical hypoalgesia (i.e. reduced mechanical sensitivity that is non-naloxone-reversible and does not show tolerance to repeated applications (Vicenzino et al., 2007)). The evidence that MWM activates endogenous inhibitory mechanisms has been reviewed in the preceding book (Sterling & Vicenzino, 2011). Interestingly, there is some suggestion that MWM-mediated changes in movement, and movement-related pain, may not be the result of these mechanisms. For example, MWM tends to both change pressure pain thresholds and improve movement; however, improvement in movement in one study did not appear to correlate with changes in pressure pain thresholds (Pearson's correlation coefficient, $r=0.29$, $p=0.17$) (Teys et al., 2008). Thus, the mechanisms responsible for changes in movement-related pain might be distinct from those responsible for the generalised pain-inhibiting effect of manual therapy. Similarly, Delgado-Gil and colleagues found improvement in movement and movement-related pain in patients with shoulder impingement syndrome 24 hours following 2 weeks of bi-weekly treatments, but no significant change in resting pain (Delgado-Gil et al., 2015). Further, improvements were specific to the movement treated: flexion and not abduction increased. Thus, a generalised inhibitory effect does not appear to explain the effects of MWM, and thus neurological, motor and cognitive processes associated with the target movement are more likely responsible for the effects of MWM that persist beyond the treatment session itself.

MWMs, placebo and reassurance

Although placebo is unlikely to play a strong role in the effect of treatment during application – as this would not easily explain the direction specificity of the improvements in pain and movement – it probably does play a role following its application. Placebo is an effect that appears to be largely dependent on a positive expectation of treatment benefit (Colloca et al., 2008). This positive expectation can be derived from a number of domains, such as verbal information, non-verbal cues and vicarious or experiential learning (i.e. past experience). One way to think about placebo is as a treatment whose active ingredient is the reassuring effect of receiving a treatment perceived as credible – which imparts a range of psychological and neurophysiological effects (Traeger et al., 2015). Interestingly, different interventions have a different degree of placebo effect (Zhang et al., 2008). For example, a placebo surgery is more effective that a needle-based placebo, which is more effective than a tablet-based placebo (Autret et al., 2012; de Craen et al., 2000; Moseley et al., 2002). This spectrum of effectiveness parallels the perceived credibility of the treatments and the associated positive expectation of recovery and reassurance that likely results from their reception. Where the application of an MWM is able to achieve pain-free movement, the perceived technique credibility is likely to be implicit and profound. This is particularly true for patients where the problem movement has been reliably associated with pain for some time. Without doubt, this experience can be profound to the client, who may feel reassured that the problem and solution has been identified. Of course caution is needed, as discovering that application of a technique reduces pain does not prove that repeated application is the panacea. None the less, even in complex cases with multiple biopsychosocial contributors, having a strategy to produce and rehearse pain-free motion during functional movements undoubtedly has utility when considered in context of a broader biopsychosocial management plan. A further note: if reassurance is the potent aspect of the placebo effect, then therapists should also consider how they can bolster the reassuring effect of MWM with other strategies – for example, reassuring patients that ongoing pain typically reflects nervous system sensitivity, rather than tissue damage, and thus movement is safe and recovery is possible. Further, framing an MWM application in terms of extinguishing learned pain and motor responses, rather than positional faults or tissue changes, might also reduce the perception of threat and facilitate reassurance.

MWMs and output (response) mechanisms

Pain and the motor system

Changes in patterns of muscle activation are a common response to pain and injury and are thought to serve a protective function in the near term. For example, facilitation of antagonist and inhibition of agonist muscles are commonly found (Hodges & Smeets, 2015). Given that these changes in activation can be caused by experimentally induced pain, it appears that pain causes changes in muscle activation, rather than the other way around (Hodges & Smeets, 2015). Of course, this does not rule out the possibility that altered muscle activation could contribute to problem persistence, or that targeting muscle activation might assist in breaking the cycle.

In a case where MWM application immediately reduces pain with movement, it can be deduced that a particular pattern, or quantity, of mechanoreceptor signalling is contributing to pain, and that altering that pattern through external force reduces it. As an external force can alter symptoms by altering mechanoreceptor activation, it is within reason that altering internal forces, by altering motor activation, might also be capable of reducing pain. Altering patterns of muscle activation through motor control training has been one approach to this aim, although with mixed reports of success (Macedo et al., 2009). It is possible that rehearsal of movements under the pain-reducing influence of MWM external forces may provide a different approach to altering muscle activation patterns. There are several reasons why rehearsal in this way might alter muscle activation. For instance, patients who are more fearful of movement tend to have greater alterations in muscle activation (Hodges & Moseley, 2003). Rehearsing movement in a less-painful manner might result in more confidence when performing the movement, and a subsequent relative normalisation of muscle activation. Further, if pain is able to perturb the motor system then rehearsal of pain-free movement might assist to restore it, although further work is clearly needed.

Mechanoreceptors and the motor system

Mechanosensory feedback serves a number of important functions underpinning motor control, such as providing information about what is occurring at articular and periarticular sites that might lead to injury, and about movement quality relative to an intended goal (Baeske, 2015; Proske & Gandevia, 2012). Muscle activation patterns are initiated centrally and are constantly modified, in real time, by complex feedback loops. Some of these operate beneath the level of consciousness, as many aspects of motor control are too complex and fast for the conscious decision-making processes. One aspect of this process is outlined in Fig. 6. For each motor command, the nervous system generates a copy of the expected sensory feedback, known as an efferent copy of the expected proprioceptive map. The actual sensory feedback, the afferent copy of the proprioceptive map, is then referenced against this efferent copy, such that fine adjustments to motor activation can be made to realign actual and expected sensory feedback (Kawato et al., 1987; Proske & Gandevia, 2012). This provides a pathway whereby changes in mechanosensory feedback might elicit changes in motor activation. That is, the application of an MWM technique might create a discrepancy between expected and actual sensory feedback, eliciting a change in motor activation intended to correct the discrepancy. If this is the case, then it is possible that repeating the MWM may cause bioplastic adaptations in motor patterning that may extend beyond technique application. Indeed, at least short-term changes in motor function have been shown following MWM in some body regions. For example, MWM at the elbow in people with lateral epicondylalgia results in an increase in grip strength when applied to the affected side, whereas a decrease occurs when applied to the non-affected side (Abbott, 2001; Vicenzino et al., 2001). Indeed, other inhibitory and facilitatory links exist between mechanoreceptors and the motor system, such as the mechanisms responsible for the well-known contract–relax phenomenon; however, only mechanisms that offer a potential for motor learning are likely to offer the potential for more than a short-term effect.

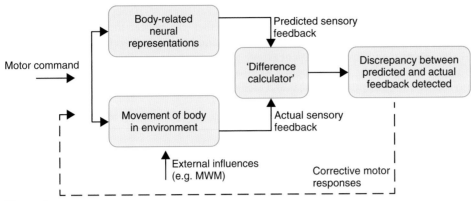

Figure 6

For each motor command, the nervous system generates a copy of the expected sensory feedback (efferent copy). The actual sensory feedback is then referenced against this efferent copy, such that fine adjustments to motor activation can be made to align actual and expected feedback.

(Adapted from Kawato et al., 1987; Proske & Gandevia, 2012.)

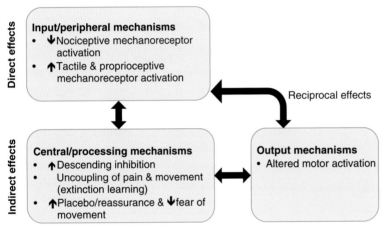

Figure 7

Summary of some of the direct and indirect effects of MWMs. The arrows highlight potential downstream and reciprocal interactions among mechanisms, providing potential pathways for improvement beyond the immediate MWM application.

The possibility of sustained benefit

Generally speaking, the duration of peripheral, central and motor changes in response to MWM remains uninvestigated. A number of characteristics of MWM distinguish it from other manual therapies, and may give it unique capacity to induce a sustained benefit in some patients. Of particular note is that MWM integrates manual therapy with active movements and, moreover, it can often render those active movements pain-free, at least for the duration of application. In this introduction we have discussed mechanisms such as reassurance, extinction learning / exposure therapy and motor learning that might result from experiencing a normally painful movement in a pain-free (or at least pain-reduced) manner. If there is sufficient rehearsal in functional contexts, then it is possible that more lasting effects might result – particularly when augmented by other biopsychosocial considerations. Further, interactions between the direct and indirect effects of MWM (Fig. 7) might contribute to a more sustained effect in well-selected clients. For example, if the reduced pain and reduced fear of movement alters motor system performance, then this may in turn change kinematic function, resulting in altered afferent sensory signalling via altered mechanoreceptor activation.

Conclusion

The positional fault hypothesis is no longer needed to explain the effects of MWM. A number of unique characteristics of MWM, among manual therapy techniques, gives it unique potential to influence patients in a way that may assist towards more lasting benefits. Specifically, in patients where MWM is able to render a normally painful movement pain-free, unique opportunities for implicit reassurance, extinction learning / exposure therapy and motor relearning may come to the fore. None the less, these ideas remain to be tested and further work is needed to elucidate the potential effects of MWM and how it can be applied to maximise these effects.

AIMS AND STRUCTURE OF THE BOOK

The primary aim of our first book (Vicenzino et al., 2011a) was to present a comprehensive and contemporary discourse on Mulligan's MWM management approach for musculoskeletal pain, injury and disability. In particular, it sought to integrate the evidence base for MWM into clinical practice, with an emphasis on explicating the underpinning clinical reasoning.

The first edition of this book (Hing et al., 2015) was a companion volume to the first book in that it covers in greater detail each technique. Each chapter covered a different area of the body carefully explaining the practitioner's body and hand positioning with respect to the patient and the treated body part. Photographs from different perspectives were widely used throughout each chapter, together with detailed text to explain each technique precisely. Alternative techniques were explored where available. In addition to practitioner techniques, there were also home exercise and taping techniques, as well as reference to relevant research.

Since this book was published in 2015, a number of new techniques have been developed, necessitating an updated and expanded version of the original first edition. In addition to new techniques, the first edition of this textbook has been updated in terms of modern evidence-based explanations for the mechanisms of action of Mulligan Concept techniques, together with updated evidence regarding each technique described. The book has also been extensively reformulated to make it easier to follow. We believe the second edition of this book provides clinicians with a valuable resource to help them manage their patients.

References

Abbott, J., 2001. Mobilization with movement applied to the elbow affects shoulder range of movement in subjects with lateral epicondylalgia. Man. Ther. 6 (3), 170–177.

Atlas, L.Y., Bolger, N., Lindquist, M.A., Wager, T.D., 2010. Brain mediators of predictive cue effects on perceived pain. J. Neurosci. 30 (39), 12964–12977.

Autret, A., Valade, D., Debiais, S., 2012. Placebo and other psychological interactions in headache treatment. J. Headache Pain 13 (3), 191–198.

Baeske, R., 2015. Mobilisation with movement: a step towards understanding the importance of peripheral mechanoreceptors. Phys. Ther. Rev. 20 (5–6), 299–305.

Bialosky, J.E., Bishop, M.D., Price, D.D., Robinson, M.E., George, S.Z., 2009. The mechanisms of manual therapy in the treatment of musculoskeletal pain: a comprehensive model. Man. Ther. 14 (5), 531–538.

Butler, D.S., Moseley, G.L., 2013. Explain Pain, 2nd ed. Noigroup, Adelaide.

Chen, C., Lu, Y., Cavanaugh, J.M., Kallakuri, S., Patwardhan, A., 2005. Recording of neural activity from goat cervical facet joint capsule using custom-designed miniature electrodes. Spine 30 (12), 1367–1372.

Chen, C., Lu, Y., Kallakuri, S., Patwardhan, A., Cavanaugh, J.M., 2006. Distribution of A-δ and C-fiber receptors in the cervical facet joint capsule and their response to stretch. J. Bone Joint Surg. 88 (8), 1807–1816.

Colloca, L., Sigaudo, M., Benedetti, F., 2008. The role of learning in nocebo and placebo effects. Pain 136 (1–2), 211–218.

de Craen, A.J., Tijssen, J., de Gans, J., Kleijnen, J., 2000. Placebo effect in the acute treatment of migraine: subcutaneous placebos are better than oral placebos. J. Neurol. 247 (3), 183–188.

Delgado-Gil, J.A., Prado-Robles, E., Rodrigues-de-Souza, D.P., Cleland, J.A., Fernández-de-las-Peñas, C., Alburquerque-Sendín, F., 2015. Effects of mobilization with movement on pain and range of motion in patients with unilateral shoulder impingement syndrome: a randomized controlled trial. J. Manipulative Physiol. Ther. 38 (4), 245–252.

Desmeules, F., Minville, L., Riederer, B., Côté, C.H., Frémont, P., 2004. Acromio-humeral distance variation measured by ultrasonography and its association with the outcome of rehabilitation for shoulder impingement syndrome. Clin. J. Sport Med. 14 (4), 197–205.

Diesch, E., Flor, H., 2007. Alteration in the response properties of primary somatosensory cortex related to differential aversive Pavlovian conditioning. Pain 131 (1–2), 171–180.

Edwards, B.C., 1999. Manual of Combined Movements: Their Use in the Examination and Treatment of Mechanical Vertebral Column Disorders. Butterworth-Heinemann, Edinburgh.

Flor, H., 2003. Cortical reorganisation and chronic pain: implications for rehabilitation. J. Rehabil. Med. 41 (41), 66–72.

Flor, H., Braun, C., Elbert, T., Birbaumer, N., 1997. Extensive reorganization of primary somatosensory cortex in chronic back pain patients. Neurosci. Lett. 224 (1), 5–8.

Gay, R.E., Nelson, C.F., 2003. Contraindications to spinal manipulative therapy. In: Alternative Medicine and Rehabilitation: A Guide to Practitioners. Demos Medical, New York.

Gifford, L., 1998. Pain, the tissues and the nervous system: a conceptual model. Physiotherapy 84 (1), 27–36.

Harvie, D.S., Broecker, M., Smith, R.T., Meulders, A., Madden, V.J., Moseley, G.L., 2015. Bogus visual feedback alters onset of movement-evoked pain in people with neck pain. Psychol. Sci. 26 (4), 385–392.

Harvie, D.S., Meulders, A., Madden, V.J., Hillier, S.L., Peto, D.K., Brinkworth, R., et al., 2016. When touch predicts pain: predictive tactile cues modulate perceived intensity of painful stimulation independent of expectancy. Scand. J. Pain 11, 11–18.

Harvie, D.S., Sterling, M., Smith, A.D., 2018. Do pain-associated contexts increase pain sensitivity? An investigation using virtual reality. Scand. J. Pain 18 (3), 525–532.

Herrington, L., 2008. The difference in a clinical measure of patella lateral position between individuals with patellofemoral pain and matched controls. J. Orthop. Sports Phys. Ther. 38 (2), 59–62.

Hing, W., Bigelow, R., Bremner, T., 2009. Mulligan's mobilization with movement: a systematic review. J. Man. Manip. Ther. 17 (2), 39E–66E.

Hing, W., Hall, T., Rivett, D., Vicenzino, B., Mulligan, B., 2015. The Mulligan Concept of Manual Therapy – Textbook of Techniques. Elsevier, Chatswood, NSW.

Hodges, P.W., Smeets, R.J., 2015. Interaction between pain, movement, and physical activity: short-term benefits, long-term consequences, and targets for treatment. Clin. J. Pain 31 (2), 97–107.

Hodges, P.W., Moseley, G.L., 2003. Pain and motor control of the lumbopelvic region: effect and possible mechanisms. J. Electromyogr. Kinesiol. 13 (4), 361–370.

Hubbard, T.J., Hertel, J., 2008. Anterior positional fault of the fibula after sub-acute lateral ankle sprains. Man. Ther. 13 (1), 63–67.

Hubbard, T.J., Hertel, J., Sherbondy, P., 2006. Fibular position in individuals with self-reported chronic ankle instability. J. Orthop. Sports Phys. Ther. 36 (1), 3–9.

Jensen, K.B., Kaptchuk, T.J., Chen, X., Kirsch, I., Ingvar, M., Gollub, R.L., et al., 2014. A neural mechanism for nonconscious activation of conditioned placebo and nocebo responses. Cereb. Cortex 25 (10), 3903–3910.

Jones, M.A., Rivett, D.A., 2004. Introduction to clinical reasoning. In: Jones, M.A., Rivett, D.A. (Eds.), Clinical Reasoning for Manual Therapists. Butterworth-Heinemann, Edinburgh, pp. 3–24.

Kaltenborn, F.M., 1980. Mobilisation of the Extremity Joints. Olaf Norlis Bokhande, Norway.

Kawato, M., Furukawa, K., Suzuki, R., 1987. A hierarchical neural-network model for control and learning of voluntary movement. Biol. Cybern. 57 (3), 169–185.

Latremoliere, A., Woolf, C.J., 2009. Central sensitization: a generator of pain hypersensitivity by central neural plasticity. J. Pain 10 (9), 895–926.

Macedo, L.G., Maher, C.G., Latimer, J., McAuley, J.H., 2009. Motor control exercise for persistent, nonspecific low back pain: a systematic review. Phys. Ther. 89 (1), 9–25.

McKenzie, R.A., May, S., 2003. The Lumbar Spine: Mechanical Diagnosis and Therapy, 2nd ed. Spinal, Waikanae, NZ.

Madden, V.J., Moseley, G.L., 2016. Do clinicians think that pain can be a classically conditioned response to a non-noxious stimulus? Man. Ther. 22, 165–173.

Madden, V.J., Harvie, D.S., Parker, R., Jensen, K.B., Vlaeyen, J.W., Moseley, G.L., et al., 2015. Can pain or hyperalgesia be a classically conditioned response in humans? A systematic review and meta-analysis. Pain Med. 17 (6), 1094–1111.

Maitland, G.D., 2005. Maitland's Peripheral Manipulation, 4th ed. Butterworth Heinemann Elsevier, Sydney.

Malisza, K.L., Gregorash, L., Turner, A., Foniok, T., Stroman, P.W., Allman, A.A., et al., 2003. Functional MRI involving painful stimulation of the ankle and the effect of physiotherapy joint mobilization. Magn. Reson. Imaging 21 (5), 489–496.

Melzack, R., Wall, P.D., 1965. Pain mechanisms: a new theory. Science 150 (3699), 971–979.

Meulders, A., Vansteenwegen, D., Vlaeyen, J.W., 2011. The acquisition of fear of movement-related pain and associative learning: a novel pain-relevant human fear conditioning paradigm. Pain 152 (11), 2460–2469.

Moseley, G.L., Arntz, A., 2007. The context of a noxious stimulus affects the pain it evokes. Pain 133 (1–3), 64–71.

Moseley, G.L., Flor, H., 2012. Targeting cortical representations in the treatment of chronic pain: a review. Neurorehabil. Neural Repair 26 (6), 646–652.

Mosley, G.L., Butler, D.S., 2017. Explain Pain Supercharged. Noigroup, Adelaide.

Moseley, G.L., Vlaeyen, J.W., 2015. Beyond nociception: the imprecision hypothesis of chronic pain. Pain 156 (1), 35–38.

Moseley, J.B., O'Malley, K., Petersen, N.J., Menke, T.J., Brody, B.A., Kuykendall, D.H., et al., 2002. A controlled trial of arthroscopic surgery for osteoarthritis of the knee. N. Engl. J. Med. 347 (2), 81–88.

Mulligan, B., 1989. Manual Therapy: 'NAGs', 'SNAGs', 'PRPs' Etc., 1st ed. Plane View Services, Wellington, NZ.

Mulligan, B., 1993. Mobilisations with movement (MWM's). J. Man. Manip. Ther. 1 (4), 154–156.

Mulligan, B., 1996. Mobilisations with movement (MWMs) for the hip joint to restore internal rotation and flexion. J. Man. Manip. Ther. 4 (1), 35–36.

Mulligan, B., 2010. Manual Therapy: 'NAGs', 'SNAGs', 'MWMs' Etc., 6th ed. Orthopedic Physical Therapy Products, Wellington, NZ.

Mulligan, B., 2019. Manual Therapy: NAGs, SNAGs, MWMs, Etc., 7th ed. Blackwell, Oxford. in press.

Myers, K.M., Davis, M., 2002. Behavioral and neural analysis of extinction. Neuron 36 (4), 567–584.

Pickar, J.G., McLain, R.F., 1995. Responses of mechanosensitive afferents to manipulation of the lumbar facet in the cat. Spine 20 (22), 2379–2385.

Proske, U., Gandevia, S.C., 2012. The proprioceptive senses: their roles in signaling body shape, body position and movement, and muscle force. Physiol. Rev. 92 (4), 1651–1697.

Sackett, D., Straus, S., Richardson, W., Rosenberg, W., Haynes, R., 2000. Evidence-Based Medicine: How to Practice and Teach EBM, 2nd ed. Churchill Livingstone, Edinburgh.

Sackett, D.L., Rosenberg, W.M.C., Gray, J.A.M., Haynes, R.B., Richardson, W.S., 1996. Evidence based medicine: what it is and what it isn't. BMJ 312 (7023), 71–72.

Sterling, M., Vicenzino, B., 2011. Pain and sensory system impairments that may be amenable to mobilisation with movement. In: Vicenzino, B., Hing, W., Rivett, D., Hall, T. (Eds.), Mobilisation With Movement: The Art and the Science. Churchill Livingstone, London, pp. 86–92.

Sterling, M., Jull, G., Wright, A., 2001. Cervical mobilisation: concurrent effects on pain, sympathetic nervous system activity and motor activity. Man. Ther. 6 (2), 72–81.

Teys, P., Bisset, L., Vicenzino, B., 2008. The initial effects of a Mulligan's mobilization with movement technique on range of movement and pressure pain threshold in pain-limited shoulders. Man. Ther. 13 (1), 37–42.

Tracey, I., 2010. Getting the pain you expect: mechanisms of placebo, nocebo and reappraisal effects in humans. Nat. Med. 16 (11), 1277.

Traeger, A.C., Hübscher, M., Henschke, N., Moseley, G.L., Lee, H., McAuley, J.H., 2015. Effect of primary care–based education on reassurance in patients with acute low back pain: systematic review and meta-analysis. JAMA Intern. Med. 175 (5), 733–743.

Vicenzino, B., Paungmali, A., Buratowski, S., Wright, A., 2001. Specific manipulative therapy treatment for chronic lateral epicondylalgia produces uniquely characteristic hypoalgesia. Man. Ther. 6 (4), 205–212.

Vicenzino, B., Paungmali, A., Teys, P., 2007. Mulligan's mobilization-with-movement, positional faults and pain relief: current concepts from a critical review of literature. Man. Ther. 12 (2), 98–108.

Vicenzino, B., Hing, W., Hall, T., Rivett, D., 2011a. Mobilisation with movement: the art and science of its application. In: Vicenzino, B., Hing, W., Rivett, D., Hall, T. (Eds.), Mobilisation With Movement: The Art and the Science. Churchill Livingstone Australia, Sydney, pp. 9–23.

Vicenzino, B., Hall, T., Hing, W., Rivett, D., 2011b. A new proposed model of the mechanisms of action of mobilisation with movement. In: Vicenzino, B., Hing, W., Rivett, D., Hall, T. (Eds.), Mobilisation With Movement: The Art and the Science. Churchill Livingstone Australia, Sydney, pp. 75–85.

Vicenzino, B., Hing, W., Hall, T., Rivett, D., 2011c. Mobilisation With Movement: The Art and the Science. Churchill Livingstone Australia, Sydney.

Wiech, K., Ploner, M., Tracey, I., 2008. Neurocognitive aspects of pain perception. Trends Cogn. Sci. 12 (8), 306–313.

Zaman, J., Vlaeyen, J.W., Van Oudenhove, L., Wiech, K., Van Diest, I., 2015. Associative fear learning and perceptual discrimination: a perceptual pathway in the development of chronic pain. Neurosci. Biobehav. Rev. 51, 118–125.

Zhang, W., Robertson, J., Jones, A., Dieppe, P., Doherty, M., 2008. The placebo effect and its determinants in osteoarthritis: meta-analysis of randomised controlled trials. Ann. Rheum. Dis. 67 (12), 1716–1723.

Zusman, M., 2004. Mechanisms of musculoskeletal physiotherapy. Phys. Ther. Rev. 9 (1), 39–49.

Cervicogenic headache

TECHNIQUES FOR CERVICOGENIC HEADACHES

INTRODUCTION

Headache is both a symptom and a disorder in its own right, hence classification of headache is important to ensure that correct treatment is administered (Dodick, 2010). The International Headache Society (IHS) has broadly classified headache as primary where there is no other causative factor, or secondary where the headache occurs in close temporal relationship to another disorder to which it is attributed (The International Classification of Headache Disorders, 2004). Cervicogenic headache (CGH) is one form of secondary headache, which arises from disorder of the cervical spine.

Current medical teaching indicates that each form of headache has a different pathological basis, the majority of which does not have a musculoskeletal cause (Dodick, 2010). Hence, it is critical that the individual presenting for treatment has their type of headache correctly identified. This is particularly important for the manual therapist's considering physical intervention for headache, where such intervention is unlikely to be effective for disorders other than those affecting the musculoskeletal system (Hall, 2011).

Mechanisms underlying CGH are those of convergence of afferent input from the upper three cervical segments with input from trigeminal afferents in the trigeminocervical nucleus (Bogduk & Govind, 2009). Hence input from sensory afferents in the cervical spine may be mistakenly perceived as pain in the head (Bogduk & Govind, 2009). Classification of headache disorders based on patient-reported symptoms and history is problematic owing to the overlap of features between CGH and migraine and other headache forms. Headache classification is therefore based on physical examination. The cervical flexion–rotation test (FRT) has been found to be a useful test to discriminate CGH from migraine or mixed headache forms (Hall et al., 2010a). The positive cut-off point is 32°–33° (Hall et al., 2010b, 2010c; Ogince et al., 2007). An MRI study revealed that a positive test primarily indicates limitation of movement at the C1/2 level (Takasaki et al., 2011). The degree of limitation on this test has been shown to correlate with the severity, frequency and duration of headache symptoms (Hall et al., 2010b), as well as being independent of other physiological and lifestyle factors (Smith et al., 2008). Consequently, the test has utility regardless of the age, gender or lifestyle of the person tested. Further study is required to identify the FRT's sensitivity to change as an outcome measure.

In the presence of a positive FRT, a C1/2 self-SNAG can be applied as a treatment technique to attempt to restore normal ROM and reduce symptoms. However, if a patient presents to the clinic experiencing a CGH at the time of consultation and has a positive FRT, then a trial of headache SNAG, reverse headache SNAG, or upper cervical traction should be administered first. On subsequent visits, if symptoms are reduced but the FRT remains positive, then a C1/2 self-SNAG should be considered at that point.

Levels of evidence

Level 2: four RCTs and one case report

The available evidence suggests that application of the SNAG technique improves cervical ROM in patients with CGH and positive FRT. The application of a self-SNAG to people with chronic CGH and a positive FRT was shown to be superior to a placebo treatment in a randomised controlled trial (RCT) (Hall et al., 2007). Hall and colleagues (Hall et al., 2007) showed that when compared with the placebo the self-SNAG improved range recorded during the FRT by 10° (95% confidence interval (CI): 4.7–15.3°) immediately after application and that at 12 months the treated group were 22 (13–31) points superior on the headache severity index (baseline headache severity index approximately 54/100). When investigating the effectiveness of different types of manual therapy techniques in information technology professionals with a positive FRT and CGH, Neeti (2017) also reported a 9.3°±2.1 improvement in cervical ROM in the group who received SNAG treatment. Such improvement was significantly superior to that of the group that received Maitland treatment (6.6°±1.6) and of the control group (2.9°±1.0) after 1 week of treatment.

Similarly, Shin and Lee (2014) demonstrated a significant reduction in pain (VAS 27.12 mm+14.66), Neck Disability Index (NDI) (3.20+1.39) and headache duration (3.20+1.39) after 4 weeks of treatment in patients who received SNAG treatment compared with the control group who received a placebo SNAG treatment. An RCT comparing the efficacy of C1–C2 SNAG with posterior anterior vertebral mobilisations (PAVMs) in the management of cervicogenic headaches revealed superior outcomes after the sixth treatment session for patients who received the SNAG treatment (Khan et al., 2014). Khan and colleagues (Khan et al., 2014) demonstrated that the group who received SNAG treatment had a 20% greater reduction in the NDI compared with the PAVMs group. The reduction in pain, assessed through the visual analogue scale (VAS), for the SNAG group was 15.5% greater than that perceived by the PAVMs group (Khan et al., 2014).

1

FLEXION–ROTATION TEST

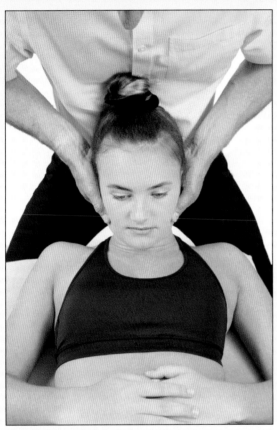

Figure 1.1
Flexion–rotation test: start position

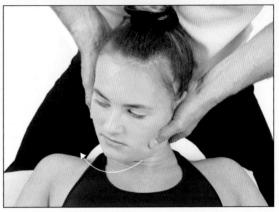

Figure 1.2
Flexion–rotation test: normal end range

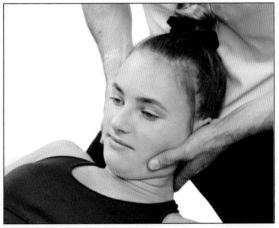

Figure 1.3
Flexion–rotation test: side view

- The patient lies supine with shoulders level with the end of the plinth.
- The patient's head is supported by the therapist's abdomen.
- The therapist passively carefully moves the patient's neck into end-range flexion, translating the head forwards.
- The patient's head is held in this position and then passively rotated to each side and the range recorded.
- See Figs 1.1–1.3.

INDICATION

Headache of possible cervical spine origin or upper cervical symptoms.

POSITIONING

Patient:	Lying supine, shoulders level with the end of the couch.
Treated body part:	Relaxed end-range cervical spine and upper thoracic spine flexion.
Therapist:	Standing at the head of the patient facing their feet with the patient's head supported on the therapist's abdomen.
Hands/contact points:	The therapist maintains end-range cervical spine flexion with hand contact on each side of the mandible together with forward pressure applied through the therapist's abdomen.

APPLICATION GUIDELINES

- End-range flexion is essential to apply the test.
- At end-range cervical spine flexion and with the head translated forwards, cervical rotation to the left and right is noted. Make sure rotation of the head/neck is as pure as possible and no lateral flexion is allowed.
- The end point is either resistance or pain, whichever comes first.
- The normal range is on average 44° to each side (Hall & Robinson, 2004).
- An estimation of loss of range more than 10° confirms a positive test (Hall & Robinson, 2004; Schäfer et al., 2018).
- When using a compass goniometer, the positive cut-off point is 32° with a mean positive predictive value of 86% (Ogince et al., 2007).
- The degree of limitation is correlated with the severity of the headache symptoms (Hall et al., 2010c).
- Typically range is restricted towards the side of the headache. However, in approximately 20% of cases the limitation may be to the opposite side of the headache.
- Range may be limited to both sides.

VARIATIONS

- The FRT may be performed actively in a seated position (Amiri et al., 2003); however, the validity of this test variant to measure upper cervical impairment has not been determined and the ROM is known to be different to that determined in supine (Bravo Petersen & Vardaxis, 2015). The supine position is also preferred because of the ease of measuring ROM, and potentially there will be less stress on the neuromeningeal system in a supine position.

COMMENTS

- Ensure that there is no axial compression force applied through the patient's head/neck. Translate the head/neck forwards, but don't lean down on the head. The purpose of holding the neck in flexion is to constrain movement to only the C1/2 vertebral level (Takasaki et al., 2011). Failure to maintain the end-range flexed position may give a false-negative finding, as movement may occur at other cervical levels.
- The ROM is much greater in children. In general there is on average 9° greater range to each side in children between the ages of 6 and 12 years (Budelmann et al., 2016). However, the FRT can still be used to identify asymmetry in those children who suffer from CGH (Budelmann et al., 2013).
- In the presence of a sensitised neuromeningeal system, it is advisable to perform the FRT with the patient's knees flexed to 90°.
- ROM during the test may be impacted by the presence of temporomandibular dysfunction (Grondin et al., 2015; von Piekartz & Hall, 2013).

C1/2 SELF-SNAG

TECHNIQUE AT A GLANCE

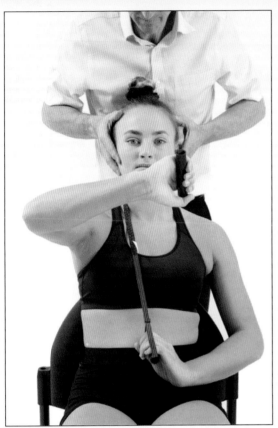

Figure 1.4
C1/2 self-SNAG: start position

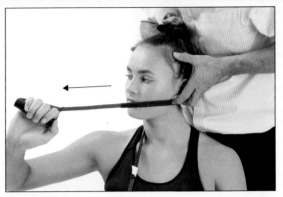

Figure 1.5
C1/2 self-SNAG: end-range position

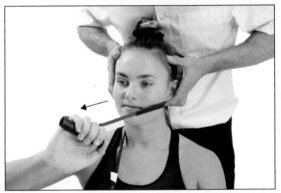

Figure 1.6
C1/2 self-SNAG: side view

- The patient sits in a chair with their back supported.
- The patient places a self-SNAG strap on the posterior arch of C1, below the mastoid process on the contralateral side of the restriction.
- With the hand on the side of the restriction, the patient pulls the strap horizontally forwards to the corner of their mouth.
- While the strap pressure is sustained, the patient rotates the head/neck towards the restricted side.
- Apply over-pressure only if symptom-free at end range.
- See Figs 1.4–1.6.

INDICATION

Headache, neck pain or restriction of C1/2 rotation, together with a unilateral or bilateral restriction on the FRT.

POSITIONING (See Figs 1.4–1.6)

Patient:	Sitting with their back supported against a hard-backed, upright chair.
Treated body part:	Relaxed neutral position of the head and neck. For a right rotation restriction, the patient holds one end of the self-SNAG strap with their right hand. The left elbow hooks over the back of the chair to stabilise the trunk and prevent trunk rotation. The left hand holds the opposite end of the strap loosely, with the left hand resting on the abdomen.
Therapist:	Standing behind the patient's left shoulder.
Hands/belt contact points:	Position the cervical strap immediately below the left mastoid process of the occiput. The strap should be directed horizontally forward, towards the corner of the patient's mouth. The strap lies on the posterior arch of C1 and then angles around the right side of the neck, and is held loosely by the patient with their left hand on their abdomen.
	The therapist directs the patient to ensure that the strap is in the correct position and the direction of force is maintained during the movement.

APPLICATION GUIDELINES

- Prior to applying the technique, the patient is advised about what to expect.

- The patient should feel a strong stretching sensation, but there should be no pain or other symptoms.

- The patient pulls on the strap with their right hand in a horizontal direction towards the corner of their mouth (Figs 1.4–1.6). The patient provides a gentle counterforce pressure with the left hand on the other end of the strap. At the same time the patient will actively rotate their head towards the right for a positive FRT to the right side. At the end of range of rotation the therapist, or as a home exercise a trusted family member, will apply gentle over-pressure to the rotation movement while the patient maintains force along the strap. The over-pressure is maintained for 1–2 seconds before the patient returns the head and neck to the neutral position.

- On the first occasion it is advisable to perform the movement only 2 times, and on subsequent visits increased repetitions can be used, but only if 2 repetitions do not produce lasting headache relief. The technique is repeated as a home exercise in the morning and evening.

- The patient is advised that no symptoms should be provoked during the technique. In addition, this technique would be contraindicated in the presence of vertebrobasilar artery insufficiency or craniovertebral ligament instability. The therapist should be familiar with routine testing procedures for vertebrobasilar artery insufficiency and craniovertebral ligament stability.

- Very occasionally the patient may feel dizziness soon after the first application of the technique. In that case it is advisable to treat the dizziness using the techniques described in Chapter 2 of this book (p. 45). This may be caused by a sudden increase in range at the C1/2 level. Hence, following a C1/2 self-SNAG to the right, as in this example, it would be advised to trial a right side C1 unilateral SNAG with right rotation as the first option to relieve dizziness.

(continued next page...)

1

- Rather than using the self-SNAG strap, it is also possible to use the selvedge edge of a towel to perform the C1/2 self-SNAG (see Fig. 1.7). Alternatively, it is also possible for the therapist to use their thumbs to exert pressure on the C1 transverse process, on the contralateral side (see Chapter 2, C1 dizziness technique, p. 45). A strap or towel is preferred, as the patient will gain optimal benefit from self-treatment, both at the time of treatment and also in the event of later recurrence.

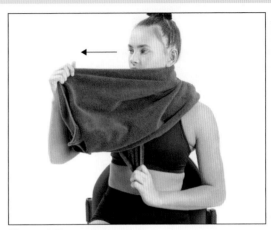

Figure 1.7
Towel C1/2 self-SNAG

COMMENTS

- If the patient presents with significant symptoms on the day of treatment, it is preferable not to use the C1/2 self-SNAG. Rather, the patient should be treated using the other headache techniques in this chapter.

- On occasions the patient may report pain or other symptoms if the strap is not located correctly, or if the angle of the strap is inappropriate. In this case, reposition the strap and correct the angle of force. If pain or other symptoms persist then stop the technique.

- The technique may induce a mild headache in the evening that the technique is first applied. It is advisable to warn the patient of this potential. If headache symptoms are aggravated by the technique on subsequent days then the patient is advised to stop doing the exercise and return for evaluation by the therapist.

- In the situation where there is bilateral restriction, the mobilisation technique is best applied to the most restricted side first and then if required to the other side after the first occasion.

- This technique has been shown to be very efficacious when compared with a placebo treatment in a clinical trial with 12-month follow-up (Hall et al., 2007). There have been three other RCTs showing the benefits of this technique over other forms of treatment including Maitland mobilisation and neck motor control exercises (Khan et al., 2014; Nambi et al., 2014; Neeti, 2017).

ANNOTATIONS

sit C1 self belt SNAG Rot R×2
sit C1 self belt SNAG Rot R +OP(therapist)×2
sit C1 self belt SNAG Rot R +OP(partner)×2
sit C1 self towel SNAG Rot R×2

HEADACHE MWM

TECHNIQUE AT A GLANCE

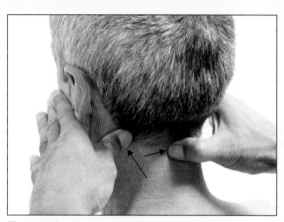

Figure 1.8
Headache MWM: start position

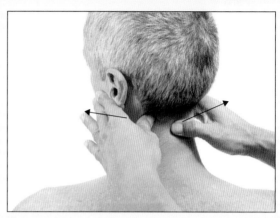

Figure 1.9
Headache MWM: end position

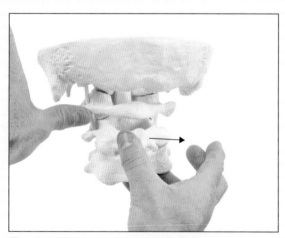

Figure 1.10
Headache MWM: bone view

- The patient sits in a chair with their back supported.
- The therapist places their left thumb on the posterior arch of C1, below the mastoid process on the ipsilateral side of restriction. The medial edge of the right thumb contacts the left side of the spinous process of C2.
- Forward pressure is exerted on C1 with counterforce against the spinous process.
- While the pressure is sustained, the patient rotates the head/neck towards the restricted side.
- Apply over-pressure only if the patient is symptom-free at end range.
- See Figs 1.8–1.10.

1

Headache, neck pain, together with a unilateral or bilateral restriction on the FRT.

POSITIONING (See Figs 1.8–1.10)

Patient:	Sitting with their back supported against a hard-backed, upright chair.
Treated body part:	Relaxed neutral position of the head and neck. Hands resting on the lap.
Therapist:	Standing behind the patient on the side of restriction.
Hands/belt contact points:	The therapist places their left thumb on the posterior arch of C1, below the mastoid process on the ipsilateral side of restriction. The medial edge of the right thumb contacts the left side of the spinous process of C2.

APPLICATION GUIDELINES

- Prior to applying the technique, the therapist advises the patient about what to expect.
- The patient should feel firm pressure on the neck but no pain or other symptoms.
- The therapist places their left thumb on the posterior arch of C1, below the mastoid process on the ipsilateral side of restriction. The medial edge of the right thumb contacts the left side of the spinous process of C2. At the same time the patient will actively rotate their head towards the left for a positive FRT to the left side. At the end of range of rotation the patient will apply gentle over-pressure to the rotation movement while the therapist maintains pressure on C1 and C2. The over-pressure is maintained for 1–2 seconds before returning the head and neck to the neutral position.
- On the first occasion it is advisable to perform the movement only 3 times; on subsequent visits increased repetitions can be used, but only if 3 repetitions do not produce lasting headache relief.
- The patient is advised that no symptoms should be provoked during the technique. In addition, this technique would be contraindicated in the presence of vertebrobasilar artery insufficiency or craniovertebral ligament instability. The therapist should be familiar with routine testing procedures for these conditions.

COMMENTS

- If the patient presents with significant symptoms on the day of treatment, it is preferable not to use this technique. Rather, the patient should be treated using the other headache techniques in this chapter.
- On occasion the patient may report pain or other symptoms if the therapist's hand contact is not applied correctly, or if the angle of the mobilisation is inappropriate. In this case, alter the contact points and correct the angle of force. If pain or other symptoms persist then stop the technique.
- In the situation where there is bilateral restriction, the mobilisation technique is best applied to the most restricted side first and then if required to the other side after the first occasion.

ANNOTATIONS

sit L C1 Ant gl+L C2 trans gl MWM Rot L×3
sit L C1 Ant gl+L C2 trans gl MWM Rot L +OP×3

HEADACHE SNAG

TECHNIQUE AT A GLANCE

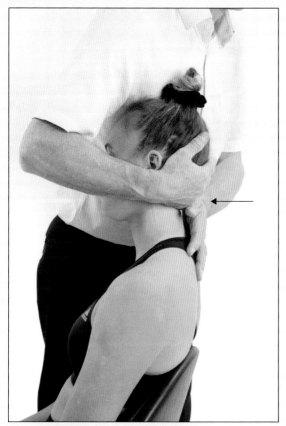

Figure 1.11
Headache SNAG

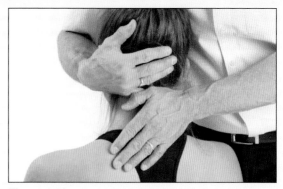

Figure 1.12
Headache SNAG: close view

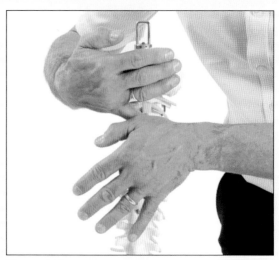

Figure 1.13
Headache SNAG: bone view

- The patient sits in a chair with the back supported and head / neck in a neutral position.
- The therapist stands to the front and side of the patient.
- The therapist stabilises the patient's head against their body.
- The therapist's middle phalanx of the little finger contacts the posterior aspect of the patient's C2 spinous process.
- The therapist's thenar eminence of the non-contact hand presses anteriorly in the horizontal plane against the little finger of the opposite hand, sustaining the force for 10 seconds.
- Headache pain should be alleviated.
- See Figs 1.11–1.13.

INDICATION

Headache or other symptoms present at the time of technique application.

POSITIONING

Patient:	Sitting with the back supported against an upright chair.
Treated body part:	Relaxed neutral position of the head and neck. Hands resting on the lap.
Therapist:	Step-stance position facing the patient, leg adjacent to patient stepped back, with the therapist's pelvis used to hold the patient's trunk against the support of the chair. The therapist can stand on the right or left side of the patient.
Hands/belt contact points:	The therapist places their contact hand around the back of the patient's head, with the middle phalanx of the little finger lying across the posterior aspect of the C2 spinous process. The thenar eminence of the therapist's other hand presses against the little finger of the contact hand.

APPLICATION GUIDELINES

- It is important to stabilise the patient's head in neutral position when applying the technique. There should be no movement of the head.
- Force is generated by the therapist pressing the little finger of the contact hand with the thenar eminence of the other hand. The direction of force should be horizontal, in the plane of the upper cervical facet joints. In this respect, the little finger of the contact hand is the locator for the application of force generated by the thenar eminence of the opposite hand (motive hand).
- Gentle force is all that is usually required for the technique to be effective.
- Maintain the applied force for 10 seconds. If the patient's headache is significantly reduced then the technique is repeated 6–10 times. If the headache is increased the technique should be abandoned and the reverse headache SNAG trialled.
- If there is contact soreness of the little finger on the spinous process then a small piece of sponge rubber can be used to soften the contact. In addition, as with a cervical natural apophyseal glide (NAG), an extremely gentle traction force may make the technique more comfortable or provide greater symptom relief to the patient.

ALTERNATIVES

- If symptoms are only marginally reduced, try applying the same technique with either more force, or a slightly different angle to the force (e.g. angled away from the side of pain to the contralateral side), or for a longer duration. The technique may also be applied to the C3 spinous process, although the angle of force will be approximately 45° to the horizontal plane, in the direction of the patient's eyes.

COMMENTS

- There is preliminary evidence that these techniques are effective when combined with other treatment modalities in patients with upper cervical symptoms (Lincoln, 2000; Richardson, 2009).

SELF-MANAGEMENT

- If symptoms are reduced then trial a self-headache SNAG (Fig. 1.14). This should be attempted early in the treatment session before all pain is alleviated, so that the patient can understand how to apply the technique and the therapist can judge the self-treatment's effectiveness. This will also improve compliance and assist in self-efficacy.

- The patient places a self-SNAG strap on the posterior aspect of the spinous process of C2 (Fig. 1.14) to affect the levels C0/1 and C1/2 and on the spinous process of C3 to affect the C2/3 level. The patient is directed to pull the strap horizontally forwards, with each side parallel to each other and to the ground. The patient retracts the head against the fixation of the strap for 10 seconds. The exercise can be repeated 6–10 times as required to alleviate the headache.

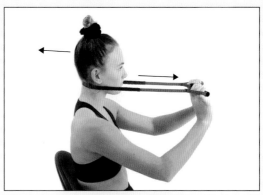

Figure 1.14
Self-headache SNAG with a strap

ANNOTATION

sit C2 HA SNAG×10 sec
sit C2 HA SNAG×10 sec (Hall et al., 2010c)
sit C3 HA SNAG×10 sec (Hall et al., 2010c)
sit C2 self strap HA SNAG×10 sec (Hall et al., 2010c)
sit C3 self strap HA SNAG×10 sec (Hall et al., 2010c)

REVERSE HEADACHE SNAG

1

TECHNIQUE AT A GLANCE

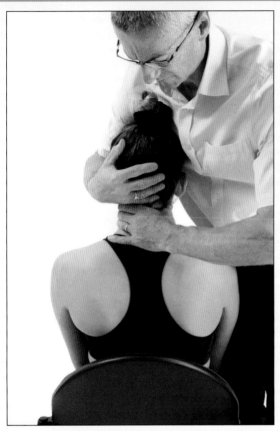

Figure 1.15
Reverse headache SNAG

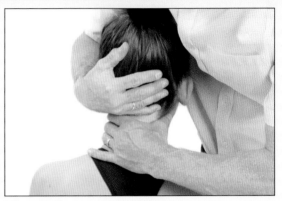

Figure 1.16
Reverse headache SNAG: close view

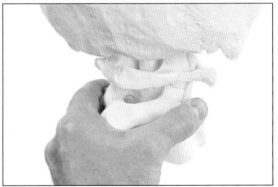

Figure 1.17
Reverse headache SNAG: bone view

- The patient sits in a chair with their back supported and head/neck in neutral position.
- The therapist stands to the front and side of the patient.
- The therapist stabilises the patient's neck by fixing the C2 vertebra with their thumb and middle fingertip in front of the transverse process or against the C2 spinous process.
- The therapist's other hand cups around the posterior aspect of the patient's occiput.
- The therapist gently pulls the head anteriorly in a horizontal plane, sustaining the force for 10 seconds.
- See Figs 1.15–1.17.

INDICATION

Headache or other symptoms present at the time of technique application. Usually the headache SNAG is trialled first and if unsuccessful the reverse headache SNAG is tested.

CONTRAINDICATION

Upper cervical ligament deficiency, particularly transverse ligament laxity.

POSITIONING

Patient:	Sitting with their back supported against a hard-backed, upright chair.
Treated body part:	Relaxed neutral position of the head and neck. Hands resting on the lap.
Therapist:	Step stance facing the patient, leg adjacent to patient stepped back, with the therapist's lower abdomen and hip used to stabilise the patient's trunk. The therapist can stand on the right or left side of the patient.
Hands contact points:	The therapist places one hand around the back of the patient's occiput with the fingers spread around the back of the occiput.
	Using the thumb and middle finger of the opposite hand, grasp around the lateral aspects of the C2 spinous and transverse processes using a lumbrical grip, if the neck of the patient is large. If the neck is small, then grasp the anterior aspect of the C2 transverse processes bilaterally.

APPLICATION GUIDELINES

- It is important to stabilise the patient's neck when applying the technique. There should be no movement of the trunk or lower neck.
- The gliding force should be in the horizontal plane, in a manner to achieve translation of the head on the neck rather than extension of the neck.
- Gentle force is all that is required.
- Maintain the applied force for 10 seconds. If the patient's headache is significantly reduced then the technique is repeated 6–10 times.

VARIATIONS

- If symptoms are only marginally reduced, then try applying the same technique with either slightly more gliding force, a slightly different angle to the force and/or for longer duration.
- The addition of minimal axial traction may also improve outcomes, as may the prescription of either a self-reverse headache SNAG (Fig. 1.18) or a self-fist traction as a home programme technique if the patient responds well to reverse headache SNAGs (see fist traction technique described in Chapter 3).

COMMENTS

- In the rare event that the patient has upper cervical instability, perhaps a damaged or absent transverse ligament, then this technique would be provocative and stress the spinal cord, and hence is contraindicated.

(continued next page...)

SELF-MANAGEMENT

- If symptoms are reduced then trial a self-reverse headache SNAG (Fig. 1.18). This should be attempted early in the treatment session before all pain is alleviated, so that the patient can understand how to apply the technique and the therapist can judge the self-treatment's effectiveness. This will also improve compliance and assist in self-efficacy.

- The patient places a self-SNAG strap on the posterior aspect of the skull. The patient is directed to pull the strap horizontally forwards, with the sides parallel to each other and to the ground. The patient retracts the neck against the fixation of the strap for 10 seconds. The exercise can be repeated 6–10 times as required to alleviate the headache.

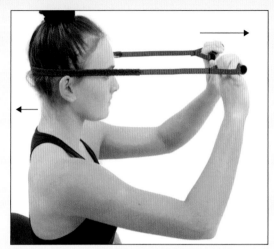

Figure 1.18
Self-reverse headache SNAG

ANNOTATIONS

sit rev HA SNAG×10 sec
sit rev HA SNAG×10 sec (Hall et al., 2010c)
sit self strap Rev HA SNAG×10 sec (Hall et al., 2010c)

UPPER CERVICAL TRACTION

TECHNIQUE AT A GLANCE

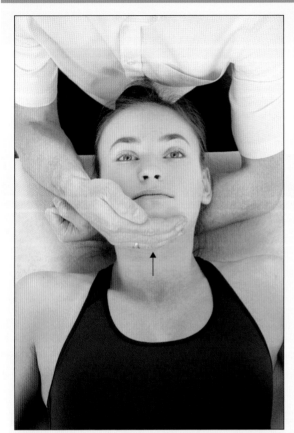

Figure 1.19
Upper cervical traction: start position

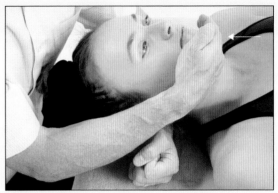

Figure 1.20
Upper cervical traction: close view

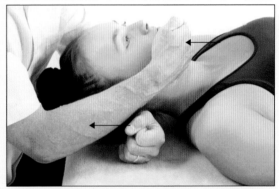

Figure 1.21
Upper cervical traction: end position

- The patient lies supine with the head/neck in neutral position.
- The therapist sits on a chair at the end of the plinth facing the patient's head.
- The therapist places their supinated forearm of the contact arm underneath the patient's neck.
- The therapist's other hand fixes underneath the patient's chin.
- The therapist's contact forearm pronates against the patient's occiput, sustaining the force for at least 10 seconds, repeating as required.
- Headache pain should be alleviated.
- See Figs 1.19–1.21.

1

INDICATION

Headache, neck pain, or other symptoms present at the time of technique application. Usually this technique could be used if there were a poor response to a headache SNAG or reverse headache SNAG.

POSITIONING

Patient:	Lying supine on a treatment plinth.
Treated body part:	Relaxed neutral position of the head with neutral to slight extension of the neck. Hands resting on the lap.
Therapist:	Sitting at the head of the patient, facing towards their feet, with the mid portion of the therapist's supinated forearm placed under the patient's upper cervical spine.
Hands/belt contact points:	The radius of the therapist's forearm under the upper cervical spine rests against the inferior aspect of the patient's occiput. The therapist's other hand stabilises under the patient's chin to prevent cervical flexion during traction.

APPLICATION GUIDELINES

- If the patient has an increased thoracic kyphosis, a small folded towel may be placed under the patient's head to keep the neck in a neutral to slight extension position.
- The therapist pronates the forearm to generate pressure against the patient's occiput.
- At the same time the therapist stabilises the patient's chin to prevent upper cervical flexion. The resultant force should be traction which is perpendicular to the long axis of the cervical spine and therefore a true traction of the upper cervical joints.
- Maintain the force for at least 10 seconds and monitor the headache symptoms. If symptoms increase then stop immediately. If symptoms reduce then the technique may be repeated several times.

VARIATIONS

- If symptoms are only marginally reduced, then try applying the same technique with either more force or a slightly longer duration.

COMMENTS

- In some patients, neck traction causes discomfort in the lumbar spine owing to sensitivity of neuromeningeal structures. In this case, flexion of the patient's hips and knees will assist in reducing this discomfort.
- In other patients who have pain from an excessive lumbar lordosis, discomfort may be alleviated again by hip and knee flexion together with posterior pelvic tilt.
- If there is any discomfort from contact over the spinous process, this may be reduced by the therapist using a slightly thicker part of their forearm so that the forearm muscles create a soft pad for contact.

SELF-MANAGEMENT

- If symptoms are reduced then trial a self-upper cervical spine traction (Fig. 1.22). This should be attempted early in the treatment session before all pain is alleviated, so that the patient can understand how to apply the technique and the therapist can judge the self-treatment's effectiveness. This will also improve compliance and assist in self-efficacy.

- The patient lies supine on a hard surface with their upper cervical spine resting on a firmly rolled small towel (Fig. 1.22). The roll must be close to the edge of the support so that the patient's head lies slightly unsupported. When the patient relaxes, the weight of the head will induce a small degree of cervical extension thereby creating a degree of upper cervical spine unloading.

- The patient remains in this position for initially 30 seconds, progressing if helpful to 2 minutes. This exercise can be repeated as required to alleviate the headache.

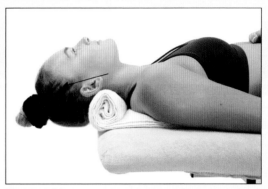

Figure 1.22
Self-upper cervical traction

ANNOTATIONS

sup ly upper Cx Fra Tr × 10 sec
sup ly upper Cx Fra Tr × 10 sec (Hall et al., 2010c)
sup ly upper Cx self towel roll Tr × 30 sec

References

Amiri, M., Jull, G., Bullock-Saxton, J., 2003. Measuring range of active cervical rotation in a position of full head flexion using the 3D Fastrak measurement system: an intra-tester reliability study. Man. Ther. 8 (3), 176–179.

Bogduk, N., Govind, J., 2009. Cervicogenic headache: an assessment of the evidence on clinical diagnosis, invasive tests, and treatment. Lancet Neurol. 8 (10), 959–968.

Bravo Petersen, S.M., Vardaxis, V.G., 2015. The flexion–rotation test performed actively and passively: a comparison of range of motion in patients with cervicogenic headache. J. Man. Manip. Ther. 23 (2), 61–67.

Budelmann, K., von Piekartz, H., Hall, T., 2013. Is there a difference in head posture and cervical spine movement in children with and without pediatric headache? Eur. J. Pediatr. 172 (10), 1349–1356.

Budelmann, K., von Piekartz, H., Hall, T., 2016. A normative study of cervical range of motion measures including the flexion–rotation test in asymptomatic children: side-to-side variability and pain provocation. J. Man. Manip. Ther. 24 (4), 185–191.

Dodick, D.W., 2010. Pearls: headache. Semin. Neurol. 30 (1), 74–81.

Grondin, F., Hall, T., Laurentjoye, M., Ella, B., 2015. Upper cervical range of motion is impaired in patients with temporomandibular disorders. Cranio. 33 (2), 91–99.

Hall, T., 2011. Cervicogenic headache: more than just a pain in the neck. Physioscience 7, 1–8.

Hall, T., Robinson, K., 2004. The flexion-rotation test and active cervical mobility – a comparative measurement study in cervicogenic headache. Man. Ther. 9 (4), 197–202.

Hall, T., Chan, H.T., Christensen, L., Odenthal, B., Wells, C., Robinson, K., 2007. Efficacy of a C1-C2 self-sustained natural apophyseal glide (SNAG) in the management of cervicogenic headache. J. Orthop. Sports Phys. Ther. 37 (3), 100–107.

Hall, T.M., Briffa, K., Hopper, D., Robinson, K., 2010a. Comparative analysis and diagnostic accuracy of the cervical flexion-rotation test. J. Headache Pain 11 (5), 391–397.

Hall, T.M., Briffa, K., Hopper, D., Robinson, K.W., 2010b. The relationship between cervicogenic headache and impairment determined by the flexion-rotation test. J. Man. Manip. Ther. 33 (9), 666–671.

Hall, T., Briffa, K., Hopper, D., 2010c. The influence of lower cervical joint pain on range of motion and interpretation of the flexion–rotation test. J. Man. Manip. Ther. 18 (3), 126–131.

Khan, M., Ali, S.S., Soomro, R.R., 2014. Efficacy of C1-C2 sustained natural apophyseal glide (SNAG) versus posterior anterior vertebral mobilization (PAVMs) in the management of cervicogenic headache. J. Basic Appl. Sci. 10, 226–230.

Lincoln, J., 2000. Case report. Clinical instability of the upper cervical spine. Man. Ther. 5 (1), 41–46.

Nambi, G., Pancholi, D., Trivedi, P., Momin, S., Patel, S., 2014. Comparative effect between c1-c2 self-sustained natural apophyseal glide (SNAG) and deep cervical flexors strength training in the management of cervicogenic headache. Int. J. Pharmacol. Screening Methods 4 (2), 69–73.

Neeti, C., 2017. Comparative study to find the effect of Mulligans SNAG technique (C1-C2) versus Maitlands technique (C1-C2) in cervicogenic headache among information technology professionals. Int. J. Physiother. 4 (3), 178–183.

Ogince, M., Hall, T., Robinson, K., Blackmore, A.M., 2007. The diagnostic validity of the cervical flexion–rotation test in C1/2-related cervicogenic headache. Man. Ther. 12 (3), 256–262.

Richardson, C., 2009. Treatment of cervicogenic headache using Mulligan SNAGs and postural re-education: a case report. Orthop. Phys. Ther. Pract. 21 (1), 33–38.

Schäfer, A., Ludtke, K., Breuel, F., Gerloff, N., Knust, M., Kollitsch, C., et al., 2018. Validity of eyeball estimation for range of motion during the cervical flexion rotation test compared to an ultrasound-based movement analysis system. Physiother. Theory Pract. 34 (8), 622–628.

Shin, E.J., Lee, B.H., 2014. The effect of sustained natural apophyseal glides on headache, duration and cervical function in women with cervicogenic headache. J. Exerc. Rehabil. 10 (2), 131–135.

Smith, K., Hall, T., Robinson, K., 2008. The influence of age, gender, lifestyle factors and sub-clinical neck pain on the cervical flexion-rotation test and cervical range of motion. Man. Ther. 13 (6), 552–559.

Takasaki, H., Hall, T., Oshiro, S., Kaneko, S., Ikemoto, Y., Jull, G., 2011. Normal kinematics of the upper cervical spine during the Flexion-Rotation test – in vivo measurements using magnetic resonance imaging. Man. Ther. 16 (2), 167–171.

The International Classification of Headache Disorders, 2004. The International Classification of Headache Disorders, 2nd ed. Cephalalgia 24 (Suppl. 1), 9–160.

von Piekartz, H., Hall, T., 2013. Orofacial manual therapy improves cervical movement impairment associated with headache and features of temporomandibular dysfunction: a randomized controlled trial. Man. Ther. 18 (4), 345–350.

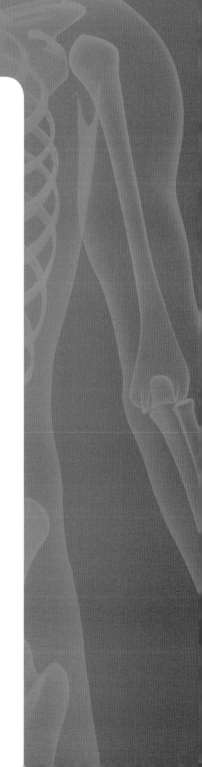

2

Cervicogenic dizziness

TECHNIQUES FOR CERVICOGENIC DIZZINESS

INTRODUCTION

Cervicogenic dizziness is characterised by imbalance or disequilibrium, which is commonly associated with cervical pain, stiffness or headache (Wrisley et al., 2000).

The genesis of this non-specific sensation of altered orientation is hypothesised to originate from abnormal afferent activity from the upper cervical mechanoreceptors creating a sensory mismatch with the visual and vestibular systems at the level of the vestibular nuclei and cerebellum (Gargano et al., 2012; Huijbregts & Vidal, 2004; Reid & Rivett, 2005; Reid et al., 2008).

Observations of immediate abolishment of these symptoms during the application of a cervical SNAG technique are used clinically to reason that the cervical spine motion segments were likely the source of the abnormal afferent activity and thus responsible for the symptoms. A gold standard clinical test does not currently exist to confirm or refute a diagnosis of cervicogenic dizziness. Cervicogenic dizziness is a diagnosis of exclusion, but is particularly common when there is a history of trauma and the reported dizziness correlates with neck pain (Huijbregts & Vidal, 2004).

Compounding the difficulties facing the practitioner when making a diagnosis is the wide range of benign and serious conditions that can cause dizziness (Sloane et al., 2001). A thorough clinical interview and history-taking including specific questions concerning health history, vascular risk factors, such as hypertension, past cervical trauma and pain distributions, are important to determine the appropriateness of a manual therapy intervention (Kerry & Taylor, 2009).

In some cases, vestibular function tests and a comprehensive neurological examination should be performed to rule out vestibular dysfunction and central nervous system involvement (Wrisley et al., 2000). This section will describe in detail the SNAG techniques commonly used to treat cervicogenic dizziness, for which there is level 2 evidence (see 'levels of evidence' below).

The order in which the following techniques are applied should be carefully considered and is detailed in the flow chart in Fig. 2.1. Technique selection is based on the symptomatic provocative movement. Once this is determined, a suggested order of testing and treatment is applied. Should the applied techniques not alter dizziness, the practitioner should reconsider the provisional diagnosis of cervicogenic dizziness.

Levels of evidence

Level 2: four RCTs

A randomised controlled trial (RCT) by Reid and colleagues (Reid et al., 2008) demonstrated that four sessions of a cervical SNAG were more effective than a placebo detuned LASER comparator at reducing dizziness at 12 weeks. The SNAG group reported great benefit on average compared with the placebo group's minimal to some benefit (on a perceived benefit scale where: 1 = no, 2 = minimal, 3 = some, 4 = a lot of, 5 = great and 6 = maximal benefit). That is, the cervical SNAG can be applied clinically in the knowledge that it has proven efficacy over 12 weeks. Further like clinical trials are required to validate this finding.

In a longitudinal study with three published RCTs, Reid and colleagues (Reid et al., 2014a, 2014b, 2015) compared the effects of Mulligan SNAG, Maitland mobilisations plus range-of-movement (ROM) exercises and placebo on both subjective measures (i.e. VAS dizziness, dizziness frequency, Dizziness Handicap Inventory (DHI), VAS pain and Global Perceived Effect (GPE)) and objective measures (i.e. cervical ROM, head repositioning accuracy and balance) related to cervicogenic dizziness. The studies found that the manual therapy groups improved the subjective measures, with no significant difference between the two. The SNAG group demonstrated greater improvement in cervical ROM post-treatment and after 12 weeks of treatment compared with the Maitland and placebo groups. However, the difference observed in ROM after 12 weeks between manual therapy groups was non-existent at the 12-month follow-up.

2

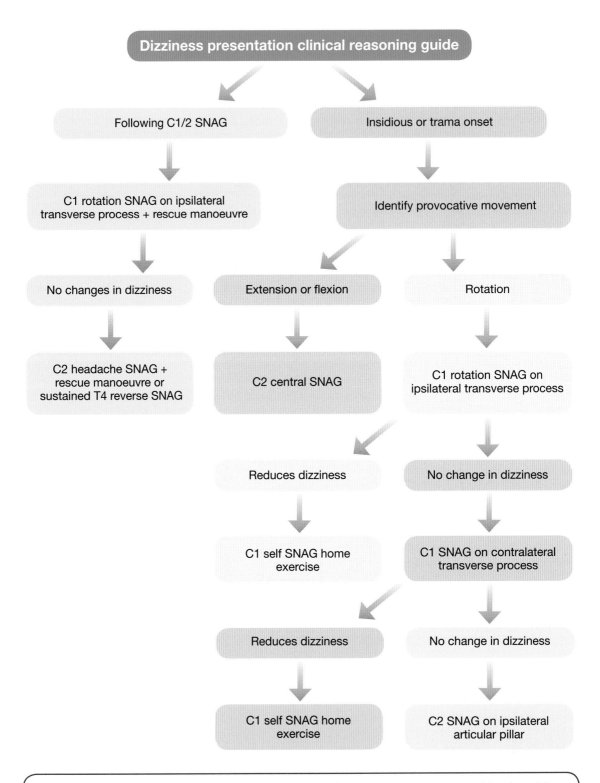

Dizziness presentation clinical reasoning guide

Following C1/2 SNAG

Insidious or trama onset

C1 rotation SNAG on ipsilateral transverse process + rescue manoeuvre

Identify provocative movement

No changes in dizziness

Extension or flexion

Rotation

C2 headache SNAG + rescue manoeuvre or sustained T4 reverse SNAG

C2 central SNAG

C1 rotation SNAG on ipsilateral transverse process

Reduces dizziness

No change in dizziness

C1 self SNAG home exercise

C1 SNAG on contralateral transverse process

Reduces dizziness

No change in dizziness

C1 self SNAG home exercise

C2 SNAG on ipsilateral articular pillar

IMPORTANT NOTE — Caution if no improvement occurs there needs to be a reconsideration of the diagnosis of cervicogenic dizziness.

Figure 2.1
Dizziness presentation clinical reasoning guide

C1 SNAG FOR CERVICAL ROTATION DIZZINESS

TECHNIQUE AT A GLANCE

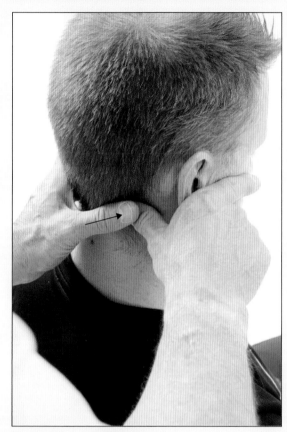

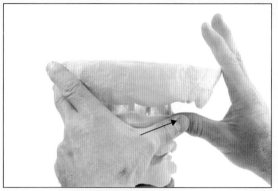

Figure 2.3
Cervicogenic dizziness: model C1 PA glide

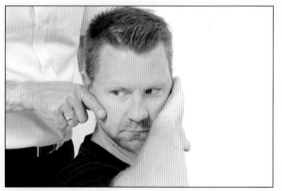

Figure 2.2
Cervicogenic dizziness: C1 PA glide

Figure 2.4
Cervicogenic dizziness: C1 right rotation SNAG with over-pressure

- The patient sits well supported in a chair.
- The cervical spine and head are set in a neutral position.
- A gentle posterior to anterior (PA) glide is applied to the transverse process of C1 on the side of the symptoms.
- While the glide is sustained the patient actively rotates their head in the direction that previously produced the dizziness.
- If symptom-free, the patient applies over-pressure to the zygomatic arch to move further into rotation.
- See Figs 2.2–2.4.

2

A sensation of dizziness, light-headedness, nausea and/or disequilibrium with head rotation.

POSITIONING

Patient:	Seated, well supported in a chair.
Treated body part:	Head and neck in neutral alignment.
Therapist:	Standing behind the patient.
Hands/contact points:	Pad of the right thumb (contact thumb) is placed on the posterior lateral aspect of the C1 transverse process. The pad of the left thumb (motive thumb) is placed over the nail of the right thumb.

APPLICATION GUIDELINES

- First ensure that the aggravating activity (right cervical rotation in this case) consistently provokes symptoms before applying the glide.
- Apply a passive PA glide on the right transverse process of C1 with the left thumb (motive thumb) pressing directly over the right thumb (contact thumb). The therapist questions the patient to assure the glide is symptom-free before adding active movement.
- The PA glide is sustained as the patient actively rotates their head in the symptomatic direction to the end range of symptom-free active motion.
- If symptom-free full range is achieved, then the patient is instructed to apply over-pressure into further right rotation using the back of their right hand against their maxilla. The back of the hand is used on the maxilla to prevent the patient from applying excessive over-pressure and to prevent lateral bending of the neck.
- The patient is questioned to ensure the over-pressure is symptom-free.
- A maximum of 3 over-pressure repetitions (rule of 3) are performed on day 1 to avoid the possibility of an adverse reaction (see comments below).

VARIATIONS

- An alternative approach for this technique is for the therapist to stand in front of the seated patient. One hand presses against the patient's forehead while the middle finger of their other hand lays across the posterior arch of C1, directing a PA glide force on the transverse process of C1 (Fig. 2.5). While maintaining a constant gliding force, the patient actively rotates the head in the symptomatic direction.
- If the symptoms do not cease with a C1 SNAG on the side of the symptoms then applying the same technique on the contralateral C1 transverse process can be attempted. If this is not successful, a final alternative is to apply the same technique on the ipsilateral C2 lamina. The therapist follows the same procedure as described above with continued close monitoring ensuring the patient is symptom-free.
- If the patient has excessive forward head posture, instruct them to slide their hips forward in the chair to reduce the suboccipital extension, allowing for effective C1 mobilisation.

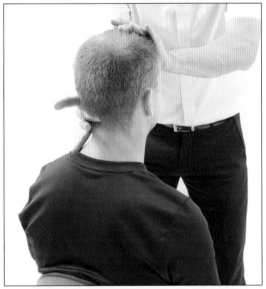

Figure 2.5
Alternative hand placement for C1 PA glide

COMMENTS

- It is important that the therapist rotates their body in conjunction with the rotation of the patient's head to ensure they maintain the correct direction and amount of pressure on the transverse process of C1.
- The rule of 3 is applicable for upper cervical SNAGs to prevent adverse symptoms that can occur despite application of the proper technique. Adverse symptoms may include dizziness, light-headedness, nausea, mild visual blurring and/or sweating. If adverse symptoms are produced the therapist has several options to address this (see rescue manoeuvre techniques p. 52).

SELF-MANAGEMENT

- The patient replicates the technique as a home exercise by using the pad of their index finger, reinforced by the middle finger, to contact the posterior lateral tip of the C1 transverse process on the side of symptoms (Fig. 2.6). A PA glide is achieved by a gentle anterior pull with their arm. The glide is sustained as they actively rotate their head towards the side of the symptoms. The motion must be symptom-free or should not be carried out. The angle and/or amplitude of the glide are adjusted to assure symptom-free active rotation.
- Over-pressure may be applied with the hand over the zygomatic arch, but only if full-range symptom-free movement can be achieved.
- Up to 3 repetitions are performed and the symptoms are then reassessed. The repetitions can be increased to 6–10 as the patient becomes accustomed to the exercise. This process is repeated 3–5 times per day until all symptoms have resolved.
- To assist in finding the transverse process of C1, the patient is shown how to palpate the mastoid process with their index finger then to move slightly medially and inferiorly.
- An alternative exercise is to use either a cervical self-SNAG strap or towel to induce C1/2 rotation, as described in the section on C1/2 self-SNAG for headache

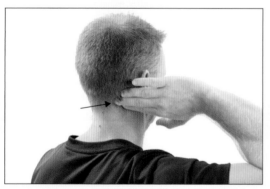

Figure 2.6A
Self-C1 PA glide: rear view

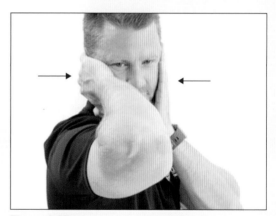

Figure 2.6B
Self-C1 PA glide: over-pressure

ANNOTATIONS

sit R C1 SNAG Rot R×3
sit stabilise forehead R C1 SNAG Rot R +OP×3
sit R C1 self SNAG Rot R +OP×3

C2 SNAG FOR CERVICAL EXTENSION DIZZINESS

TECHNIQUE AT A GLANCE

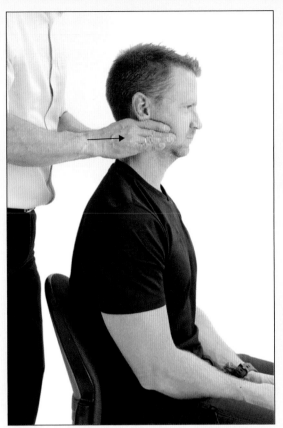

Figure 2.7
Cervicogenic dizziness: C2 PA glide

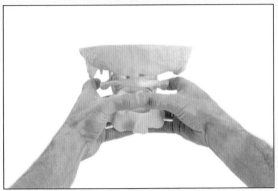

Figure 2.8
Cervicogenic dizziness: model C2 PA glide

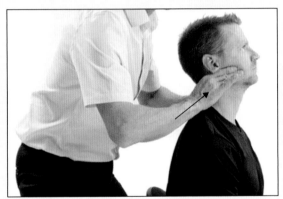

Figure 2.9
Cervicogenic dizziness: C2 extension SNAG

- The patient sits well supported in a chair.
- The cervical spine and head are set in a neutral position.
- A painless passive PA glide is applied to the spinous process of C2, in the horizontal plane.
- While the glide is sustained the patient actively extends their neck in the direction that previously produced the dizziness.
- See Figs 2.7–2.9.

INDICATION

A sensation of dizziness, light-headedness, nausea and/or disequilibrium with cervical extension.

POSITIONING

Patient:	Seated, well supported in a chair.
Treated body part:	Head and neck in neutral alignment.
Therapist:	Standing behind the patient.
Hand contact:	The pad of the thumb is placed on the spinous process of C2 and the opposite thumb is placed over the first thumb. The index fingers are in contact with the zygomatic arches.

APPLICATION GUIDELINES

- The therapist first ensures that the aggravating activity consistently provokes symptoms before applying the glide (i.e. cervical extension in this case). A PA glide is applied to the spinous process of C2.

- While sustaining the PA glide the patient is instructed to extend the cervical spine.

- The therapist must ensure that they maintain a consistent and constant PA pressure on the spinous process of C2 as the patient extends their neck. This will require the therapist to extend their wrists an equal amount to the cervical movement.

- The patient is instructed to extend the cervical spine to the end range of movement, ensuring no symptoms are provoked. If a symptom is produced the movement is stopped and adjustments to the amplitude and/or direction of glide should be made. Movement is again attempted until the cervical extension is symptom-free or no change is elicited.

- Over-pressure with this technique is gained solely by the weight of the head moving past vertical allowing gravity to assist the motion. In some cases, restrictions in the lower cervical spine limit the ROM in the upper cervical spine, eliminating the benefit of gravity. In these cases, the patient can apply a gentle pressure under the chin into extension to achieve the over-pressure.

- Up to 3 repetitions are performed.

(continued next page...)

2

- If the comparable symptoms are produced in standing or with the patient reaching their arms overhead, the technique is easily adapted to this position (see Figs 2.10 and 2.11).

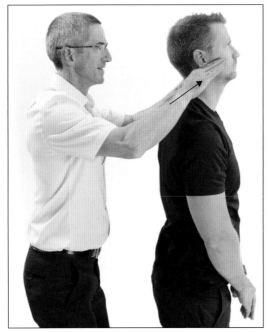

Figure 2.10
Cervicogenic dizziness: C2 extension SNAG (standing)

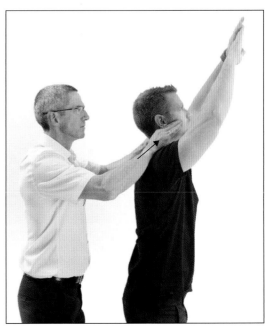

Figure 2.11
Cervicogenic dizziness: C2 extension SNAG with arm elevation (standing)

COMMENTS

- If the symptoms are of cervical origin they may be immediately abolished with the application of the C2 SNAG.
- If the symptoms are of other origin they may worsen with the mobilisation and/or extension movement and the technique should be immediately abandoned.
- If the symptoms do not abolish with the first 3 attempts the technique is not indicated.

SELF-MANAGEMENT

- The patient is instructed to locate the C2 spinous process by palpating the first midline prominence below the skull (see Fig 2.12A and B).

- PA pressure is applied through the distal pads of the middle fingers of each hand with the verbal cue to 'push the pads of your fingers towards the tip of your nose' (see Fig 2.12C).

- A consistent glide is sustained as the patient is instructed to extend their neck to the point of symptom onset. If the movement is not symptom-free, then the patient is instructed on how to make small changes to the direction of the glide to attain a symptom-free movement. The verbal cue, 'push the tips of your fingers towards your left (or right) nostril' will be easily understood by the patient and achieve the small change that may now render the movement symptom-free.

- Up to 3 repetitions are performed when the patient first trials the exercise, increasing to 6–10 as the patient becomes accustomed to the exercise. This process is repeated 3–5 times per day until all of the symptoms have resolved without the need for the C2 SNAG to be applied.

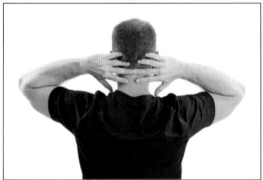

Figure 2.12A
Self-C2 PA glide: back view start position

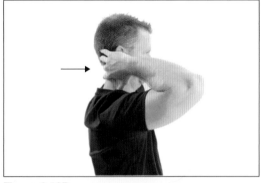

Figure 2.12B
Self-C2 PA glide: side view start position

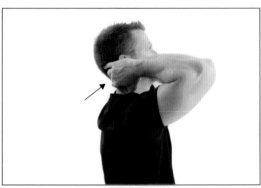

Figure 2.12C
Self-C2 PA glide: end position

(continued next page...)

2

- An alternative exercise is to use either a cervical self-SNAG strap or towel to induce C2 PA glide force during active cervical extension. In this technique, the patient's fingers on the C2 spinous process are replaced by the self-SNAG strap or towel (Fig. 2.13). The exercise is carried out in the same way as described above.

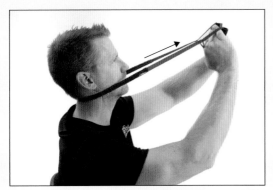

Figure 2.13A
Strap C2 self-SNAG

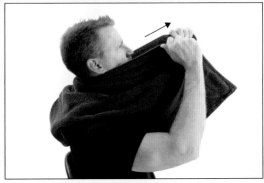

Figure 2.13B
Towel C2 self-SNAG

ANNOTATIONS

sit C2 SNAG E×3
st C2 SNAG E×3
st bilat Sh El C2 SNAG E×3
sit C2 self SNAG E×3
sit C2 self towel SNAG E×6
sit C2 self strap SNAG E×10

C2 SNAG FOR NAUSEA, LIGHT-HEADEDNESS OR VISUAL DISTURBANCES (RESCUE MANOEUVRE)

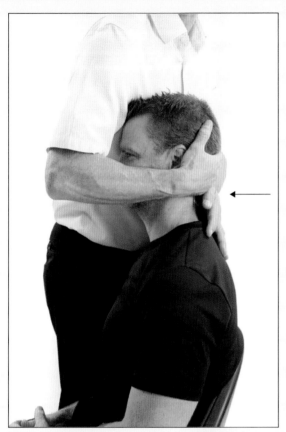

Figure 2.14
Rescue manoeuvre: side view

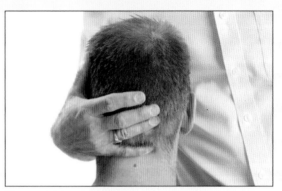

Figure 2.15
Rescue manoeuvre: hand placement

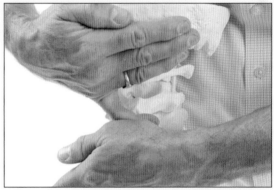

Figure 2.16
Rescue manoeuvre: anatomical model C2 PA glide

- The patient sits well supported in a chair, with cervical spine and head in neutral position.
- The therapist stands in front of patient, stabilising the patient's trunk.
- One hand cradles the head, with middle phalanx of little finger hooked around C2 spinous process.
- The C2 PA glide is generated by the thenar eminence of the opposite hand. The glide is horizontal and sustained for 30 seconds, or the patient actively extends their neck.
- See Figs 2.14–2.16.

2

INDICATION

The patient reports a sensation of dizziness, light-headedness, nausea and/or visual disturbances at rest or after the application of a manual technique, exercise or movement to the cervical spine.

POSITIONING

Patient:	Seated, well supported in a chair.
Treated body part:	Head and neck in neutral alignment.
Therapist:	Stands facing the seated patient with the anterior hip supporting the patient's anterior shoulder.
Hands/contact points:	The right hand cradles the patient's head contacting the spinous process with the mid-phalanx of the fifth digit. The thenar eminence of the left hand is placed directly over the right mid-phalanx.

APPLICATION GUIDELINES

- A PA glide is applied to the C2 spinous process using the left thenar eminence applying force through the contact point of the mid-phalanx of the fifth digit.
- If the symptoms are abolished by the PA pressure then the glide is held for 30 seconds, released and then symptoms reassessed.
- If the symptoms do not change with the C2 PA glide then the patient is instructed to slowly extend their cervical spine, while the PA glide force is maintained, until the patient reaches a point where the symptoms abolish.
- This position is held and the patient is asked to inhale slowly and then slowly completely exhale. Repeat the 'rescue breathing' 3 times then release the SNAG and reassess.

VARIATIONS

- If the adverse symptom produced is visual such as *blurred vision* the technique is modified by changing the therapist position to standing behind the patient as described in **C2 SNAG for cervical extension dizziness** (see Fig. 2.7). The patient focuses on a clearly defined object directly in front of them while the therapist applies a C2 PA glide. The patient is questioned whether the glide abolished the blurry vision (see Fig. 2.7). If the symptoms are abolished the glide is held for 30 seconds, released and then reassessed.
- If the symptoms do not change with a straight C2 PA glide the patient is instructed to slowly extend their cervical spine while continuing to focus intently on the object until they reach the position where the object is now clearly in focus. The position is held for 30 seconds, released and reassessed (see Fig. 2.9).

COMMENTS

- Clinical experience with patients who present with dizziness, light-headedness, nausea and/or visual disturbances at rest or after the application of a manual technique, exercise or movement to the cervical spine has shown that the use of 'rescue breathing' can provide an added benefit to the C2 PA SNAG (rescue manoeuvre) technique. The moderate inhalation followed by a long, extended exhalation, performed 3 times for approximately 30 seconds each time, may provide a calming effect on the patient by slowing their respiratory rate. This is particularly useful when a patient is quite distressed by their symptoms and can also enable them to further actively contribute to their management as part of collaborative clinical reasoning.

SELF-MANAGEMENT

- The exercise for the C2 self-SNAG rescue manoeuvre is similar to the self-C2 PA glide (Fig. 2.12)

- The patient applies a constant PA pressure through their middle fingers to the C2 spinous process with the verbal cue to 'push the pads of your fingers towards the tip of your nose'. If the symptoms are abolished then this position is held for 30 seconds, released and reassessed.

- If the symptoms do not change with a C2 PA glide, the patient is instructed to slowly extend their cervical spine until they reach the point where the symptoms are abolished. At this position, the glide is maintained with no further movement.

- An alternative exercise is to use either a cervical self-SNAG strap or towel to induce C2 PA glide force (Fig. 2.13). In this technique, the patient's fingers on the C2 spinous process are replaced by the self-SNAG strap or towel. The exercise is carried out in the same way as described above.

ANNOTATIONS

sit C2 HA SNAG×30 sec
sit C2 HA SNAG E+3 breaths×30 sec
sit C2 HA SNAG visual focus×30 sec
sit C2 HA SNAG visual focus+E×30 sec
sit C2 self HA SNAG×30 sec
sit C2 self towel HA SNAG×30 sec
sit C2 self strap HA SNAG×30 sec

References

Gargano, F., Hing, W., Cross, C., 2012. Vestibular influence on cranio-cervical pain: a case report. N. Z. J. Physiother. 40 (2), 51–58.

Huijbregts, P., Vidal, P., 2004. Dizziness in orthopaedic physical therapy practice: classification and pathophysiology. J. Man. Manip. Ther. 12 (4), 199–214.

Kerry, R., Taylor, A.J., 2009. Cervical arterial dysfunction: knowledge and reasoning for manual physical therapists. J. Orthop. Sports Phys. Ther. 39 (5), 378–387.

Reid, S.A., Rivett, D.A., 2005. Manual therapy treatment of cervicogenic dizziness: a systematic review. Man. Ther. 10 (1), 4–13.

Reid, S.A., Rivett, D.A., Katekar, M.G., Callister, R., 2008. Sustained natural apophyseal glides (SNAGs) are an effective treatment for cervicogenic dizziness. Man. Ther. 13 (4), 357–366.

Reid, S.A., Callister, R., Katekar, M.G., Rivett, D.A., 2014a. Effects of cervical spine manual therapy on range of motion, head repositioning, and balance in participants with cervicogenic dizziness: a randomized controlled trial. Arch. Phys. Med. Rehabil. 95 (9), 1603–1612.

Reid, S.A., Rivett, D.A., Katekar, M.G., Callister, R., 2014b. Comparison of Mulligan sustained natural apophyseal glides and Maitland mobilizations for treatment of cervicogenic dizziness: a randomized controlled trial. Phys. Ther. 94 (4), 466–476.

Reid, S.A., Callister, R., Snodgrass, S.J., Katekar, M.G., Rivett, D.A., 2015. Manual therapy for cervicogenic dizziness: long-term outcomes of a randomised trial. Man. Ther. 20 (1), 148–156.

Sloane, P.D., Coeytaux, R.R., Beck, R.S., Dallara, J., 2001. Dizziness: state of the science. Ann. Intern. Med. 134 (9 Pt 2), 823–832.

Wrisley, D.M., Sparto, P.J., Whitney, S.L., Furman, J.M., 2000. Cervicogenic dizziness: a review of diagnosis and treatment. J. Orthop. Sports Phys. Ther. 30 (12), 755–766.

Cervical spine

TECHNIQUES FOR THE CERVICAL SPINE

CERVICAL SNAGS
C2–7 SNAGs for cervical motion restriction – flexion, extension, lateral, flexion and rotation
- Mid cervical spine central SNAG
- Unilateral SNAG
- Self-SNAG

C5 / 6 or C6 / 7 transverse (positional) SNAG
- Self-C5 transverse SNAG

FIST TRACTION

NATURAL APOPHYSEAL GLIDES (NAGS) (CENTRAL AND UNILATERAL)
Central NAG
Unilateral NAG

REVERSE NAGS (CENTRAL AND UNILATERAL)
Central reverse NAG
Unilateral reverse NAG

CERVICOTHORACIC JUNCTION MOBILISATION: BRIDGE TECHNIQUE
- Self-management following the cervicothoracic junction bridge mobilisation technique

CERVICAL TRACTION: UPPER EXTREMITY PAIN

SPINAL MOBILISATION WITH ARM MOVEMENT (SMWAM)
Shoulder abduction
- Self-SMWAM for abduction

SMWAM: horizontal extension and neurodynamic dysfunction
- Self-SMWAM neurodynamic technique

INTRODUCTION

The application of an MWM in the spine is referred to as a Sustained Natural Apophyseal Glide (SNAG) and consists of a passive glide force applied to a specific motion segment together with active movement. Determination of the appropriate segmental level to which to apply the SNAG is achieved through a thorough interview and physical examination. The glide force is performed parallel to the perceived facet plane, with the degree of glide force determined by the patient's active movement response. Failure to achieve a good response may indicate a subtle variation in the glide direction or a higher force applied, but only if the technique remains pain-free (remembering force should only be as much as required to effect change).

The choice of applying the SNAG centrally at the spinous process or unilaterally on the articular pillar is determined by a process of iterative clinical reasoning steps in the evaluative process. Two examples are provided, but are not meant to be restricted to other possible clinical thought processes. If the clinician has hypothesised that motion is restricted owing to a loss of both left and right facet hypomobility at a given motion segment then a central SNAG on the spinous process may be tried. Brian Mulligan suggests that the initial application is on the side of the symptoms or pain. If rotation to the right produced pain on the right at a particular motion segment then a unilateral SNAG is applied on the right and the patient moves to the right, provided that when applied both the glide and motion to the right is pain-free.

As with all MWMs, final minor adjustments to the glide direction and angle may be required in order to make the glide and movement pain-free. When an immediate improvement in active range of motion (AROM) is achieved with a SNAG then the patient is instructed to assist by applying over-pressure further into the restricted direction, making sure that the movement is still pain-free. Reassessment of the restricted motion without the SNAG in situ is undertaken after several pain-free repetitions of the SNAG have been performed. Self-SNAGs should be taught to the patient early in the treatment session to enable self-management.

Indications for applying a cervical SNAG can simply be to improve pain-free AROM. A typical clinical presentation might be of an individual with cervical spondylosis in the lower cervical spine who has pain with moving their neck in one direction. However, some patients may have a more complex movement restriction. For example, an individual may report cervical pain at end-range cervical rotation and extension with a follow-through swing in golf. This individual's outcome to a cervical SNAG may be determined only if a SNAG is applied during a combination of both rotation and extension.

Levels of evidence

Level 2: eight RCTs, one case report and two laboratory-based studies

There is an agreement between the available RCTs regarding the effects of Mulligan treatment in decreasing pain, disability indexes and improving cervical ROM in patients with cervical-related conditions.

Kumar (2013) reported an RCT of natural apophyseal glides (NAGs) in 100 patients who had neck pain without radiculopathy. All patients received a hot pack for 12 minutes and a set of active exercises per session over a 12-day period. Patients were then randomly allocated to 3 groups involving NAG treatment (NAGs administered on each of the 12 days, only the first 6 days or only the last 6 days) or a control group (hot pack and active exercises). On pain, ROM and neck disability index, all NAG groups were statistically superior to the control group at the final outcome time (42 days). NAGs applied over the first 6 days were as beneficial as 12 days of application, while being superior to delaying NAG treatment for 6 days.

Studies highlight that the application of manipulation therapy in treating cervical conditions of mechanical origin with no radiculopathy is superior to the use of conventional physiotherapy (Buyukturan et al., 2018; Said et al., 2017) and exercise only. When comparing the Mulligan technique with either Maitland mobilisation (Ganesh et al., 2015; Gautam et al., 2014) or high-velocity low-amplitude manipulation (Abdelgalil et al., 2015), the application of SNAGs was superior to both interventions in minimising pain and increasing ROM.

A case report of a 47-year-old female patient with cervical radiculopathy highlighted the efficacy of the use of SNAGs and neurodynamic mobilisation in improving pain, cervical ROM and functional abilities. After application of 3 sets (6 repetitions) of unilateral superior glide in combination with ipsilateral cervical rotation and elbow extension, the patient's right cervical rotation increased from 25° to 65° and upper limb neurodynamic testing-1 measuring elbow extension range up to symptom reproduction improved from 70° to 10°.

Apart from this clinical trial there are two laboratory-based studies exploring underlying mechanisms of the Mulligan cervical treatments. A biomechanical analysis of a cervical spine SNAG proposed that it is highly unlikely to create its effects through a biomechanical action (Hearn & Rivett, 2002). A neurophysiological study reported sympathoexcitation to occur during the application of the SNAG (Moulson & Watson, 2006), and it was proposed that this effect was similar to that reported for spinal manual therapy (Vicenzino et al., 1998) and a lateral glide MWM of the elbow (Paungmali et al., 2003), which have been used to develop a mechanistic model of MWM that involves a periaqueductal grey-coordinated endogenous inhibitory system (Vicenzino et al., 2011). There is an obvious need to rationalise the apparent contradiction between hypothesised mechanisms, which usually relate to a mechanical joint effect, and the evidence that does not appear to support the hypothesis. Further research is required for this to occur.

CERVICAL SNAGS

C2–7 SNAGs for cervical motion restriction – flexion, extension, lateral flexion and rotation

TECHNIQUE AT A GLANCE

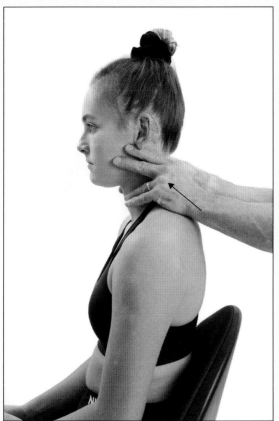

Figure 3.1
Mid cervical spine central SNAG: finger placement

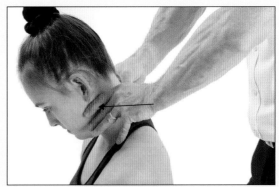

Figure 3.2
Mid cervical spine central SNAG: flexion end range

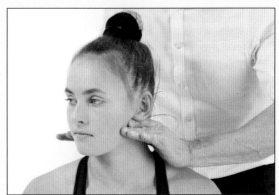

Figure 3.3
Mid cervical spine central SNAG: rotation end range

- The patient sits well supported in a chair.
- The cervical spine and head are set in a neutral position.
- A painless passive posterior to anterior (PA) glide is applied in the plane of the facets on either the spinous process or the articular pillar/cervical lamina.
- While the glide is sustained the patient actively moves their neck in the direction that previously produced the symptoms.
- If symptom-free, the patient applies over-pressure further into the movement restriction.
- Self-SNAGs are taught when clinically relevant changes occur in pain and motion.
- See Figs 3.1–3.3.

INDICATION

Loss of cervical AROM due to pain or stiffness.

POSITIONING

Patient:	Seated, well supported in a chair.
Treated body part:	The position of the cervical spine should be to allow for effective mobilisation of the cervical segment.
Therapist:	Standing behind the patient.
Hands/contact points:	The medial border of the right thumb (contact thumb) is placed on the posterior aspect of the spinous process. The pad of the left thumb (motive thumb) is placed perpendicular to the nail of the right thumb (in line with the facet plane).

APPLICATION GUIDELINES

- Apply a passive PA glide along the plane of the facets via the spinous process for any of the motion segments between C2 and C7 with the left thumb (motive thumb) through the right thumb (contact thumb). Question the patient to ensure the glide is symptom-free before adding active movement.
- The facet-inclined PA glide is sustained as the patient is asked to actively move their neck in the symptomatic direction to the end range of active motion.
- If the patient is symptom-free they are instructed to apply over-pressure (Fig. 3.4).
- Extension over-pressure is not usually required, owing to the weight of the head moving past vertical to assist motion. In some cases where assistance to achieve full ROM is required, the patient can apply a gentle pressure under the chin into extension to achieve the over-pressure.
- The patient is questioned to ensure the over-pressure is symptom-free.
- Typically 3–6 repetitions are performed and then AROM into cervical flexion is reassessed.
- The use of the rule of 3 is recommended (3 repetitions only) in the first session in the presence of more severe and irritable disorders.
- On subsequent treatment occasions, if AROM has a clinically meaningful improvement, then an additional 3–5 sets of 6–10 repetitions may be applied.

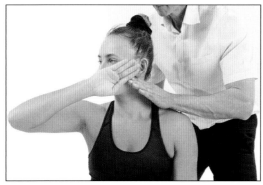

Figure 3.4A
Over-pressure: rotation

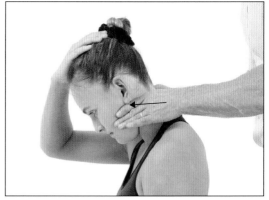

Figure 3.4B
Over-pressure: flexion

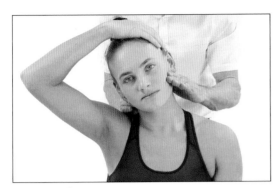

Figure 3.4C
Over-pressure: lateral flexion

VARIATIONS

- If the symptoms do not abolish with a central SNAG through the spinous process, then applying the technique with the contact thumb on the lamina may be successful (Fig. 3.5).

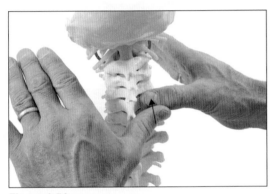

Figure 3.5A
Unilateral SNAG: model view

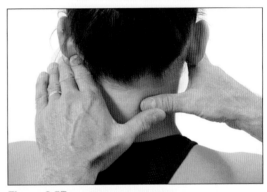

Figure 3.5B
Unilateral SNAG: finger placement

- Typically a unilateral SNAG is applied to the lamina on the side that is painful. If tenderness with lamina contact point is excessive (i.e. unacceptable to the patient), the therapist would attempt the SNAG to either the spinous process of the same vertebra or the lamina of the superior vertebra on the opposite side of pain.
- Ensure the contact thumb is as close as possible to the spinous process for maximum comfort.
- If the initial unilateral contact is painful the therapist may use foam to decrease soft tissue sensitivity.
- Additional adjustments may be to change the angle of the glide, such as slightly laterally, or alter the degree of force.

COMMENTS

- It is important that the therapist adjusts the angle of the glide during the application of the technique, as the facet plane angle will decrease during flexion.
- The therapist must maintain the glide parallel to the facet plane during the MWM.

(continued next page...)

3

SELF-MANAGEMENT

- If a cervical SNAG has proven effective, then typically a self-mobilisation should be taught to the patient early in the treatment session on day 1 if the condition is not irritable or as the therapist's clinical decision/treatment plan indicates. Figure 3.6 shows some examples.

- The patient places a self-SNAG strap on the lamina of C2 (for a C2/3 problem), just lateral to the spinous process.

- With the hand on the side of the restriction, the patient pulls the strap along the plane of the facet joints towards their eyes. Both hands pull along the facet plane for flexion and extension. For rotation and lateral flexion, only the hand on the side of limitation pulls along the facet plane. The other hand holds the strap loosely against the chest (see Fig. 3.6).

- While the strap pressure is sustained, the patient moves the head/neck towards the restricted direction.

- 6–10 repetitions are performed and this process is repeated 3–5 times per day until all symptoms have resolved.

- Rather than using the self-SNAG strap, it is also possible to use the selvedge edge of a towel to perform the self-SNAG.

- If the patient has benefited from cervical flexion SNAG then a fist traction (see the fist traction technique later in this chapter) self-mobilisation may be added as a treatment in the clinic or a home exercise. This can be added on day 1 if the condition is warranted as not irritable or as therapist's clinical decision/treatment plan indicates.

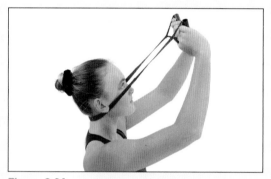

Figure 3.6A
Self-SNAG: strap extension

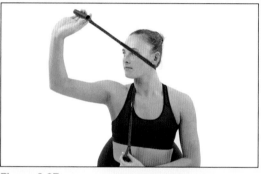

Figure 3.6B
Self-SNAG: strap rotation

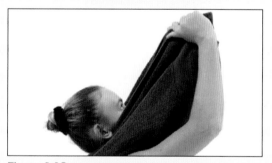

Figure 3.6C
Self-SNAG: using a towel

ANNOTATIONS

sit C4 SNAG F×3
sit C4 SNAG Rot R×3
sit C4 SNAG Rot R +OP×6(3)
sit C4 SNAG F +OP×6(3)
sit R C4 SNAG LF R×3
sit C2 self strap SNAG E×3
sit C2 self strap SNAG Rot R×6
sit C2 self towel SNAG Rot R×10

C5/6 or C6/7 transverse (positional) SNAG

TECHNIQUE AT A GLANCE

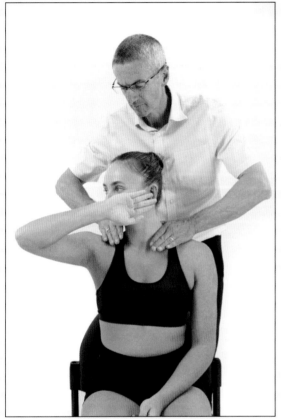

Figure 3.7
C5/6 transverse SNAG: end-range position with over-pressure

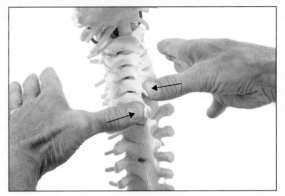

Figure 3.8
C5/6 transverse SNAG: model view

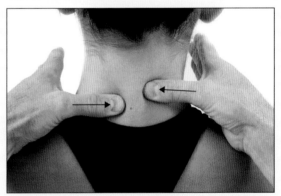

Figure 3.9
C5/6 transverse SNAG: hand placement

- The patient sits well supported in a chair.
- The cervical spine and head are set in a neutral position.
- The therapist applies a transverse glide with their right thumb to the right side of the spinous process (i.e. C5) of the superior vertebra and at the same time applies a transverse glide with their left thumb on the left side of the spinous process of the lower vertebra (C6).
- While the glide is sustained the patient actively moves their neck in the direction that previously produced the symptoms.
- If symptom-free, the patient applies over-pressure further into the movement restriction.
- See Figs 3.7–3.9.

INDICATION

Loss of motion or pain at the C5/6, C6/7 and C7/T1 may benefit from a specific type of SNAG. The patient reports pain or stiffness arising from the above motion segments. Patients typically report unilateral pain and may have a loss of combined motion, including extension, lateral flexion and rotation.

POSITIONING

Patient:	Seated, well supported in a chair.
Treated body part:	The position of the cervical spine should be neutral to allow for effective mobilisation of the cervical segment. The patient is looking forwards.
Therapist:	Standing close behind the patient.
Hands/contact points:	The position of the cervical spine should be neutral to allow for effective mobilisation of the cervical segment. The therapist's right thumb contacts the right side of the spinous process of the superior vertebra and the left thumb contacts the left side of the spinous process of the lower vertebra.

APPLICATION GUIDELINES

- A transverse glide is applied to both spinous processes.
- The therapist maintains the glide through both the left and right thumbs.
- The transverse glide is sustained as the patient is asked to actively move their neck in the symptomatic direction to the end range of active motion. Restore pain-free range of single plane movement before combined movement.
- If the patient is symptom-free they are instructed to apply over-pressure into the restricted motion.
- Soft tissue tenderness is frequently encountered with this technique, and discerning between soft tissue tenderness and the patient's pain is important. The use of a foam pad on the skin is advocated to minimise soft tissue tenderness.

COMMENTS

- It is important that the therapist adjusts the angle of the glide during the active movement. Minor adjustments are often critical to a successful technique, and the therapist may need to adjust glides when the patient reports that the pain or movement is better but not pain-free. As with all SNAGs, glide adjustment is always a treatment variable to be considered.
- This was formerly called a positional SNAG or cervical MWM.

SELF-MANAGEMENT

- The patient is instructed in locating the spinous process at the affected level (Fig. 3.10).
- Transverse pressure is applied to the side of the spinous process through the pad of the index finger with one hand, reinforced with the middle finger of the same hand.
- A consistent transverse glide is sustained as the patient is instructed to move their neck towards the restricted direction. If the movement is not symptom-free, then the patient is instructed on how to make small changes to the direction of the glide and force applied to attain a symptom-free movement.
- 6–10 repetitions may be performed as the patient becomes accustomed to the exercise. This process is repeated 3–5 times per day until all of the symptoms have resolved without the need for the SNAG to be applied.

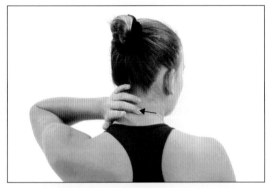

Figure 3.10A
Self-C5 transverse SNAG: rear view start position

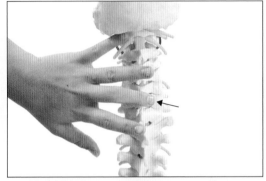

Figure 3.10B
Self-C5 transverse SNAG: rear view end position, model view

ANNOTATIONS

sit R C5/L C6 Trans SNAG Rot R +OP×3
sit R C5/L C6 Trans SNAG F×3
sit R C5/L C6 Trans SNAG E×3
sit R C5/L C6 Trans SNAG LF R×3
sit self R C5 Trans SNAG Rot R×6

FIST TRACTION

TECHNIQUE AT A GLANCE

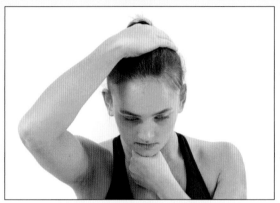

Figure 3.12
Fist traction: start position front view

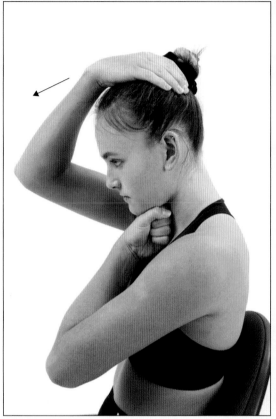

Figure 3.11
Fist traction: start position side view

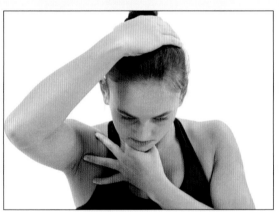

Figure 3.13
Fist traction: end position front view

- The patient sits in neutral upright posture.
- The patient makes a fist and places it under their chin, thumb side up.
- The patient flexes their neck forwards until their chin makes contact with their fist.
- If there is no pain, the patient uses their other hand on the back of their head to apply over-pressure into flexion.
- The patient holds the pain-free over-pressure for 10 seconds.
- See Figs 3.11–3.13.

INDICATION

Loss of cervical flexion due to pain or stiffness.

POSITIONING

Patient:	Seated, well supported in a chair.
Treated body part:	The position of the cervical spine should be in neutral alignment.
Hand position:	The patient makes a fist and places it under their chin, thumb side up.

APPLICATION GUIDELINES

- The patient places a tight fist with the thumb side up resting on the chest underneath their chin to block cervical flexion movement.
- The patient then flexes their neck until their chin makes contact with their fist.
- If the patient is symptom-free, they reach up with their other hand and contact the back of their head to pull the back of the head up to create the flexion movement and create flexion over-pressure.
- If symptom-free, the patient will hold the flexion with over-pressure for 10 seconds.
- Repeat the process 3 times.

VARIATIONS

- If the symptoms are not abolished when the patient flexes, they may need to increase the effective size of the fist by adding a small folded towel between the fist and the chest and re-test to see if symptoms are now abolished. This towel can be used for 1–2 10-second repetitions, before trying to progress the technique again without the towel. Similarly, if flexion improves, but a small degree of limitation remains, then the size of the patient's fist can be reduced by removing 1, 2 or 3 fingers from the fist.

COMMENT

- Note: there should be no neck, head, teeth or jaw pain or dizziness with this technique.

ANNOTATION

 sit self fist Tr×10 sec (3)

NATURAL APOPHYSEAL GLIDES (NAGS) (CENTRAL AND UNILATERAL)

TECHNIQUE AT A GLANCE

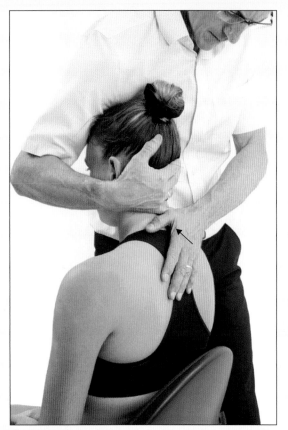

Figure 3.14
Central NAG: posterior view

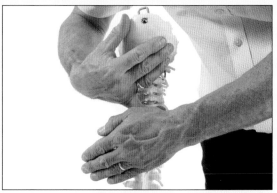

Figure 3.15
Central NAG: model view

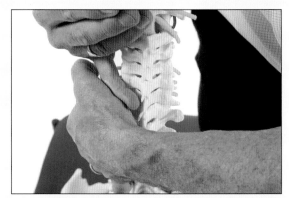

Figure 3.16
Unilateral NAG: left unilateral model view

- The patient sits well supported in a chair.
- The therapist stands facing the patient in step-stance posture stabilising the patient's shoulder/trunk.
- Painless oscillatory mid- to end-range mobilisation is applied in the plane of the facet joints on the spinous process or articular pillar.
- This technique can be applied between C2 and C7.
- See Figs 3.14–3.16.

INDICATION

Patient with multidirectional or multilevel movement loss due to pain or stiffness from C2 to C7.

POSITIONING

Patient:	Seated, well supported in a chair.
Treated body part:	Cervical spine slightly flexed without rotation or lateral flexion, head resting against the therapist's trunk or upper arm.
Therapist:	Standing facing the patient's right shoulder (step-stance posture), with the therapist's hip blocking the patient's shoulder.
Hands/contact points:	Middle phalanx of the therapist's right little finger is placed under the spinous process or on the articular pillar of the superior vertebra of the mobilised segment. The other fingers of that hand are wrapped around the occiput, stabilising the head. The lateral border of the thenar eminence of the left hand partially covers the little finger of the therapist's right hand. The therapist typically needs to take up the slack in the soft tissue to come into contact with the vertebrae to be moved.

APPLICATION GUIDELINES

- Mid- to end-range glides are performed along the cervical spine facet plane via the fifth digit of the right hand by pushing up and forwards with the therapist's left hand (motive hand) towards the patient's eyes.
- Prior to mobilisation, the therapist takes up the skin slack to ensure good bone contact.
- Mobilisation is applied to the spinous process for bilateral or central pain, or unilaterally on the side of pain.
- Ensure the fifth digit is relaxed so it is being moved only by the therapist's motive hand during the oscillations.
- Keep the head stationary during the mobilisation.
- Ensure the mobilisation is symptom-free. If symptoms are provoked, try applying traction with the mobilisation. In step-stance position, the therapist shifts their weight to their rear leg, which induces a gentle distraction to the cervical spine.
- Mobilise at all vertebral levels causing symptoms.
- Glides are rhythmical and at a rate of 1–2 per second.
- Mobilisations should be repeated 6–10 times (i.e. oscillate for 5–10 seconds) at each level, working from superior to inferior vertebral levels.
- Repeat the mobilisation 3–5 times per vertebral level, if reassessment indicates a positive response.

VARIATIONS

- A gentle glide should be trialled in acute pain and a stronger glide for more chronic stiffness-related disorders. If pain is elicited try a more gentle glide, cushioning with a foam pad, or applying traction combined with mobilisation.
- A foam pad also helps to avoid excessive sliding on the skin.

COMMENTS

- It is important that the glide is applied along the facet plane. This plane may vary from person to person and from level to level. So if pain is provoked try to alter the direction of the glide.
- In the patient with a deep cervical lordosis, try flexing the neck more to reduce the lordosis and separate the spinous process to enable easier contact for mobilisation.
- If the patient is unable to tolerate NAGs due to pain, despite these modifications, then their condition is too irritable and they are not suitable for manual therapy at this time.

ANNOTATIONS

sit C2–7 NAG×5 sec (3)
sit L C2–7 NAG×5 sec (3)
sit R C2–7 NAG×10 sec (5)

REVERSE NAGS (CENTRAL AND UNILATERAL)

TECHNIQUE AT A GLANCE

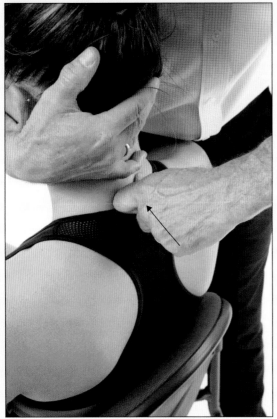

Figure 3.17
Central reverse NAG C5/6 and C6/7: posterior view

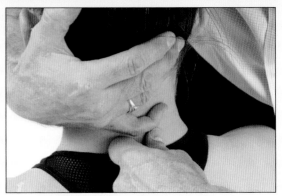

Figure 3.18
Central reverse NAG C5/6 and C6/7: close view

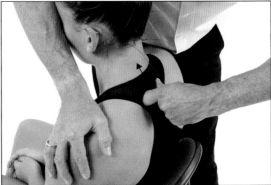

Figure 3.19
Unilateral reverse NAG: thoracic levels: posterior view

- The patient sits well supported in a chair.
- The therapist stands facing the patient in step-stance posture stabilising patient's shoulder/trunk.
- Painless oscillatory mid- to end-range mobilisation is applied in the plane of the facet joints on the spinous process or articular pillar.
- This technique can be applied between C6 and the upper thoracic spine.
- See Figs 3.17–3.19.

INDICATION

End-range loss of neck movement, typically associated with a forward head posture, as well as a degenerative lower cervical or upper thoracic spine.

POSITIONING

Patient:	Seated, well supported in a chair.
Treated body part:	Cervical spine slightly flexed without rotation or lateral flexion.
Therapist:	Standing facing the patient's right shoulder (step-stance posture), cradling the patient's head.
Hands/contact points:	Right (stabilising) hand: distal interphalangeal (IP) joint of the fifth finger hooks around the spinous process of the superior vertebra.
	Mobilising left hand: third, fourth and fifth metacarpophalangeal (MCP) joints are flexed; IP joints of the index finger are flexed and MCP joints of the thumb and index finger are extended.
	Note: spreading the thumb and index finger will allow the therapist to make contact with the transverse processes.

APPLICATION GUIDELINES

- Mobilisation is applied through the spinous process or bilaterally through the articular pillars of the inferior segment. For a unilateral technique, greater pressure is applied through the index finger or thumb.

- Mid- to end-range oscillatory glides are performed along the plane of the facet joints.

- Prior to mobilisation, the therapist takes up the skin slack to ensure good bone contact.

- Glides are rhythmical, 1–2 per second.

- Keep the head and trunk stationary during the mobilisation.

- Ensure the mobilisation is symptom-free. If symptoms are provoked, try applying traction with the mobilisation. In step-stance position, the therapist shifts their weight to their rear leg, which induces a gentle distraction to the cervical spine.

- Mobilise at all vertebral levels causing symptoms.

- Mobilisations should be repeated 6–10 times (or 5–10 seconds) at each level, working from inferior to superior vertebral levels.

(continued next page...)

VARIATIONS

- A gentle glide should be trialled in acute pain and a stronger glide for more chronic stiffness-related disorders. If pain is elicited try a more gentle glide, cushioning with a foam pad, or applying traction combined with mobilisation.
- A foam pad also helps to avoid excessive sliding on the skin.
- For those with small hands, reverse NAGs applied bilaterally can be difficult. Using the thumb or flexed first interphalangeal joint of the index finger (Fig. 3.20), the therapist can apply a reverse NAG on the side of pain, or if the pain is bilateral a reverse NAG to each side separately can be used.

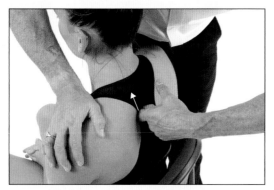

Figure 3.20A
Unilateral reverse NAG using the index finger

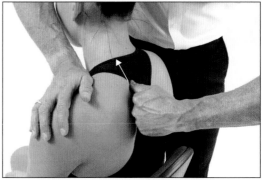

Figure 3.20B
Unilateral reverse NAG using the thumb

COMMENTS

- It is important that the glide is applied along the facet plane. This plane may vary from person to person and from level to level. So if pain is invoked try to alter the direction of the glide.
- In the patient with a deep cervical lordosis, try flexing the neck more to reduce the lordosis and separate the spinous process.
- Avoid compressing the cervical spine by ensuring that the patient's forehead rests in the therapist's arm.

ANNOTATIONS

sit C6–T4 rev NAG×5 sec (3)
sit L C6–T4 rev NAG×5 sec (3)
sit R C6–T4 rev NAG×10 sec (5)

CERVICOTHORACIC JUNCTION MOBILISATION: BRIDGE TECHNIQUE

TECHNIQUE AT A GLANCE

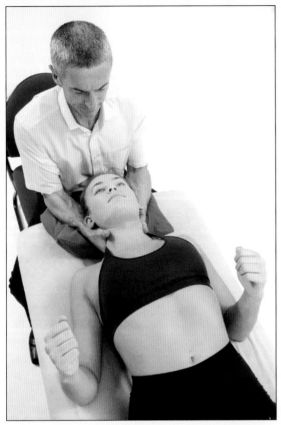

Figure 3.21
Bridge technique: end position

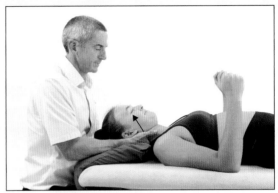

Figure 3.22
Bridge technique: start position

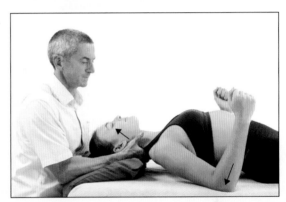

Figure 3.23
Bridge technique: end position lateral view

- The patient lies supine, head resting on a pillow, knees flexed.
- The therapist sits at the head of the table stabilising the occiput with both hands while the index and middle finger contact the articular pillar at the cervicothoracic junction.
- Painless oscillatory mid- to end-range extension mobilisation is applied to the cervicothoracic junction while the patient lifts their chest, pushing down through their elbows.
- This technique can be applied between C7 and the upper thoracic spine.
- See Figs 3.21–3.23.

INDICATION

Pain and limitation of cervical extension.

POSITIONING

Patient:	Supine, head resting on a pillow.
Treated body part:	Cervical spine relaxed in neutral, head resting on a pillow.
Therapist:	Sitting at the head of the table.
Hands/contact points:	Hands supporting both sides of the head through the thenar eminence on each side. Fingers in contact with the C7, T1 or T2 articular pillar bilaterally.

APPLICATION GUIDELINES

- The therapist contacts the articular pillars of the cervicothoracic junction on each side.
- The eminence stabilises the head. Keeping the hands rigid helps the therapist to stabilise the mid and upper cervical spine during the mobilisation.
- Mid- to end-range mobilisation of the cervicothoracic junction takes place when the patient actively lifts their chest by pushing down through their elbows while the therapist stabilises the neck above the level of hand contact.
- Mobilisation is rhythmical, with a pause at the end-range position.
- Perform 6 repetitions in one set, with 2–4 sets per treatment session if reassessment indicates a positive response.

COMMENTS

- The technique can be performed with the therapist standing.
- The hand contact can be moved from level to level to achieve variations in effect at different cervico-thoracic spinal levels.

SELF-MANAGEMENT

- Improved range in pain-free cervicothoracic mobility can be maintained with the aid of a mobilisation belt or small towel/scarf placed under the occiput.
- While sitting with their back supported, the patient pulls the belt vertically, supporting the weight of the head while moving the neck into extension (see Fig. 3.24).
- Repeat the exercise 5 times on each occasion, twice per day.

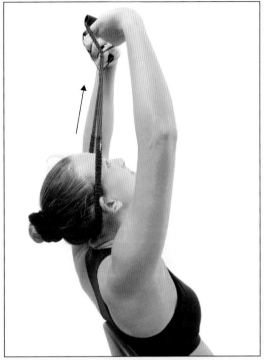

Figure 3.24
Self-management following the Bridge mobilisation technique

ANNOTATIONS

sup ly C7–T2 Bridge×6(4)
sit occiput self strap SNAG E×6

CERVICAL TRACTION: UPPER EXTREMITY PAIN

TECHNIQUE AT A GLANCE

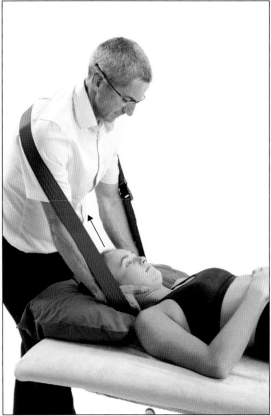

Figure 3.25
Belt traction to relieve arm pain

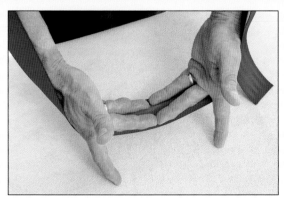

Figure 3.26
Belt traction to relieve arm pain: hand placement

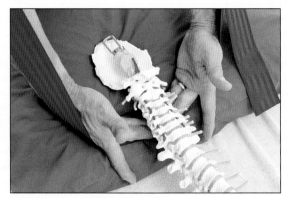

Figure 3.27
Belt traction to relieve arm pain: model view

- The patient is lying supine with the therapist standing at the patient's head.
- Traction is provided by a mobilisation belt applied at a specific cervical vertebral segment, localised by the therapist's hand position.
- The direction of traction is along the facet plane.
- Traction is sustained while the patient lies in a pain-free position, or the patient may move their arm through their previously pain-provocative motion.
- See Figs 3.25–3.27.

INDICATION

Cervical pain, cervical radiculopathy, or upper limb pain with a suspected cervical spine origin.

POSITIONING

Patient:	Patient lies supine.
Treated body part:	Cervical spine is positioned in the maximum pain-free position.
Therapist:	Standing at the patient's head, with belt around therapist's upper back/shoulders.
Hands/contact points:	Therapist's middle fingers are placed inside the belt, leaving the fingertips gapped to accommodate the spinous process.
	The therapist's hands are placed under the patient's neck with the middle fingers along the cervical articular pillar. The spinous process lies between the middle fingers. As the therapist leans back the tension on the belt is carried through the fingers to the cervical vertebra, causing traction.

APPLICATION GUIDELINES

- The therapist leans back into the belt. The belt will tighten around the hands, making active gripping of the neck unnecessary.
- Apply gentle traction, just enough to relieve the patient's pain.
- There should be an immediate significant reduction in pain.
- Hold initially for 30 seconds. Longer durations of up to 2 minutes can be sustained, depending on the patient's response.
- Perform 3–5 repetitions.
- Move slowly in and out of the traction to avoid sudden movement at the symptomatic level, which may provoke pain.

VARIATIONS

- The therapist may apply traction at different spinal levels as necessary to gain the optimum effect.
- The therapist may influence the direction of the glide by changing the belt angle from the hand to the shoulders, or by flexing or extending the cervical spine. In some cases, positioning the shoulder in abduction reduces the arm symptoms (see Fig. 3.28).
- A greater effect on increasing the size of the intervertebral foramen may be achieved by rotating, laterally flexing and flexing the patient's cervical spine to the contralateral side of the arm symptoms.

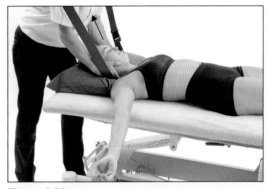

Figure 3.28
Belt traction with the shoulder resting in abduction

COMMENTS

- It is better to under-treat than over-treat on the first day, particularly with a more painful, irritable condition affecting the spine.
- The therapist should strive to remain in an upright, balanced position to ensure consistent tension on the belt.
- Keeping the hands relaxed will result in a more consistent traction throughout the application of the technique.

ANNOTATIONS

sup ly C4 belt Tr×30 sec
sup ly in R Sh Ab 80 degrees C4 belt Tr×2 min
sup ly in R Sh Ab 80 degrees C4 belt Tr+Cx Rot L/LF R/F×30 sec (5)

SPINAL MOBILISATION WITH ARM MOVEMENT (SMWAM)

Shoulder abduction

TECHNIQUE AT A GLANCE

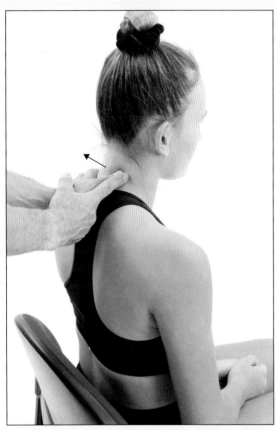

Figure 3.29
SMWAM: start position

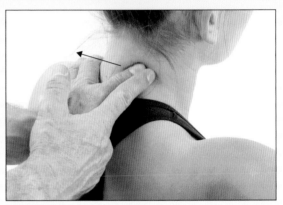

Figure 3.30
SMWAM: hand placement close view

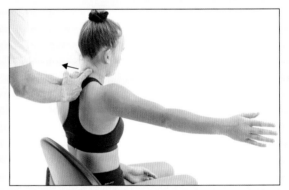

Figure 3.31
SMWAM: abduction

- The patient is seated.
- The therapist contacts the length of the spinous process with the medial aspect of the thumb.
- A transverse glide is applied by the therapist's index finger against the thumb contacting the spinous process.
- The direction of the glide is to the contralateral side of the pain.
- While the mobilisation is sustained the patient moves their arm through a pain-free abduction range.
- See Figs 3.29–3.31.

INDICATION

Pain with shoulder abduction that is of suspected cervical or upper thoracic spine origin.

POSITIONING

Patient:	Seated with the shoulder relaxed.
Treated body part:	Arm resting at side or supported on the lap.
Therapist:	Standing behind the patient.
Hands/contact points:	Contact hand: medial border of the thumb along the spinous process of the symptomatic vertebral level. Use some of the patient's soft tissue (cervical extensors) to soften the contact point and reduce contact pain. The remaining fingers relax around the base of the neck.
	Gliding hand: index finger pushes transversely through the contact thumb, away from the painful side. The thumb of the mobilising hand rests on the dorsum of the hand while the third to fifth fingers are placed in the palm of the contact hand.

APPLICATION GUIDELINES

- Apply a transversely directed glide of the superior spinous process at the involved cervical vertebral segment away from the painful side. This is thought to mobilise the involved vertebral segment.
- While sustaining the transverse glide, have the patient repeat the shoulder abduction, which should now have greater pain-free range.
- Maintain the glide throughout the active abduction movement as well as the return to neutral.
- Apply 3 repetitions only on the first day; 3–5 sets of 6–10 repetitions may be performed on subsequent treatment sessions, but only if there has been a positive response to the first treatment session and there are no latent pain responses.
- Over-pressure may be applied at end range but only if it is pain-free. Alternatively, loading may be achieved by applying resistance to abduction using a resistance band or a small weight.
- It is important that the patient's head is kept relaxed in a neutral position.

VARIATIONS

- The mobilisation may also be applied by the non-contact (motive) thumb of the opposite hand. The position of the contact finger on the spinous process remains unchanged (see Fig. 3.32).
- This method may be found useful when more glide force is needed to achieve the desired result of full, pain-free arm motion by the patient.

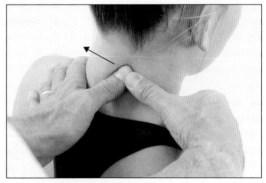

Figure 3.32
Alternative hand placement for SMWAM

(continued next page...)

COMMENTS

- Ensure that some soft tissue such as the cervical extensor muscle group is used to soften the contact between the spinous process and the contact thumb. This improves patient comfort and helps to align the thumb along the entire length of the spinous process.
- The contact thumb does not provide the glide. The glide is applied by the motive index finger applying pressure through the thumb.
- Keeping the hands relaxed but firm will result in a more consistent glide through the application of the technique.

SELF-MANAGEMENT

- This technique may be converted to a home exercise. The patient places the index finger of the contralateral hand on the superior spinous process at the involved vertebral segment pulling away from the painful side. While maintaining the glide the patient abducts the shoulder through the pain-free range (see Fig. 3.33).

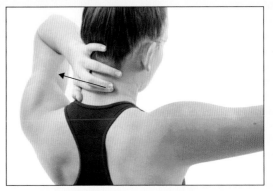

Figure 3.33
Self-SMWAM for abduction

ANNOTATIONS

sit R C3 SMWAM R Sh Ab×3
sit R C3 SMWAM R Sh Ab +OP×6
sit R C3 SMWAM res R Sh Ab (1 kg)×10(3)
sit R C3 self SMWAM R Sh Ab×6

SMWAM: HORIZONTAL EXTENSION AND NEURODYNAMIC DYSFUNCTION

TECHNIQUE AT A GLANCE

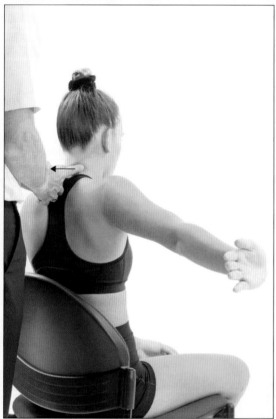

Figure 3.34
SMWAM: horizontal extension

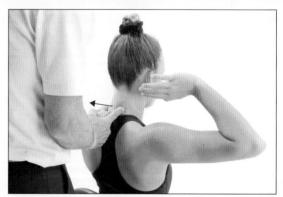

Figure 3.35
SMWAM: ulnar nerve neurodynamic movement

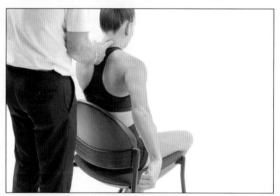

Figure 3.36
SMWAM: radial nerve neurodynamic movement

- The patient is seated.
- The therapist contacts the spinous process with the medial edge of their thumb.
- A transverse glide is applied by the therapist's index finger pressing onto their thumb in contact with the spinous process.
- The direction of glide is away from the painful side.
- While the mobilisation is sustained the patient moves their arm through a pain-free horizontal extension range or neurodynamic movement.
- See Figs 3.34–3.36.

INDICATION

Pain with shoulder horizontal extension or neurodynamic test movement that is of suspected cervical or thoracic spine origin.

POSITIONING

Patient:	Seated with the shoulder relaxed.
Treated body part:	Arm resting at side or supported on the lap.
Therapist:	Standing behind the patient.
Hands / contact points:	Contact hand: medial border of the thumb along the spinous process of the symptomatic vertebral level. Use some of the patient's soft tissue (cervical extensor muscle) to soften the contact point and reduce contact pain. The remaining fingers relax around the base of the neck.
	Gliding hand: index finger pushes transversely through the contact thumb, away from the painful side. The thumb of the mobilising hand rests on the dorsum of the hand while the third to fifth fingers are placed in the palm of the contact hand.

APPLICATION GUIDELINES

- Apply a transversely directed glide of the superior spinous process at the involved cervical vertebral segment away from the painful side. This is thought to mobilise the affected vertebral segment, eliminating pain provoked by shoulder movement.

- While sustaining the transverse glide, have the patient repeat the shoulder horizontal extension or neurodynamic test movement (median, radial or ulnar neurodynamic test movement in sitting), which should now have greater pain-free range.

- Maintain the glide throughout the active shoulder and arm movement as well as the return to neutral.

- Apply 3 repetitions only on the first day; 3–5 sets of 6–10 repetitions may be performed on subsequent treatment sessions, but only if there has been a positive response to the first treatment session and there are no latent pain responses.

- Over-pressure for horizontal extension only may be applied at end range but only if it is pain-free. Alternatively, loading to horizontal extension may be achieved by applying resistance using a resistance band.

VARIATIONS

- When treating neurodynamic dysfunction, the active movement could begin with cervical spine movements (lateral flexion, rotation or flexion) with the arm positioned in a mildly provocative neurodynamic position. Following this, progress to more extreme ranges of arm movement.

COMMENTS

- Ensure that some soft tissue such as the cervical extensor muscle group is used to soften the contact between the spinous process and the contact thumb. This improves patient comfort and helps to align the thumb along the entire length of the spinous process.

- The contact thumb itself does not provide the glide. The glide is applied by the mobilising index finger through the thumb.

- Keeping the hands relaxed but firm will result in a more consistent application of glide through the application of the technique.

SELF-MANAGEMENT

- This technique can also be taught as a home exercise (Fig. 3.37) as per SMWAM for abduction above. The patient places the index finger of the contralateral hand on the superior spinous process at the involved vertebral segment pulling away from the painful side. While maintaining the glide, the patient performs horizontal extension or the neurodynamic movement through the pain-free range.

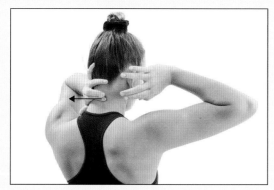

Figure 3.37A
Self-SMWAM: ulnar neurodynamic technique

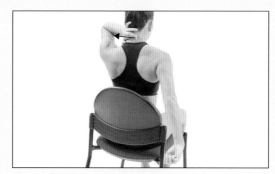

Figure 3.37B
Self-SMWAM: radial neurodynamic technique

ANNOTATIONS

sit R C3 SMWAM R Sh HE×3
sit R C7 SMWAM R ulnar nerve slide×6
sit R C6 SMWAM R radial nerve slide×6(3)
sit R C6 SMWAM median nerve slide×6(3)
sit L C3 self SMWAM L Sh HE×10

References

Abdelgalil, A., Balbaa, A.A., Elazizi, H.M., Abdelaal, A., Abdelaal, M., 2015. High velocity low amplitude manipulation versus sustained apophyseal glides on pain and range of motion in patients with mechanical neck pain: an immediate effect. Int. J. Adv. Res. 3 (6), 503–513.

Buyukturan, O., Buyukturan, B., Sas, S., Kararti, C., Ceylan, I., 2018. The effect of Mulligan mobilization technique in older adults with neck pain: a randomized controlled, double-blind study. Pain Res. Manag. 2018, 2856375.

Ganesh, G.S., Mohanty, P., Pattnaik, M., Mishra, C., 2015. Effectiveness of mobilization therapy and exercises in mechanical neck pain. Physiother. Theory Pract. 31 (2), 99–106.

Gautam, R., Dhamija, J.K., Puri, A., 2014. Comparison of Maitland and Mulligan mobilization in improving neck pain, ROM and disability. Int. J. Physiother. Res. 2 (3), 482–487.

Hearn, A., Rivett, D.A., 2002. Cervical SNAGs: a biomechanical analysis. Man. Ther. 7 (2), 71–79.

Kumar, D. A study on the efficacy of Mulligan concept in cervical spine pain and stiffness [PhD Thesis]. Guru Nanak Dev University, India, 2013.

Moulson, A., Watson, T., 2006. A preliminary investigation into the relationship between cervical SNAGS and sympathetic nervous system activity in the upper limbs of an asymptomatic population. Man. Ther. 11 (3), 214–224.

Paungmali, A., O'Leary, S., Souvlis, T., Vicenzino, B., 2003. Hypoalgesic and sympathoexcitatory effects of mobilization with movement for lateral epicondylalgia. Phys. Ther. 83 (4), 374–383.

Said, S.M., Ali, O.I., Elazm, S.N.A., Abdelraoof, N.A., 2017. Mulligan self mobilization versus Mulligan SNAGS on cervical position sense. Int. J. Physiother. 4 (2), 93–100.

Vicenzino, B., Collins, D., Benson, H., Wright, A., 1998. An investigation of the interrelationship between manipulative therapy-induced hypoalgesia and sympathoexcitation. J. Manipulative Physiol. Ther. 21 (7), 448–453.

Vicenzino, B., Hall, T., Hing, W., Rivett, D., 2011. A new proposed model of the mechanisms of action of Mobilisation with Movement. In: Vicenzino, B., Hing, W., Rivett, D., Hall, T. (Eds.), Mobilisation With Movement: The Art and the Science. Churchill Livingstone, Australia, Chatswood, NSW, pp. 75–85.

3

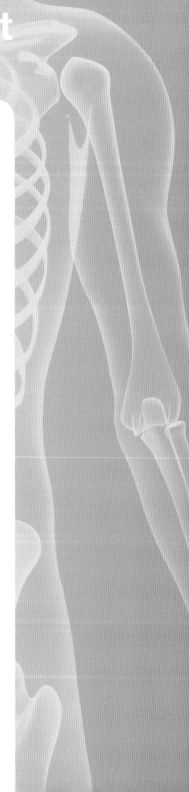

Temporomandibular joint

TECHNIQUES FOR THE TEMPOROMANDIBULAR JOINT

TEMPOROMANDIBULAR JOINT: MWM

INTRODUCTION

The treatment of temporomandibular joint (TMJ) dysfunction requires an understanding of the anatomy and pathophysiology of the region. In addition, when treating long-standing temporomandibular dysfunction (TMD) it is critical to have an accurate diagnosis and, if necessary, appropriate radiological imaging.

TMJ MWM techniques were developed for specific presentations including TMJ internal derangements, acute malocclusions and long-standing TMJ hypomobility. As for all MWM techniques, it is important to understand the need to apply TMJ MWM in a pain-free manner and to apply end-of-range over-pressure judiciously. Using inappropriate stretching techniques may cause permanent elongation of the inferior and superior retrodiscal lamina, which will disturb the normal mandibular condyle–articular disc relationship through the loss of the slight posterior retractive force usually exerted on the disc by the superior retrodiscal lamina (Okeson, 2003). A TMJ with a reducible disc displacement may thus be damaged and result in permanent disc displacement.

TMJ MWM techniques are also useful for re-education of poor mandibular movement patterns due to altered muscle activity, are ideal for use as self-treatment procedures and can be integrated into existing TMJ exercise routines. It is important that TMJ self-MWM and exercise rehabilitation exercises do not permit abnormal compensatory movements to occur as this will lessen the effectiveness of the activity and may even contribute to the problem. Examples of simple TMJ MWM techniques are provided in this chapter and a case study illustrating their use for a complex temporomandibular dysfunction is provided elsewhere (Oliver, 2011).

Principles of application are the same as for MWM for other joints (Vicenzino et al., 2011). However, a unique feature is that TMJs move as a pair and are very mobile, such that applying a mobilisation technique to one TMJ will usually influence the contralateral joint. There is an upper (superior) and lower (inferior) joint within a single TMJ, each having its own joint plane. The joint plane of the upper joint (determined by the slope of the articular eminence) is variable between individuals and between sides, and can change with age (Yamada et al., 2004). The impact of this variation in joint plane is that the treatment plane (Vicenzino et al., 2011), which is parallel to the joint plane, will vary in orientation. Thus, to determine the optimal angle of application of an anteroinferior glide the clinician will need to vary the orientation of the glide angle to ascertain the angle that produces the maximal amount of translation.

Identification of the individual patient's treatment plane (predominantly in the sagittal plane) by the clinician will then serve as a basis from which to determine the individual's medial or lateral glide components of an MWM or to serve as a frame from which to perform more-complex movements (e.g. laterotrusal motion, which involves both TMJs differently). Medial or lateral glide components of an MWM will be performed perpendicular to the treatment plane and, if anatomy of the joint is relatively normal, the condylar–disc complex will move as a unit in relation to the articular eminence.

If a laterotrusal movement of the jaw is required, there is greater glide of the condylar–disc complex on one side so that the jaw swings to the contralateral side. This movement will occur parallel to the articular eminence so that the glide component in the superior joint is obliquely anterior and inferior on opening. When the MWM is performed with a component of laterotrusion the glide is usually directed from one mandibular head to the other. If the mandible is swinging to the left, the axis will swing obliquely left as the right condyle slides further down and forwards on the articular eminence.

TMJ behaviour on mouth closure and occlusion of the teeth are intimately related. Pain originating from an injured TMJ may contribute to malocclusion and painful limitation of jaw movement by altering masticatory muscle function (Broton & Sessle, 1988; Lund & Olsson, 1983; Smith, 1981; Stohler et al., 1985). If inflammation and pain of the TMJ have been present for a long period, secondary central nervous system effects including referred pain and secondary muscle symptoms such as tenderness and co-contraction of the masticatory muscles may occur (Okeson, 1995).

There appears to be an important neurophysiological link between the cervical spine and the TMJ that influences TMD. Constant afferent nociceptive activity to the trigeminocervical nucleus from the cervical spine can excite adjacent interneurons from the trigeminal fields. If the central excitatory effect involves efferent trigeminal (motor) interneurons, there may also be a resulting alteration in orofacial muscular activity (Okeson, 1995). Consequently, the cervical spine should be considered as a likely contributing factor to orofacial pain and temporomandibular dysfunction.

There also appear to be other significant links between the cervical spine and the TMJ. A clinical example is provided by individuals who have whiplash-associated disorders – they have decreased range of jaw-opening compared with healthy individuals (Zafar et al., 2006), and jaw movements and muscle activity during normal function occur simultaneously with movement and muscle activity of the cervical spine (Eriksson et al., 2000; Zafar, 2000). Furthermore, a study by Motta and colleagues (Motta et al., 2012) found that subjects with TMD had different head posture compared with asymptomatic people. Consequently, when performing the TMJ MWM techniques the position of the spinal column should be taken into account.

If the Mulligan Concept guidelines and principles of PILL and CROCK are followed (see the introduction to this book), then the TMJ MWM techniques are a very specific, safe and effective treatment tool to assist in management of temporomandibular dysfunction and orofacial pain.

Levels of evidence

Level 4: one case series and one case report

There are no readily identifiable clinical trials and only one case series that report on the efficacy or effects of the TMJ MWM. The case series of 15 patients with TMJ disorder who were treated with thoracic and cervical spine manipulation, trigger point dry needling and TMJ MWM reported, amongst other significant improvements, an improvement of 36.1 mm on a 100 mm visual analogue scale for pain severity at the 2-month follow-up (González-Iglesias et al., 2013). The case series highlights the notion that treatment might need to target the vertebral column as well as the TMJ. A recent case report of a 23-year-old female with clinical observations of tinnitus, bilateral jaw pain, limited maximal mouth opening (MMO), flattened thoracic kyphosis, prominent C7 spinous process and mildly forward head posture supports the combined treatment of TMJ and cervical spine (Sault et al., 2016). The patient was treated with a combination of Maitland, MWM and exercise. The MWM consisted of anterior glide TMJ (2–3 minutes, 2–3 × daily), SNAG C2/3 left rotation (3 minutes, 2 × daily), SNAG C0/1 PA with flexion (3 minutes, 2 × daily). After six sessions, Sault and colleagues (Sault et al., 2016) reported an increase in MMO from 30 mm to 45 mm and improvement in pain pressure thresholds at the thenar eminence and right/left masseter, as well as decreases in jaw pain and improved function measured by questionnaire and the Tampa Scale of Kinesiophobia for temporomandibular disorders.

TEMPOROMANDIBULAR JOINT: MWM

MWM for reduction of internal derangement limiting mandibular depression

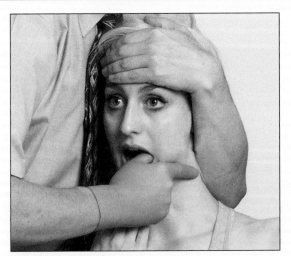

Figure 4.1
MWM for reduction of internal derangement limiting
mandibular depression: hand placement

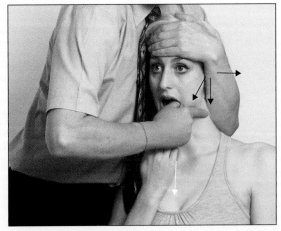

Figure 4.2
MWM for reduction of internal derangement limiting
mandibular depression: wide view

- The therapist cradles the patient's head with the left arm so that the hand is wrapped around the forehead and the forearm is positioned over the left side of the head (see Figs 4.1 and 4.2).
- The thumb of the gloved right hand is placed intraorally along the top of the left lower teeth with the fingers wrapped gently around the mandible.
- If a transverse glide (medial or lateral) is required, apply it first and then apply the inferior glide (traction).
- Inferior glide (traction) is at 90° to the treatment plane. The patient then actively opens their mouth.
- The patient applies end-of-range over-pressure using a hand on the chin, but only if pain-free and there is no lateral deviation.
- Over-pressure is maintained for 2–3 seconds and the jaw is slowly closed while the therapist maintains the applied corrections.

Limited mandibular depression with or without pain due to reducible TMJ internal derangement.

(continued next page...)

POSITIONING

Patient:	Sitting facing mirror with TMJ in relaxed rest position.
Therapist:	Standing beside the patient on the opposite side to the joint to be treated.
Hands/contact points:	Stabilising hand: if mobilising the left TMJ, cradle the head with the left arm so that the hand is wrapped around the forehead and the forearm is positioned over the left side of the head. The head is cradled to the therapist's chest.
	Mobilising hand: the thumb of the gloved right hand is placed intraorally along the top of the left lower teeth with the fingers wrapped gently around the mandible (see Fig. 4.1).

APPLICATION GUIDELINES

- If a transverse glide is required as part of the correction, it is applied initially.
- Traction is then applied at 90° to the treatment plane, and the patient is asked to actively open the mouth. As the patient opens the mouth, the traction and any lateral correction is maintained while the therapist controls the amount of anteroinferior translation occurring in the affected TMJ.
- The amount of anteroinferior translation must match that occurring in the opposite TMJ.
- The jaw must remain in the midline while opening; if this is not possible, mouth opening is permitted only to the point that any movement away from the midline can be controlled.
- The patient applies end-of-range over-pressure using a hand on the chin.
- Over-pressure is applied only if there is no lateral deviation, and if the movement is painless.
- Over-pressure is maintained for 2–3 seconds and the jaw is slowly closed while the therapist maintains the applied corrections.
- The mobilisation is performed 3 times then reassessed.
- 2–3 sets of 6 movements can be applied but, in the case of a reducible derangement, often only 3–6 movements are required to bring about a significant change.

VARIATIONS

- If pain cannot be relieved using this technique, the manoeuvre may need to be entirely passive and performed as described elsewhere (Okeson, 2013, p. 325).
- The traditional passive mobilisation technique can often be made more effective by correcting any positional faults as described for this technique.
- The technique can be adapted for restriction of laterotrusion due to a reducible internal derangement.

COMMENTS

- For this technique, use of a mirror is necessary so that the therapist and patient can observe the movement pathway of the mandible while performing the technique.
- If the opposite TMJ is hypermobile, unstable or demonstrating extra movement due to the limitation of movement in the involved joint, the non-affected joint should be protected by controlling the amount of anterior translation occurring at that joint during the technique (as described in the application guidelines for MWM for painful limitation of mandibular depression).
- If muscular forces exerted by the masticatory muscles are too great to overcome, techniques directed at lessening muscle over-activity are used first and may include dry needling, massage, release techniques and use of modalities including laser and ultrasound.
- Using the hand located over the chin, the patient can help to control deflection or deviation from the midline as well as applying end-of-range over-pressure.
- The patient must be instructed to avoid pushing the jaw posteriorly when applying end-of-range over-pressure.
- To become comfortable with the techniques, the clinician can place the hands and fingers in the appropriate positions and practise 'swinging' the jaw to the left and right while the 'patient' is relaxed. End of range is avoided when rehearsing these techniques.

ANNOTATION

sit L TMJ Lat gl/Ant-inf gl MWM Depr +OP×6

MWM for painful limitation of mandibular depression

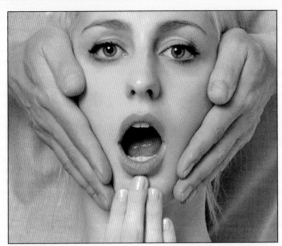

Figure 4.3
MWM for painful limitation of mandibular depression: close view

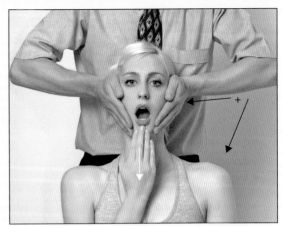

Figure 4.4
MWM for painful limitation of mandibular depression: wide view

- With the patient facing a mirror, the therapist places their hands over the temporalis muscles with the fingers pointing down with thumbs over the zygomatic arches (see Figs 4.3 and 4.4).
- The hands and thumbs are used to stabilise the head. The index fingers lie parallel to and just in front of the posterior border of the mandible passing over the TMJ. The left third and fourth fingers are placed behind the posterior border of the ramus of the mandible just above the angle of the mandible.
- The purpose of the technique is to maintain a midline position and maintain correct anatomical relationships of the TMJ components as the patient fully opens the mouth.
- The patient applies over-pressure at end of range into depression with the fingers of one hand on the chin, while the patient also assists in controlling deflection or deviation from the midline. The midline position is maintained as the patient releases the over-pressure and closes the jaw.

INDICATIONS

Painful or non-painful limitation of mandibular depression with or without lateral deviation or deflection.

The limitation may:

- be caused by a mild TMJ internal derangement without reduction
- remain after spontaneous or therapist reduction of moderate–severe internal derangement
- be due to capsular and/or intra-articular adhesions or masticatory muscle dysfunction.

(continued next page...)

4

POSITIONING	
Patient:	Sitting facing mirror with TMJ in relaxed rest position.
Therapist:	Standing behind the patient.
Hands/contact points:	The hands lie over the temporalis muscles with the fingers pointing down so that the thumbs lie over the zygomatic arches. The hands and thumbs are used to stabilise the head. The left index finger lies parallel to and just in front of the posterior border of the mandible passing over the TMJ. The left third and fourth fingers are placed behind the posterior border of the ramus of the mandible just above the angle of the mandible. The right fingers can be located the same as the left, or the index and middle fingers can be placed on the lateral aspect of the body of the mandible just in front of the anterior border of the masseter muscle (see Figs 4.3 and 4.4).

APPLICATION GUIDELINES

- The technique described here illustrates use of the technique for the following presentations:
  - deflection of the mandible to the left when opening the jaw with restricted ROM and pain in the left TMJ
  - limited anterior gliding of the left mandibular head and excessive anterior gliding of the right mandibular head on jaw-opening and on accessory movement testing
  - left mandibular head slightly posterior in the mandibular fossa
  - displacement of the mandibular heads transversely to the left so that on palpation the left head is prominent laterally in the mandibular fossa, and the right mandibular head is recessed medially into the right mandibular fossa.
- The purpose of the technique is to maintain a midline position and maintain correct (or 'best possible' in the case of a permanently deranged joint) anatomical relationships of the TMJ components as the patient opens the mouth fully.
- This is achieved by moving the mandible sideways to correct any transverse displacement of the mandibular heads, applying a forward gliding force on the side of the limited anterior glide and controlling the unrestricted side so that excessive forward gliding is not permitted.
- If there is no problem with mouth closure, the patient is then asked to gently clench and relax the jaw several times to lessen muscle tension.
- The palmar aspect of the left index finger gently glides the mandible to the right to correct the transverse displacement of the mandibular heads.
- While this position is maintained, the patient is instructed to open the jaw while the third and fourth fingers of the left hand apply an anterior translation force (directed anteroinferiorly along the treatment plane of the superior joint) to the left TMJ and the fingers of the right hand prevent excessive anterior gliding of the right TMJ. The combined forces keep the mandible in the midline as it opens.
- At end of range, the patient applies over-pressure into depression with the fingers of one hand on the chin. No lateral excursion is permitted. The midline position is maintained as the patient releases the over-pressure and closes the jaw.
- Using the hand located over the chin, the patient can assist by helping to control deflection or deviation from the midline as well as applying over-pressure.
- The mobilisation is initially performed 3 times then reassessed; 2–3 sets of 6 repetitions will often produce a significant change in unassisted movement.

VARIATIONS

- The technique can also be performed in supine lying. In some cases, it is easier for the therapist and patient to control components of the movement in this position.

COMMENTS

- If a reducible derangement is not recognised, application of an inappropriate technique may cause permanent damage to the joint.
- A stretching sensation may be reported in the hypomobile joint but, as with all MWMs, no pain should be produced during the technique.
- The MWM technique protects the normal or hypermobile joint while allowing fairly strong mobilisation of the limited joint.
- It is important to use just enough force to control movement of the opposite normal or hypermobile TMJ, because if excessive posterior force is applied the technique may be painful, particularly if the retrodiscal tissue is sensitive.
- If clicking is present in the hypermobile or hypomobile joint, it will often be significantly lessened or eliminated when the technique is being performed and there may be long-term lessening of the clicking.
- As the technique is repeated, the amount of effort required to control the aberrant movements often lessens.
- If muscular forces exerted by the masticatory muscles are too great to be controlled, techniques directed at lessening muscle overactivity may need to be used before applying the MWM technique.
- A mirror is very useful for the therapist and patient to monitor the movement of the mandible. It also prepares the patient for home exercises using a mirror.
- If the correct movement pathway cannot be maintained, the ROM during the MWM must be limited to that which can be controlled.
- The patient must be instructed to avoid pushing the jaw posteriorly when applying end-of-range over-pressure.
- Once good range has been achieved, the patient may be able to use a self-mobilising technique (MWM for movement limitation and pain on mandibular depression home exercise or MWM scream stretch).
- If the movement limitation is caused by a moderate–severe reducible joint derangement, this must be treated first using the MWM for internal derangement (MWM for reduction of internal derangement limiting mandibular depression) or another reduction technique such as that described by Okeson (2013, p. 325).

SELF-MANAGEMENT

- After the severe or persistent limitation or pain has been addressed by the therapist (using this MWM or other procedures), the technique can be performed as a home exercise (see Fig. 4.5).
- As a home exercise, the patient is seated facing a mirror. The hands are placed so that the fingers are pointing cephalad with the distal interphalangeal joints of the thumbs placed around the angle of the mandible, the thenar and hypothenar eminences under the edge of the mandibular ramus, and the tips of the index fingers just making contact with the anterosuperior aspect of the ears. The jaw can be lightly held between the hands and a gentle traction force applied by letting the arms 'go heavy'. If more force is required, an active pull can be applied.
- The hands are used to gently apply the appropriate mobilisations to the TMJs.
- The patient actively opens the mouth while maintaining a midline opening pathway using appropriate pressure from the hands. Another person is required to apply end-of-range over-pressure.
- An alternative technique which can be used as a home exercise for movement limitation and pain on mandibular depression is the scream stretch shown in Fig. 4.6.

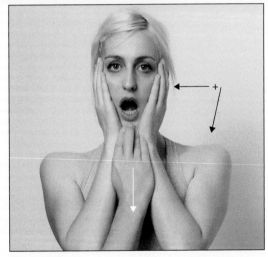

Figure 4.5
MWM for painful limitation of mandibular depression, home exercise: white arrow indicates the direction of the physiological component of the MWM; black arrows indicate the accessory movement components

ANNOTATIONS

sit L TMJ Med gl/Ant-inf gl MWM Depr +OP×6(3)
sup ly L TMJ Med gl/Ant-inf gl MWM Depr +OP×6(3)
sit L TMJ self Med gl/Ant-inf gl MWM Depr +OP (partner)×6

MWM scream stretch: movement limitation and pain on mandibular depression

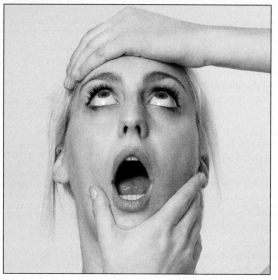

Figure 4.6A
MWM scream stretch for movement limitation and pain on mandibular depression: close view

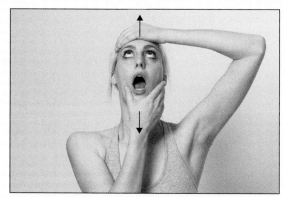

Figure 4.6B
MWM scream stretch for movement limitation and pain on mandibular depression: wide view

- The patient sits facing a mirror with jaw in relaxed rest position, and places one hand over the chin and the other horizontally over the forehead (Fig. 4.6).
- The jaw is opened to comfortable end of range and held in position by the hand over the jaw.
- The patient then looks up with the eyes and actively extends the upper cervical spine so that the jaw opens further.
- The hand on the forehead is used to apply gentle end-of-range over-pressure into cervical extension and maintained for 2–3 seconds.
- After maintaining the stretch for 2–3 seconds, the patient looks down, and lowers the head to close the jaw before releasing the hold on the chin and closing the mouth fully.

INDICATION

Limited mandibular depression with or without pain due to intra-articular adhesions or muscular dysfunction and minimal lateral deviation from the midline.

POSITIONING

Patient:	Sitting facing a mirror with TMJ in relaxed rest position.
Patient's hand position:	One hand is placed over the mandible so that the deepest part of the first web-space is in the midline just above the chin. The lateral border of the index finger is placed just above the edge of the mandible on one side and the medial aspect of the thumb is just above the edge of the opposite side. The other hand is placed horizontally over the forehead.

APPLICATION GUIDELINES

- With the anterior half of the tongue resting gently on the hard palate, the mouth is opened actively as far as possible. This should allow no more than 20 mm of opening.
- When this point is reached, the tongue is lowered and the jaw is opened to comfortable end of range.
- The hand around the chin is used to correct any deviation from the midline.
- If movement cannot be maintained in the midline, do not proceed to the next stage of the MWM.
- When end-of-range mandibular depression has been reached, the mandible is held in position by the hand over the jaw.
- The patient then looks up with the eyes and actively extends the upper cervical spine so that the jaw opens further.
- If no pain is experienced and the movement can still be maintained in the midline, the hand on the forehead is used to apply gentle end-of-range over-pressure into cervical extension.
- This stretch is maintained for 2–3 seconds; the patient then looks down, and lowers the head to close the jaw.
- When the head has been lowered to the start position, the patient releases the hold on the chin, and closes the mouth fully.
- The stretch is repeated 3–4 times. If intra-articular adhesions are limiting jaw-opening, the stretch can be repeated 2–3 times per day with 3–6 repetitions each time.

VARIATIONS

- If significant difficulty is experienced controlling deviation from the midline when opening, other MWW techniques such as the MWM for painful limitation of mandibular depression may be more appropriate.

COMMENTS

- The patient must be instructed to avoid pushing the jaw posteriorly when applying end-of-range over-pressure.
- If cervical problems are present, they must be treated before this technique can be used.
- The scream stretch utilises upper cervical extension to produce a true end-of-range stretch that cannot be achieved by just opening the mouth. It can be regarded as a progression of the home exercise described in the MWM for painful limitation of mandibular depression technique.
- If a reducible joint derangement is present, this must be reduced first using the MWM for internal derangement (MWM for reduction of internal derangement limiting mandibular depression).

ANNOTATION

sit bilat TMJ self Scream Stretch×3 sec(3)

MWM for pain on jaw closure

TECHNIQUE AT A GLANCE

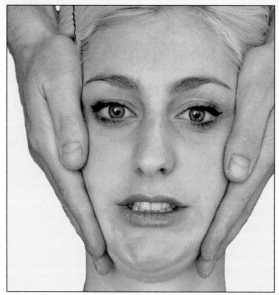

Figure 4.7A
MWM for pain on jaw closure: close view

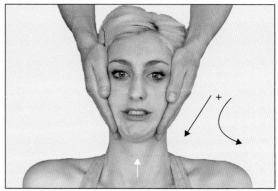

Figure 4.7B
MWM for pain on jaw closure: wide view; white arrow indicates the direction of the physiological component of the MWM; black arrows indicate the accessory movement components MWM for pain on jaw closure

- The therapist places the palms of their hands on either side of the head and the fingers over the jaw so that the fingertips point inferiorly (see Fig. 4.7).
- The therapist's palms are used to stabilise the head while the proximal parts of the fingers are used to position the mandible to restore comfortable jaw closure when the patient clenches.
- Subtle changes in the position of the mandibular head in any direction can be made until a position that renders the movement painless is found. This may include medial or lateral translation, anterior or posterior translation, and medial or lateral rotation.
- When the mobilisation forces have been applied and maintained, the patient is asked to close the jaw more firmly and if normal occlusion is possible and pain-free then over-pressure can be applied by the patient clenching the jaw lightly.

INDICATION

Pain on closure of mouth with or without acute malocclusion. This technique is used for acute malocclusion caused by muscular dysfunction or by acute TMJ derangement, but not for malocclusion caused by dental malalignment.

POSITIONING

Patient:	Supine lying or sitting facing a mirror with TMJ in rest position.
Therapist:	Standing at the head of the plinth if the patient is lying supine or behind the chair of a seated patient.
Hands/contact points:	The hands rest with the palms on either side of the head and the fingers over the jaw so that the fingertips point inferiorly with the fourth fingers resting just behind the mandibular ramus.

APPLICATION GUIDELINES

- The therapist's palms are used to stabilise the head while the proximal parts of the fingers are used to position the mandible to restore comfortable jaw closure when the patient clenches the jaw.
- The mandibular head of the painful joint may be moved in any direction that renders jaw closure pain-free and restores comfortable occlusion. This may include medial or lateral translation, anterior or posterior translation, and medial or lateral rotation.
- Subtle changes in the position of the mandibular head in any direction can be made until a position that renders the movement painless is found.
- Mobilisation directions are performed with respect to the treatment planes of the superior and inferior TMJ.
- When the mobilisation forces have been applied and maintained, the patient is asked to close the jaw more firmly.
- If normal occlusion is possible and pain-free, end-of-range over-pressure is effectively applied by asking the patient to clench the jaw lightly.
- As a trial treatment, 2 sets of 3 movements are performed, and jaw closure is then reassessed.
- If the trial treatment is successful, a further 2–3 sets of 6 movements are performed.

VARIATIONS

- If the occlusion is poor or the teeth are painful, the patient can close against a tongue depressor or a bite plate, but it is important to note that on occasion using the bite plate or the depressor alone (without the MWM) will render the movement pain-free.
- If the opposite joint is symptomatic, it may be necessary to apply gentle anterior force to prevent the mandibular head from moving into the painful posterior part of that joint.

COMMENTS

- If painful jaw closure has occurred in association with an acute malocclusion, the pain-easing position should coincide with restoration of a comfortable normal 'bite'.
- Minimal pressure is required for this technique.
- If pain is produced in the posterior aspect of a TMJ as the patient closes the jaw, it may be due to the mandibular head pushing into painful retrodiscal tissue (Okeson, 2013, p. 249).
- To prevent this pain occurring, as the patient slowly closes the jaw the therapist's fingers on the painful side are used to move the left mandibular head slightly anterior in the mandibular fossa (less than 1 mm). Sufficient pressure is used to prevent the mandibular head from moving posteriorly into the painful retrodiscal tissue as the patient slowly closes the jaw.
- TMJ MWM techniques often require only very small positional corrections particularly when treating acute malocclusions due to the involvement of the teeth.

(continued next page...)

4

SELF-MANAGEMENT

- The technique can be performed as a home exercise (see Fig. 4.8). The patient's hands are positioned over each mandible so that the distal phalanx of the thumb is resting behind the mandibular ramus with the interphalangeal joint at the angle of the jaw and the lower border of the mandible resting between the thenar and hypothenar eminences. The fingers will then be pointing in a posterosuperior direction so that the index fingers pass over the TMJs. The patient uses the left hand to move the jaw slightly forwards and inferiorly on the left, while using the right hand to prevent the right mandibular condyle from moving backwards in the right glenoid fossa.

- The patient is then instructed to follow the guidelines used for the therapist-administered technique to render jaw closure painless.

- If symptoms are acute, initially the home exercise may be performed up to 6 times per day with 6 movements each time, progressively reducing the frequency as the condition improves.

- The home exercise may be used as a maintenance technique 3–4 times per week in chronic conditions.

- If pain is experienced on jaw closure when eating, 1 set of 6 self-MWMs should be performed just before each meal.

- If pain is experienced when eating, the patient can also apply and maintain gentle forward pressure or lateral pressure on the mandibular ramus while chewing.

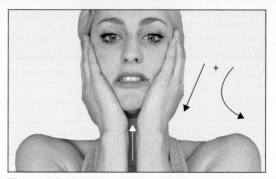

Figure 4.8
MWM for pain on jaw closure home exercise: white arrow indicates the direction of the physiological component of the MWM; black arrows indicate the accessory movement components

ANNOTATIONS

sit L TMJ Med gl/Ant-inf gl MWM Occl or El×6(3)
sup ly L TMJ Lat gl/Post g MWM Occl×6(3)
sit L TMJ self Ant-inf gl/ER MWM Occl×6

References

Broton, J.G., Sessle, B.J., 1988. Reflex excitation of masticatory muscles induced by algesic chemicals applied to the temporomandibular joint of the cat. Arch. Oral Biol. 33 (10), 741–747.

Eriksson, P.O., Haggman-Henrikson, B., Nordh, E., Zafar, H., 2000. Co-ordinated mandibular and head-neck movements during rhythmic jaw activities in man. J. Dent. Res. 79 (6), 1378–1384.

González-Iglesias, J., Cleland, J.A., Neto, F., Hall, T., Fernández-de-las-Peñas, C., 2013. Mobilization with movement, thoracic spine manipulation, and dry needling for the management of temporomandibular disorder: a prospective case series. Physiother. Theory Pract. 29 (8), 586–595.

Lund, J.P., Olsson, K.A., 1983. The importance of reflexes and their control during jaw movement. Trends Neurosci. 6, 458–463.

Motta, L.J., Fernandes, K.P.S., Mesquita-Ferrari, R.A., Biasotto-Gonzalez, D.A., Bussadori, S.K., 2012. Temporomandibular dysfunction and cervical posture and occlusion in adolescents. Brazil J. Oral Sci. 11 (3), 401–405.

Okeson, J.P., 1995. Bell's Orofacial Pains. Quintessence, Carol Stream IL.

Okeson, J.P., 2003. Management of Temporomandibular Disorders and Occlusion, fifth ed. Mosby Year Book, St Louis, MO.

Okeson, J.P., 2013. Management of Temporomandibular Disorders and Occlusion, seventh ed. Elsevier, St Louis, MO.

Oliver, M.J., 2011. Temporomandibular joint function: an open and shut case. In: Vicenzino, B., Hing, W.A., Rivett, D., Hall, T. (Eds.), Mobilisation with Movement: The Art and the Science. Churchill Livingstone, Edinburgh, pp. 123–133.

Sault, J.D., Emerson Kavchak, A.J., Tow, N., Courtney, C.A., 2016. Regional effects of orthopedic manual physical therapy in the successful management of chronic jaw pain. Cranio. 34 (2), 124–132.

Smith, A.M., 1981. The coactivation of antagonist muscles. Can. J. Physiol. Pharmacol. 59 (7), 733–747.

Stohler, C., Yamada, Y., Ash, M.M., 1985. Antagonistic muscle stiffness and associated reflex behaviour in pain-dysfunctional state. Helv. Odontol. Acta 29, 719–726.

Vicenzino, B., Hing, W., Hall, T., Rivett, D., 2011. Mobilisation with Movement: the art and science of its application. In: Vicenzino, B., Hing, W., Rivett, D., Hall, T. (Eds.), Mobilisation with Movement: The Art and the Science. Churchill Livingstone, Australia, Chatswood, NSW, pp. 9–23.

Yamada, K., Tsuruta, A., Hanada, K., Hayashi, T., 2004. Morphology of the articular eminence in temporomandibular joints and condylar bone change. J. Oral Rehabil. 31 (5), 438–444.

Zafar, H., 2000. Integrated jaw and neck function in man. Studies of mandibular and head-neck movements during jaw opening-closing tasks. Swed. Dent. J. Suppl. 143, 1–41.

Zafar, H., Nordh, E., Eriksson, P.O., 2006. Impaired positioning of the gape in whiplash-associated disorders. Swed. Dent. J. 30 (1), 9–15.

4

Shoulder complex

TECHNIQUES FOR THE SHOULDER COMPLEX

MWM TO SHOULDER GIRDLE
Scapular depression, retraction and downward rotation with clavicle and scapular approximation for shoulder girdle elevation
Shoulder girdle MWM with an assistant
Scapular depression, retraction and downward rotation with clavicle and scapular approximation for shoulder girdle flexion, abduction or scaption in four-point kneeling

ACROMIOCLAVICULAR JOINT

MWM FOR SHOULDER FLEXION / ABDUCTION / SCAPTION AND / OR ELEVATION
Mid-range mobilisation in sitting: posterolateral glide
Shoulder posterolateral glide: modification
Self-shoulder posterolateral glide for abduction or scaption
Mid-range elevation mobilisation in sitting: posterolateral–inferior glide with a belt
End-range elevation mobilisation in sitting: posteroinferior glide
Shoulder posterolateral–inferior glide in supine

MOVEMENT LIMITATION: HAND BEHIND BACK
Inferior glide MWM to restore a loss of hand-behind-back (HBB) movement
Belt 'accelerator' technique to improve shoulder hand-behind-back movement

MOVEMENT LIMITATION: INTERNAL OR EXTERNAL ROTATION
Inferior glide MWM to restore a loss of internal rotation and HBB movement
Inferior glide MWM for external rotation
Sleeper stretch MWM to restore a loss of internal rotation
Contraction combined with MWM to restore a loss of internal or external rotation

INTRODUCTION

The shoulder complex involves the glenohumeral (GH), acromioclavicular, sternoclavicular and scapulothoracic joints. Such multitude of articulations working in combination to provide a single movement poses a challenge to the practitioner considering the treatment plan. The disproportional size of the humeral head compared with the glenoid articular surface permits great ROM for the upper limb. To counter such a mismatch, static (i.e. capsule, ligaments, labrum) and dynamic (i.e. muscles) stabilisers are required, as they often resist translation and maintain tension throughout different ROM.

Mulligan's MWM concept of applying a sustained glide to member elements of an articulation while evaluating alterations in symptoms lends itself well to a multi-segment joint complex such as the shoulder joint. This should resonate well with clinicians who manage shoulder conditions, as they frequently have to deal with issues in relation to the questionable validity of physical examination and diagnostic tests (Hanchard et al., 2013) and a lack of understanding of the underlying pathoaetiology and inadequate evidence of efficacious treatments (Lewis, 2009).

Interestingly, the symptom modification approach implicit within MWM has also been independently advocated by Lewis (2009) as a means to overcome the issues of diagnosis, pathoaetiology and treatment selection. Central to the Mulligan approach for this region is the range of treatment options and modifications available to the clinician. For example, a patient who is having difficulty elevating the arm might well have a primary problem in either the spine, scapulothoracic, acromioclavicular or sternoclavicular joints that requires addressing rather than a GH movement dysfunction.

The decision as to which part of the shoulder joint complex to target will usually involve clinical reasoning skills and the information gathered from the interview (history, area and type of symptoms) and the physical examination. The addition of the Mulligan MWM approach to the physical examination will not only help confirm which joint or joints need to be treated, but also provide a clear indication as to which manual therapy technique and exercises will likely benefit the patient. This approach is consistent with a contemporaneous consensus statement on scapular dyskinesis, which recommends observing changes to symptoms and movement while manually correcting scapular position (Kibler et al., 2013). The poor relationship between any physical tests of the scapula (e.g. scapular dyskinesis test, winging scapula, tilting scapula, kinetic medial rotation test, lateral scapular slide test) and shoulder disorders (Wright et al., 2013) further reinforces the need for the clinician to apply the MWM techniques on the basis of improvements in pain / symptom-free shoulder motion and not on preconceived determined movement dysfunctions of the scapula.

The application of MWM and observation of symptom modification during movement is likely to be specific to each individual patient (especially as the shoulder complex possesses many degrees of freedom during movement). For one, scapular kinematics are influenced by the plane in which the arm is elevated, the angle to which it is elevated, the type of activity being observed, different populations and different shoulder conditions, as a recent meta-analysis showed (Timmons et al., 2012). Secondly, Tate and colleagues (Tate et al., 2008), in a study of college level athletes who engaged in repetitive overhead sports, reported that the scapular reposition test (uniformly emphasising posterior tilt and external rotation of the scapula but avoiding full retraction) was able to significantly reduce symptoms on clinical impingement tests (Jobe, Hawkins-Kennedy and Neer tests) in 46 athletes (47%). The lack of customisation of the scapular reposition test components on an individual athlete basis might have contributed to the 47% success in symptom modification response. It would be interesting to speculate that the success rate might have been higher if the scapular reposition test was allowed to be modified by the clinician on an individual athlete basis.

While the clinician will be guided by the modification of symptoms on movement to apply the MWM techniques, it is salient to note for MWM applied to the scapula that Mulligan (2003) has reported substantial benefits following the application of shoulder girdle depression, downward rotation, adduction and external rotation of the scapula. For the glenohumeral joint (GHJ) during elevation of the arm it is usually a posterolateral glide along the plane of the glenoid (the glenoid orientation being a function of thoracic spine, rib cage and scapular boney morphology) that is beneficial. At the acromiohumeral joint the glide is best directed caudally and posteriorly. Mulligan hypothesises that with each glide component that is used in a MWM there will return a biomechanical efficiency of the axial skeleton thorax–scapula–humerus during movement thereby restoring or allowing more normal symptom-free scapulohumeral rhythm.

Levels of evidence

Level 2: five RCTs, one pilot RCT, one multi-case series, one case report

There are five RCTs providing level 2 evidence (Howick et al., 2011) for shoulder MWM (Boruah et al., 2015; Delgado-Gil et al., 2015; Doner et al., 2013; Romero et al., 2015; Satpute et al., 2015). Overall their findings support the use of MWM in a variety of shoulder pathologies, as the results of most of the RCTs herein demonstrate increased ROM and decreased pain at the end of the treatment.

In the study by Doner and colleagues (Doner et al., 2013), 40 subjects with shoulder pain (>3 months) who were diagnosed with adhesive capsulitis were randomly allocated to either receive traditional treatment (transcutaneous nerve stimulation, hot pack and stretching) or the same treatment combined with MWM. Treatment was given over 15 sessions and follow-up was over 3 months. MWM led to significantly better improvements in terms of pain, ROM, shoulder disability scores, and patient and physiotherapist satisfaction.

Boruah and colleagues (Boruah et al., 2015) compared the effectiveness of MWM with scapular mobilisation on ROM and pain reduction in 50 patients diagnosed with adhesive capsulitis. At the end of 3 weeks of treatment, the MWM group had gained on average 21.2° in GH external rotation and 45.9° in GH flexion, whereas the scapular mobilisation group had gained on average 11.4° and 26.1° respectively (Boruah et al., 2015).

Delgado-Gil and colleagues (Delgado-Gil et al., 2015) compared the immediate effects of MWM with a sham technique in 42 patients with shoulder impingement syndrome (SIS). This group reported a between-group difference of 34.2° (95% CI 25.0–43.4) for pain-free shoulder flexion, 19.3° (95% CI 10.7–27.9) for maximum shoulder flexion and 8.2° (95% CI 1.8–14.6) for shoulder external rotation in favour of the group who received MWM treatment. Such improvements were not, however, supported by findings from a cross-over experimental design by Guimarães and colleagues (Guimarães et al., 2016) who reported MWM technique to be no more effective than sham intervention in patients with SIS in improving ROM for shoulder external rotation and abduction, pain and function.

The efficacy of the hand-behind-back (HBB) MWM technique on acute shoulder pain, impairment and disability was substantiated by Satpute and colleagues (Satpute et al., 2015). The group who underwent MWM with exercise had on average 9.31° (95% CI 7.38–11.27) of HBB ROM and 7.75° (95% CI 5.71–9.80) of internal rotation ROM more than the group treated with hot pack/exercise. The MWM+exercise group also enjoyed a greater reduction in shoulder pain with maximal HBB (quantified through a VAS) and presented a lower Shoulder Pain and Disability Index score than the hot pack+exercise group.

Regarding the influence of MWM on muscular activity, Youngjoon and colleagues (Youngjoon et al., 2015) found that the use of spinal mobilisation with arm movements was efficient in increasing shoulder muscle strength for flexion, extension and adduction immediately post-session in 12 healthy male university students. Interestingly, Ribeiro and colleagues (Ribeiro et al., 2016) found that shoulder scaption with sustained GH posterolateral glide and shoulder abduction with sustained GH posterolateral glide caused greater reduction to supraspinatus, infraspinatus, middle and posterior deltoid (abduction group only) activity than the control group, who performed the shoulder actions without the glide. It is clear that the effects of MWM in muscle activity warrant further investigation, as it may contribute to correcting pathological neuromuscular patterns often present in shoulder dysfunctions.

In addition, there are a number of other reports of varying quality investigating the Mulligan Concept for the shoulder. In a comprehensive review of MWM, six studies that assessed the effects of the technique in patients with shoulder pain were identified (Bisset et al., 2011). The issue of diagnostic heterogeneity was identified as a major limitation to data pooling. Notwithstanding the issues of quality, on balance these studies show: (a) an immediate post-MWM improvement in limited ROM in a group with shoulder pain-limited elevation (Teys et al., 2013) and (b) an MWM and end-range mobilisation to similarly improve shoulder ROM in frozen shoulder syndrome (Yang et al., 2007). These findings are consistent with reports from case studies (DeSantis & Hasson, 2006; Mulligan, 2003). In contrast, a study of a 6-week programme of MWM and passive mobilisations compared with a control reported no statistically significant superiority of the manual therapy techniques, which was probably due to a type II error (sample size=33, in a three-arm study) (Kachingwe et al., 2008). However, there was a tendency for the manual therapy-treated patients to have better outcomes (pain, function, ROM).

A study that was conducted after the abovementioned comprehensive review showed that taping the shoulder (as shown in Fig. 5.17) maintained the gains in range of shoulder elevation (scaption) over a 7-day period to a greater extent than if no tape was applied (Teys et al., 2013).

MWM TO SHOULDER GIRDLE

Scapular depression, retraction and downward rotation with clavicle and scapular approximation for shoulder girdle elevation

TECHNIQUE AT A GLANCE

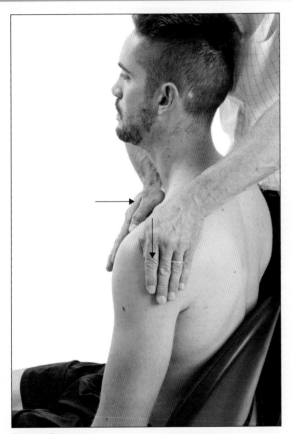

Figure 5.1
MWM to shoulder girdle: hand placement

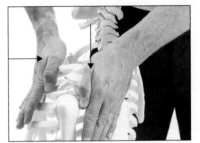

Figure 5.2
MWM to shoulder girdle: model view

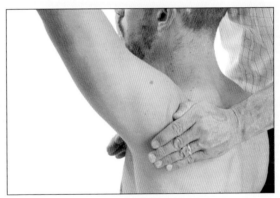

Figure 5.3
MWM to shoulder girdle: end position

- The patient is seated on a chair with arms at the side.
- The therapist stands on the opposite side to the involved shoulder of the patient with one hand over the medial third of the clavicle and the thenar eminence and thumb of the other hand over the outer end of the spine of the scapula.
- The therapist uses the hand on the spine of the scapula to depress (also termed inferior glide), adduct (also termed medial glide or retraction) and limit upward rotation.
- Simultaneously the clavicle and scapula are approximated (also termed external rotation) between the two hands of the therapist correcting scapular winging and facilitating more appropriate scapulothoracic relations (Fig. 5.2).
- The patient now actively elevates the arm through flexion, abduction or elevation in the plane of the scapula (scaption).
- See Figs 5.1–5.3.

INDICATION

Pain and/or limitation of shoulder elevation on abduction, flexion or scaption/elevation.

POSITIONING

Patient:	Sitting on a chair or a stool.
Treated body part:	Relaxed with the arm resting by the side.
Therapist:	Standing on the opposite side of the involved shoulder.
Hands/contact points:	If applying the technique to the left shoulder girdle, the therapist reaches across the patient's upper trunk and places the heel of the right hand over the medial third of the clavicle.
	The thenar eminence and thumb of the left hand are placed over the outer end of the spine of the scapula.

APPLICATION GUIDELINES

- The therapist uses the thenar eminence of the left hand on the spine of the scapula to push the outer end of the scapula down (correcting elevation and upward rotation) and retracting (correcting protraction).
- Simultaneously the clavicle and scapula are approximated between the two hands, reducing the scapuloclavicular angle and correcting excessive winging.
- The movements required in each direction are often minimal and require little force.
- While maintaining these corrections, the patient is asked to actively elevate their arm through flexion, abduction or 'scaption' (Fig. 5.3).
- All corrections are maintained until the arm is returned to the start position.
- This technique often requires subtle adjustments of applied force (more force in one direction, less in another) so as to maximise effectiveness.
- The shoulder movement may be applied passively in the case of severe limitation of active movement.
- A foam pad may be used between the hand and the clavicle as this region is often tender.

VARIATIONS

If an assistant is available:

- In this case (Fig. 5.4A, option 1) the assistant places the heel of the right hand in front of the lateral border of the scapula to assist correction of upward rotation and protraction and the left hand clasps the arm around the elbow to posteriorly translate the humerus in relation to the glenoid fossa. The GH repositioning is applied in line with the shaft of the humerus throughout the movement.
- The assistant can also apply over-pressure at the end of range.
- Alternatively, the assistant can use both hands to apply posterior translation along the line of the shaft of the humerus (Fig. 5.4B, option 2).
- Subtle changes can be made to the plane of elevation. If it is difficult to achieve pain-free elevation in the restricted plane, perform the MWM initially in a slightly different plane, then progress by attempting the original plane of restriction as the movement eases.

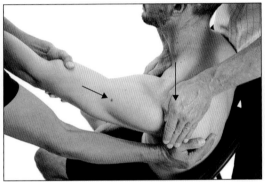

Figure 5.4A
Shoulder girdle MWM with an assistant: option 1

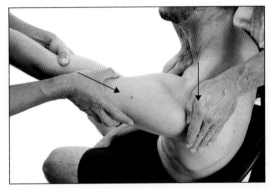

Figure 5.4B
Shoulder girdle MWM with an assistant: option 2

COMMENTS

- MWM in the plane of scaption is often the best option for acute shoulder pain.
- The technique often requires an assistant to be effective when treatment is first started, but can often be progressed quickly to four-point kneeling (see MWM to shoulder girdle in four-point kneeling in the next section).
- With this technique, it is very important to maintain the scapula position until the arm is returned to the start position.
- Up to 6 repetitions can be undertaken on the initial treatment. Subsequent treatments can be 3–5 sets of 6–10 repetitions.
- This technique is often effective for what appears to be painful limitation of shoulder movement abduction and/or flexion due to GHJ dysfunction. This is applicable from acute stage shoulder injuries to long-standing painful limitations.

ANNOTATIONS

sit L Scapulothoracic Depr/Ad/Downw Rot/Approx MWM F×6
sit L Scapulothoracic Depr/Ad/Downw Rot/Approx MWM Ab×6
sit L Scapulothoracic Depr/Approx/Ad/Downw Rot+Post gl GH MWM F +A +OP(A)×6(3)
NB List corrective forces in order of application in annotation. The first force applied is the most corrective. Please note: the corrective forces have been renamed to correlate to current terms used to describe scapular repositioning.

Scapular depression, retraction and downward rotation with clavicle and scapular approximation for shoulder girdle flexion, abduction or scaption in four-point kneeling

TECHNIQUE AT A GLANCE

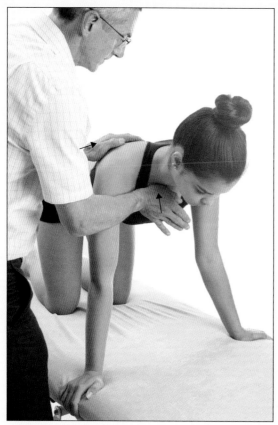

Figure 5.5
Shoulder girdle hand placement in four-point kneeling

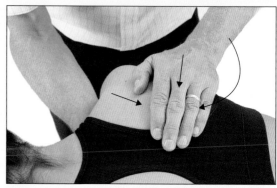

Figure 5.6
Close view of hand placement

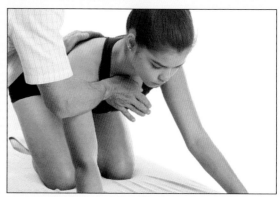

Figure 5.7
End position

- The patient is positioned into four-point kneeling.
- The therapist uses one hand on the scapula to depress, retract and downwardly rotate the scapula while approximating the scapula and clavicle.
- While the therapist maintains the scapular position, the patient is asked to sit back towards their heels keeping their hands on the plinth, thus flexing the shoulder.
- Six repetitions are sufficient on the initial treatment.
- See Figs 5.5–5.7.

INDICATION

Pain and/or limitation of shoulder elevation on abduction, flexion or scaption.

POSITIONING

Patient:	Four-point kneeling on treatment plinth.
Treated body part:	Shoulder flexed to 90°.
Therapist:	Standing alongside and facing the patient's involved shoulder.
Hands/contact points:	For the right shoulder the therapist's reaches over the top of the shoulder to place their right hand over the medial end of the left clavicle.
	The thenar and hypothenar eminence of the left hand are placed along the lateral border of the scapula with the fingers hooked onto the medial border of the scapula to grasp the scapula.

APPLICATION GUIDELINES

- The therapist uses the left hand on the scapula to depress, retract and downwardly rotate the scapula.
- While maintaining the scapula position, the clavicle and scapula are approximated between the two hands, reducing the scapuloclavicular angle and correcting any excessive winging.
- While the therapist maintains these corrections, the patient is asked to sit back towards their heels keeping their hands firmly on the plinth, thus flexing the shoulder.
- The patient indirectly applies a posterior translation of the head of the humerus in relation to the glenoid by leaning onto their hands.
- The patient returns to the start position and repeats the movement.
- Six repetitions are sufficient on the initial treatment; 3–5 sets of 6–10 repetitions can be undertaken in subsequent treatment sessions.
- A foam pad may be used between the hand and the clavicle as this region is often tender.

VARIATIONS

- Subtle changes to the various glides may be necessary to achieve a totally pain-free technique.
- If a patient is unable to four-point kneel and flex hips and knees, the technique can be modified by having the patient stand alongside the plinth with the affected hand on the plinth.

COMMENT

- The patient must be sufficiently mobile in the hips and knees to perform the active movement.

ANNOTATION

4 point kneel R Scapulothoracic Depr/Add/Downward rot/Approx MWM F×6(3)

ACROMIOCLAVICULAR JOINT

TECHNIQUE AT A GLANCE

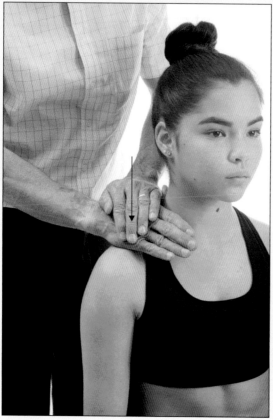

Figure 5.8
Acromioclavicular joint treatment: hand placement

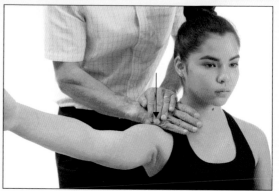

Figure 5.9
Acromioclavicular joint treatment: with abduction or scaption – mid range

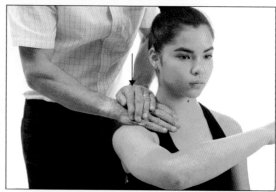

Figure 5.10
Acromioclavicular joint treatment: with horizontal adduction

- The patient sits well supported in a chair, arm resting by their side.
- The therapist applies a caudal and/or posterior or anterior glide to the outer end of the clavicle.
- While the glide is sustained the patient actively moves into the previously restricted or pain-provocative direction. (This could be, for example, shoulder flexion or scaption, into elevation or horizontal adduction.)
- See Figs 5.8–5.10.

INDICATION

Limitation of shoulder movement due to pain or stiffness of the acromioclavicular joint (especially end-range flexion or horizontal adduction).

CONTRAINDICATIONS

Total shoulder arthroplasty, non-united clavicle fracture and marked instability of the joint are absolute contraindications.

POSITIONING

Patient:	Sitting well supported in a chair.
Treated body part:	Arm resting by the side.
Therapist:	Standing behind the patient on the affected side.
Hands/contact points:	Hypothenar eminence of therapist's lateral-most hand is placed on the lateral end of the affected clavicle. The other hand is placed on top of this hand to reinforce.

APPLICATION GUIDELINES

- The therapist applies pressure in a caudal combined with posterior or anterior direction on the outer end of the patient's clavicle.
- The patient performs shoulder movement (using momentum for the hypomobile joint) to reach the end range of shoulder flexion/elevation or horizontal adduction as the case may be.
- The therapist sustains the glide and allows normal shoulder movement.
- Ensure mobilisation is pain-free at all times.
- Use a foam pad to avoid discomfort.
- The therapist stands well clear of the patient's arm, to avoid arm contact.
- If the patient cannot move their arm quickly, passive pain-free over-pressure to achieve end-range motion can be applied.
- The therapist's contact and glide must maintain mobilisation and not prevent or block the patient's shoulder movement.
- Perform 3 repetitions in a set, with 3 sets in a session.

VARIATIONS

- In the case of joint laxity or partial subluxation, gentle pressure should be applied to the clavicle during active movement.

COMMENT

- The caudal and posterior or anterior force imparted by the therapist induces a mobilisation of the acromioclavicular joint. Expect to feel crepitation under the mobilising hand during the shoulder movement.

(continued next page...)

SELF-MANAGEMENT

- The patient can perform self-treatment (Fig. 5.11) by placing the ulnar border of their hand over the outer end of the clavicle, reaching across from the contralateral side. The patient holds the clavicle directly with their hand. While maintaining the glide on the clavicle, the patient will use the same rapid flexion movement of the affected shoulder to gain end-of-range flexion. This exercise should be pain-free.

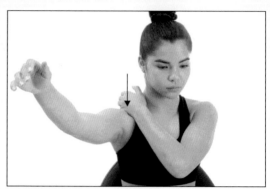

Figure 5.11
Acromioclavicular joint self-treatment for shoulder elevation

ANNOTATIONS

sit R ACJ Inf gl MWM F×6
sit R ACJ Inf gl/Post gl MWM HF×6
sit R ACJ self Inf gl/Post gl MWM Ab×6(3)

MWM FOR SHOULDER FLEXION / ABDUCTION / SCAPTION AND / OR ELEVATION

Mid-range mobilisation in sitting: posterolateral glide

TECHNIQUE AT A GLANCE

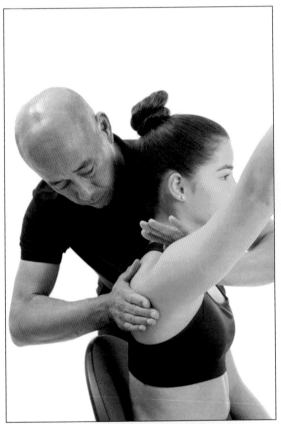

Figure 5.12
Posterolateral glide: hand placement side view

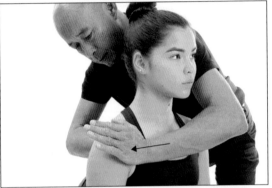

Figure 5.13
Posterolateral glide: hand placement anterior view

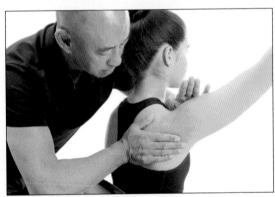

Figure 5.14
Shoulder posterolateral glide with abduction: end position

- The patient is sitting.
- The therapist stands on the contralateral side of pain, stabilising the scapula posteriorly with one hand.
- The head of the humerus is translated posteriorly and laterally with the other hand, along the plane of the glenoid fossa.
- While the glide is sustained, the patient actively elevates their arm through the plane of abduction or scaption (elevation).
- See Figs 5.12–5.14.

INDICATION

Painful limitation of active range of GH abduction and/or elevation.

POSITIONING

Patient:	Sitting upright.
Treated body part:	Arm resting by side.
Therapist:	Standing facing patient on the contralateral side to the affected shoulder.
Hands/contact points:	Stabilising hand: reaching across the patient's back to stabilise the scapula with a broad open-palm grip. Note this hand stabilises but does not fixate the scapula. The normal scapulothoracic rhythm is allowed to occur. Gliding hand: reaching across the patient's chest to cup the head of humerus with the thenar eminence. Note: care is taken to not impinge the coracoid process.

5

APPLICATION GUIDELINES

- Apply a pain-free posterolaterally directed glide in the plane of the glenoid fossa. The mobilisation force should be sufficient to reorient the head of the humerus within the glenoid such that this mobilisation is itself pain-free and facilitates a functional improvement in pain-free elevation of the arm.

- While sustaining the posterolateral glide force, ask the patient to abduct the arm through scaption or the frontal plane to the onset of pain only. Initial repetitions may be performed with the elbow in relative flexion to reduce the leverage force with progression of leverage resistance as irritability reduces.

- Maintain the glide through the movement until the arm returns to the start position.

- Apply 6–10 repetitions in a set, with 3–5 sets in a treatment session.

VARIATIONS

- An alternative grip is where the therapist stands on the ipsilateral side reaching between the patient's arm and chest to contact the head of the humerus. With the other hand stabilising the scapula, the head of the humerus may be pulled posterolaterally by contact with the hypothenar eminence (Fig. 5.15).

- Progression of forces for patients with a pain-through range may be achieved by the use of resistance weights or bands.

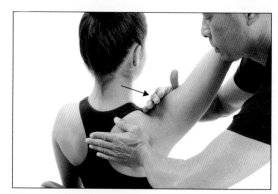

Figure 5.15
Shoulder posterolateral glide: modification

COMMENTS

- Do not block the normal scapulothoracic rhythm; allow the scapula to upwardly rotate during abduction.
- A moderate caudal orientation to the glide may be required as the patient approaches normal end-range elevation.
- Correction of the scapula position may be required in addition to correction of the GHJ position. This can be achieved with the posterior hand on the scapula. For example, if the scapula is protracted or anteriorly tilted then the correction would be retraction and posterior tilt.
- If the range of pain-free elevation does not improve, experiment with various orientations of the glide from pure posterior to posterolateral. The grade of mobilisation force may also be varied based on the patient's symptomatic response.
- Soft tissue tenderness over the head of the humerus may be reduced by the use of a foam pad.
- Attempt no more than 4 trials to elicit a positive response in any one treatment session, as failure to relieve pain over this number of trials will prove counterproductive.
- Do not release the sustained posterolateral glide before the patient returns to neutral.

SELF-MANAGEMENT

- A home exercise for this technique is shown in Fig. 5.16. A resistance band looped around the shoulder and trapped at the other end in a door may be used instead of the treatment belt. Alternatively a thin strap can be used, lassoed around the medial aspect of the humeral head.

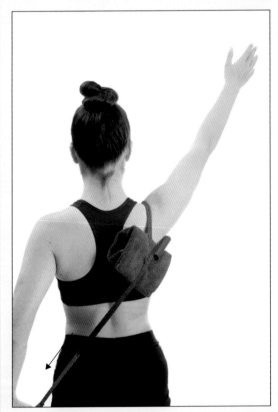

Figure 5.16A
Self-shoulder posterolateral glide for abduction or scaption: strap

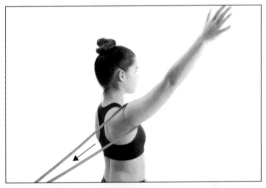

Figure 5.16B
Self-shoulder posterolateral glide for abduction or scaption: stretch cord

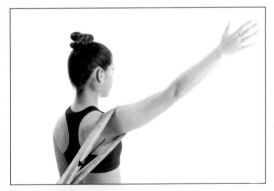

Figure 5.16C
Self-shoulder posterolateral glide for abduction or scaption: strap band

(continued next page...)

TAPING

- Tape may also be used to sustain the glide force on the humeral head and is shown in Fig. 5.17.

- Use 30-mm non-stretch sports tape or flexible tape at greater than 50% elongation.

- Start the tape on the anterior aspect of the humeral head crossing the acromion lateral to the acromioclavicular joint, and ending at the inferior border of the scapula. The therapist glides the humeral head posteriorly while applying the tape. Take care not to apply excessive tension initially at the humeral head as the skin is liable to break down.

- Apply two layers in the same location.

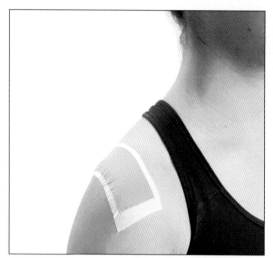

Figure 5.17A
Shoulder tape following MWM: front view

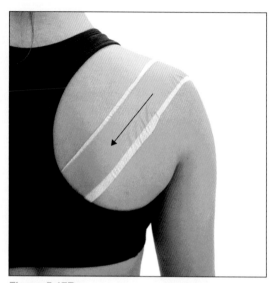

Figure 5.17B
Shoulder tape following MWM: posterior view

ANNOTATIONS

sit R GH Post-lat gl MWM El×3
sit R GH Post-lat gl MWM Ab×3
sit R GH ipsi Post-lat gl MWM El×6(3)
sit R GH self strap Post-lat gl MWM El×3
sit R GH self stretch cord Post-lat gl MWM El×6
R GH Post-lat tape

Mid-range elevation mobilisation in sitting: posterolateral–inferior glide with a belt

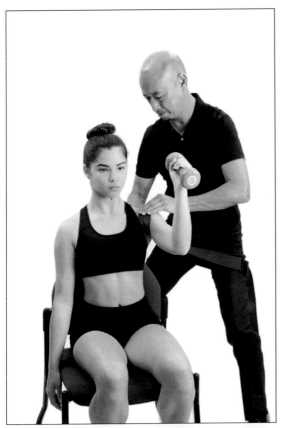

Figure 5.18
Shoulder posterolateral–inferior glide: start position

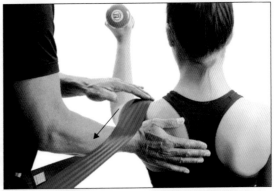

Figure 5.19
Shoulder posterolateral–inferior glide with scaption: rear close view

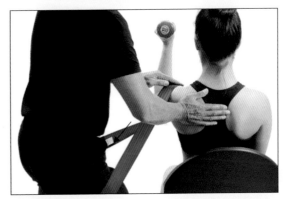

Figure 5.20
Shoulder posterolateral–inferior glide with scaption: alternative hand placement

- The patient is sitting with their trunk supported in a chair, arm by side and elbow flexed.
- The therapist uses a manual therapy belt to glide the humerus at the GHJ in a posterolateral–inferior direction.
- The patient performs repeated shoulder flexion, punching forwards with the arm.
- A 1–2-kg weight in the hand improves control of the movement.
- The therapist moves their body rhythmically, transferring their weight from back to front foot, in step with the patient's arm movement, to ensure the belt remains clear of the axilla (Fig. 5.20).
- See Figs 5.18–5.20.

INDICATION

Mid-range restriction of shoulder elevation movement (flexion, scaption or abduction).

POSITIONING

Patient:	Patient seated with trunk supported.
Treated body part:	The shoulder to be treated is relaxed with the arm by their side and elbow flexed.
Therapist:	Standing obliquely posterior and lateral to the shoulder of the patient to be treated. The therapist's posterior hand stabilises and controls the scapula.
Hands and belt application:	Belt is placed around the anteromedial aspect of patient's GHJ just lateral to the joint line. Belt is positioned diagonally from the shoulder, down around therapist's hips or upper thigh. The therapist stabilises the scapula with the stabilising hand inside or outside the belt (Figs 5.19 and 5.20) ensuring the belt does not slip off the patient's shoulder. The fingertips of the therapist's hand control the position of the belt on the anteromedial aspect of the head of the humerus.

APPLICATION GUIDELINES

- The therapist's posterior hand controls and stabilises the scapula, preventing retraction and depression.
- The therapist applies a gentle glide by gently leaning back through the belt; the glide is posterolateral and slightly downwards with respect to the glenoid fossa.
- The patient performs repeated flexion, punching forwards with the arm, extending the elbow with shoulder flexion, reaching a point just short of the limitation of movement. Alternatively, scaption movement can also be used.
- Perform 6–10 repetitions in a set before re-evaluating the patient-specific outcome measure. If the movement is improved then repeat 3–5 sets.
- The therapist maintains the glide throughout the active shoulder movement, always allowing some movement of the scapula and keeping the belt free of the anterior wall of the axilla by moving the body as the patient moves.

VARIATIONS

- The technique can be progressed through range between treatment sessions as the patient's movement improves through the earlier range.

COMMENTS

- The therapist's hand on the scapula is important. This hand can control the scapula movement and thereby improve motor control of the shoulder.
- The preferred active movement is flexion, but scaption can also be used; avoid abduction due to the possibility of subacromial impingement.
- Ensure the belt pulls downwards, backwards and laterally. This ensures that the humeral head does not ride up in the glenoid fossa.
- Ensure excessive glide force is not used as this could cause excessive posterior glide and potentially increase symptoms.

SELF-MANAGEMENT

- See Fig. 5.16 for self-management options following successful application of the mid-range mobilisation in sitting.

ANNOTATIONS

sit R GH belt Post-lat/Inf gl MWM El×6
sit R GH belt Post-lat/Inf gl MWM F×6
sit R GH belt Post-lat/Inf gl MWM Abv 6
sit R GH belt Post-lat/Inf gl MWM res punch (2 kg)×6(3)

End-range elevation mobilisation in sitting: posteroinferior glide

TECHNIQUE AT A GLANCE

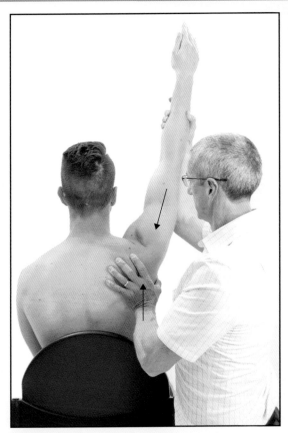

Figure 5.21
Shoulder posterior and inferior glide MWM: start position

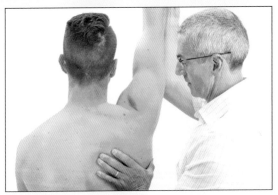

Figure 5.22
Shoulder posterior and inferior glide MWM: start position close view

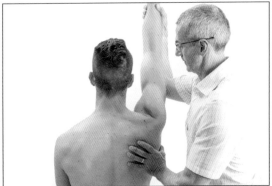

Figure 5.23
Shoulder posterior and inferior glide MWM: end range

- The patient elevates the arm, just short of the limitation.
- The therapist kneels behind the patient and imparts a gentle painless posterior–inferior glide of the head of the humerus while stabilising the scapula. The patient simultaneously elevates the shoulder.
- The patient then performs repeated pain-free arm movement, or over-pressure can be included if necessary.
- Alter the position of the shoulder if pain-free movement cannot be achieved.
- See Figs 5.21–5.23.

INDICATION

Limitation of shoulder elevation due to pain and/or stiffness occurring towards the end range.

The technique can be performed with elevation, or involve specific functional impairments that may be associated with activities such as a loading movement.

POSITIONING

Patient:	Patient sits upright on a chair.
Treated body part:	Shoulder is moved to the onset of pain or limitation of movement.
Therapist:	Therapist stands behind and on the same side of the restriction (kneel if necessary).
Hands/contact points:	The left hand is placed on the inferior aspect of the patient's right scapula.
	The right hand grasps the patient's arm, maintaining the elbow in extension and applies the gliding force along the line of the humerus.

APPLICATION GUIDELINES

- The patient elevates the affected arm and stops just short of symptom provocation.
- The therapist's left hand stabilises the scapula and prevents depression and downward rotation.
- The therapist's right hand grasps the patient's arm. A caudal and posterior glide is applied along the line of the humerus.
- While sustaining the glide, the patient performs active elevation, which should now be rendered symptom-free.
- If greater symptom-free movement cannot be achieved, the therapist should first subtly vary the amount and direction of glide force.
- Perform 6–10 repetitions per set, with 3–5 sets at each treatment session.

VARIATIONS

- If symptom-free movement cannot be achieved, the therapist should first vary the position of GH rotation (internal or external) while repeating the same mobilisation. Failing this, varying the abduction position may also be tested.
- If the patient has a stiff shoulder, then the technique in Fig. 5.24, with the hands on a wall, may be more appropriate.
- The belt must be placed around the humeral head while the therapist stabilises the scapula with their other hand, maintaining pressure to keep the hand in contact with the wall.
- The patient achieves increased arm elevation by flexing at the hips. The shoulder rotation and abduction position can be varied according to pain response.

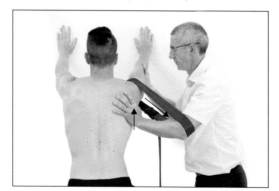

Figure 5.24A
Shoulder posterolateral–inferior glide using a belt: option 1

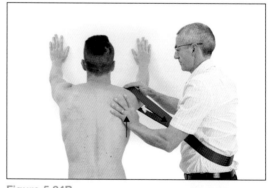

Figure 5.24B
Shoulder posterolateral–inferior glide using a belt: option 2

- Alternatively the technique may be performed in supine position (Fig. 5.25), where the scapula is stabilised by the bed and the humerus can be repositioned with respect to the scapula while the patient's shoulder is flexed. The humeral glide can be achieved through both the therapist's hands. Many variations in the direction of the humeral head glide can be achieved with this technique.

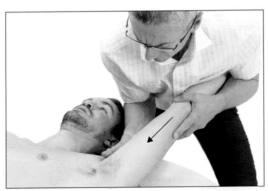

Figure 5.25A
Shoulder posterolateral–inferior glide in supine: start position

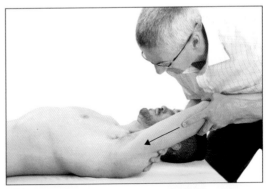

Figure 5.25B
Shoulder posterolateral–inferior glide in supine: lateral view

COMMENT

- The degree of humeral glide will depend on the chronicity of the condition, laxity of the joint and other factors. Hence it is best to trial the technique with minimal force. Greater force can then be used if required.

ANNOTATIONS

sit R GH Post-inf gl (long lever) MWM F×6
sit R GH Post-inf gl (long lever) MWM Ab×6
sit R GH Post-inf gl (long lever) MWM El×6
st hands on wall L GH belt Post-lat/Inf gl MWM F×6(3)
sup ly R GH Post gl/Lat gl/Inf gl MWM F×6

MOVEMENT LIMITATION: HAND BEHIND BACK

Inferior glide MWM to restore a loss of hand-behind-back (HBB) movement

TECHNIQUE AT A GLANCE

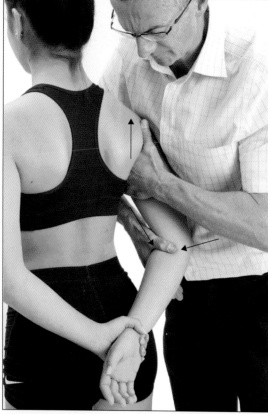

Figure 5.26
Shoulder hand behind back: hand placement

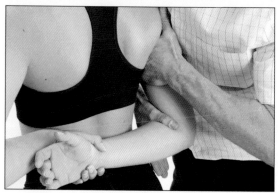

Figure 5.27
Shoulder hand behind back: end-range position

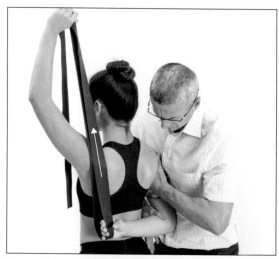

Figure 5.28
Hand behind back: with belt assistance

- The patient is in standing position, reaching up behind their back.
- The therapist stabilises the scapula with one hand, preventing depression, while gliding the humerus with the other hand.
- The therapist glides the head of the humerus in a caudal direction with respect to the glenoid fossa and simultaneously adducts the humerus with their abdomen while the patient performs the HBB movement.
- See Figs 5.26–5.28.

INDICATION

Limitation of shoulder internal rotation and HBB movement due to pain or stiffness.

POSITIONING

Patient:	Standing.
Treated body part:	Position the patient's hand behind their back just prior to the movement limitation or pain onset.
Therapist:	Step standing on the same side as the affected shoulder and facing the patient.
Hands/contact points:	Stabilising hand: place the first web-space of the left hand up into the patient's axilla to stabilise the scapula, preventing depression.
	Gliding hand: the first web-space of the therapist's right hand is placed in the cubital fossa of patient's flexed elbow, with the palm facing towards the therapist.

APPLICATION GUIDELINES

- Position the patient's hand behind their back just prior to the movement limitation or pain onset.
- The therapist applies a caudal glide along the line of the humerus with the right hand to glide the humeral head inferiorly in the glenoid fossa.
- Then the patient reaches higher up their back, while the therapist assists. The therapist pushes the arm across the patient's body with their abdomen, creating shoulder adduction and potentially joint separation.
- Maintain the caudal humeral glide during the MWM technique.
- Perform 6–10 repetitions for one set, with 3–5 sets per treatment session.

(continued next page...)

5

VARIATIONS

- A manual therapy belt can be used to achieve the humeral caudal glide. A figure of eight is created with the belt to loop around the humerus and forearm. Ankle plantarflexion imparts caudal gliding to the humerus. In this case, the therapist uses two hands to apply GHJ distraction as well as stabilisation of the scapula (Fig. 5.29).

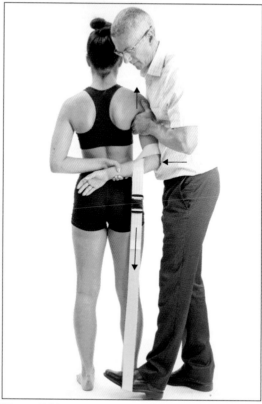

Figure 5.29
Belt 'accelerator' technique to improve shoulder hand-behind-back movement

COMMENTS

- The patient can assist the movement and ultimately apply over-pressure using their other hand or a belt to achieve greater range of hand behind back (see Fig. 5.28).

ANNOTATIONS

st R Sh Inf gl/E/Ad MWM HBB×6
st R Sh Inf gl/E/Ad MWM HBB +OP (belt)×10(3)
st R Sh belt Inf gl/E/Ad MWM HBB +OP×10(3)

MOVEMENT LIMITATION: INTERNAL OR EXTERNAL ROTATION

Inferior glide MWM to restore a loss of internal rotation and HBB movement

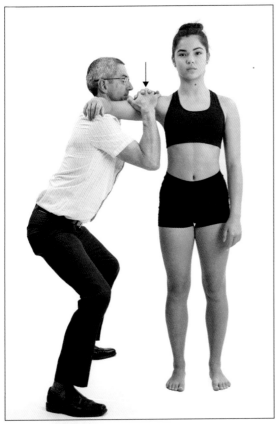

Figure 5.30
Shoulder internal rotation in abduction: start position

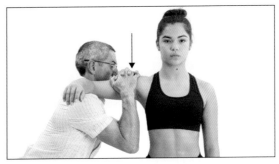

Figure 5.31
Shoulder internal rotation in abduction: front close view

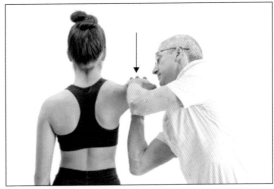

Figure 5.32
Shoulder internal rotation in abduction: end range

- The patient is standing with their arm at 90° shoulder abduction.
- The therapist links both hands over the superior aspect of the humeral head, while supporting the elbow on their shoulder.
- The therapist glides the head of the humerus in a caudal direction while the patient performs the movement of GHJ internal rotation.
- See Figs 5.30–5.32.

INDICATION

Limitation of shoulder internal rotation and HBB movement due to pain or stiffness.

POSITIONING

Patient:	Standing.
Treated body part:	Position the patient's shoulder to 90° abduction, elbow flexed.
Therapist:	Standing on the same side as the affected shoulder and facing the patient.
Hands/contact points:	Gliding hands: linked fingers of both hands placed on the superior aspect of the proximal end of the humerus.

APPLICATION GUIDELINES

- The therapist positions the patient's shoulder at 90° abduction with the elbow flexed to 90° and elbow resting on the shoulder of the therapist.
- The therapist applies a caudal glide towards the floor with both hands to glide the humeral head caudally in the glenoid fossa.
- Then the patient actively internally rotates the GHJ, while the therapist assists.
- Maintain the caudal humeral glide during the MWM technique.
- Perform 6–10 repetitions for one set, with 3–5 sets per treatment session.

VARIATIONS

- If the patient is unable to achieve 90° abduction in the frontal plane, then the technique can be performed in a position of scaption, with less abduction.
- The same technique may be trialled for external rotation starting from the same position (Fig. 5.33).

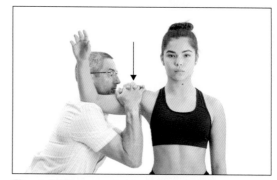

Figure 5.33
Inferior glide MWM for external rotation

COMMENTS

- The patient can apply over-pressure using their other hand to achieve full range without pain.
- If a caudal glide fails to improve range, then trial a posterior glide with the anterior hand while stabilising the scapula with the posterior hand.

ANNOTATIONS

st R GH (in 90 degrees Ab) Inf gl MWM IR×6
st R GH (in 90 degrees scaption) Inf gl MWM ER×6(3)

Sleeper stretch MWM to restore a loss of internal rotation

TECHNIQUE AT A GLANCE

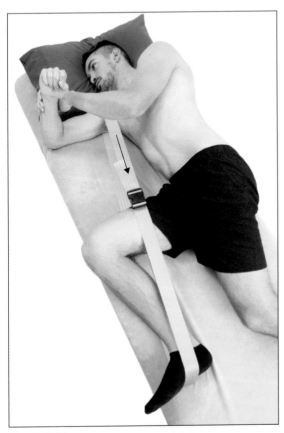

Figure 5.34
Sleeper stretch MWM: start position

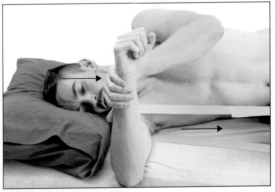

Figure 5.35
Sleeper stretch MWM: start position side view

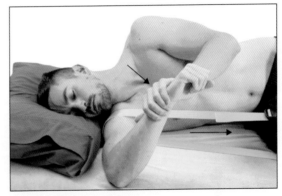

Figure 5.36
Sleeper stretch MWM: end position

- Patient is in side lying, arm in 90° shoulder flexion and elbow flexed to 90°.
- A manual therapy belt is looped around the humeral head and the heel.
- The patient extends their hip to glide the head of the humerus in a caudal direction while performing the movement of GHJ internal rotation.
- See Figs 5.34–5.36.

INDICATION

Limitation of shoulder internal rotation due to pain or stiffness.

POSITIONING

Patient:	Side lying.
Treated body part:	Position the patient's shoulder to 90° flexion, with elbow flexed to 90°.
Self-glide description:	Extend the hip to tension the belt, gliding the head of the humerus in a caudal direction while performing the movement of GHJ internal rotation.

EXERCISE GUIDELINES

- The patient tensions the belt by extending their hip and knee inducing caudal glide of the humerus in the glenoid.
- Then the patient actively internally rotates the GHJ.
- Maintain the caudal humeral glide during the MWM technique.
- Repeat 10 times in a session.

COMMENTS

- The patient can apply over-pressure using their other hand to achieve full range.
- If a caudal glide fails to improve range, then trial small differences in the glide force or subtly changing the arm position.

ANNOTATIONS

R side ly R GH self belt Inf gl MWM IR×10
or R side ly R GH self belt Inf gl MWM Sleeper Stretch×10

Contraction combined with MWM to restore a loss of internal or external rotation

TECHNIQUE AT A GLANCE

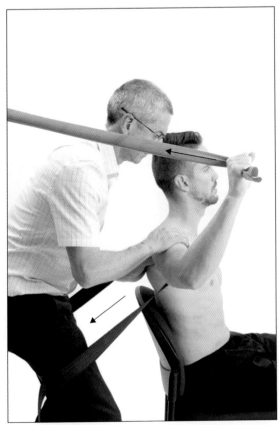

Figure 5.37
Shoulder internal rotation in abduction: with resistance start position

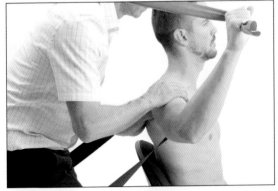

Figure 5.38
Shoulder internal rotation in abduction: with resistance close view

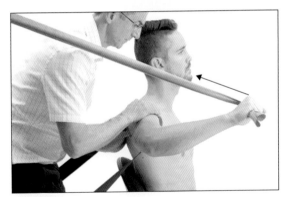

Figure 5.39
Shoulder external rotation in abduction: with resistance mid position

- The patient in sitting with their trunk supported in a chair, with their arm in 90° shoulder abduction and the elbow flexed.
- The therapist uses a manual therapy belt to glide the humerus at the GHJ in a posterolateral–inferior direction.
- The patient performs the movement of GHJ internal rotation against resistance such as a stretch band.
- See Figs 5.37–5.39.

INDICATION

Limitation of shoulder internal rotation and HBB movement due to pain or stiffness.

POSITIONING

Patient:	Patient is seated with trunk supported.
Treated body part:	Position the patient's shoulder to 90° abduction, elbow flexed.
Therapist:	Stands obliquely posterior and lateral to the shoulder of the patient to be treated.
	The therapist's posterior hand stabilises and controls the scapula.
Hands/contact points:	Belt is placed around the anteromedial aspect of patient's GHJ just lateral to the joint line. Belt is positioned diagonally from the shoulder, down around therapist's hips or upper thigh.
	The therapist stabilises the scapula with the stabilising hand inside or outside the belt (Figs 5.37–5.39) ensuring the belt does not slip off the patient's shoulder.
	The fingertips of the therapist's hand control the position of the belt on the anteromedial aspect of the head of the humerus.

APPLICATION GUIDELINES

- Position the patient's shoulder at 90° abduction with the elbow flexed to 90°.
- The therapist's posterior hand controls and stabilises the scapula, preventing retraction and depression.
- The therapist applies a posterolateral–inferior glide with the belt while stabilising the scapula.
- Then the patient actively internally rotates the GHJ, working against the resistance of the stretch band.
- The therapist maintains the humeral glide throughout the active shoulder movement, always allowing some movement of the scapula and keeping the belt free of the anterior wall of the axilla by moving the body as the patient moves.
- Perform 6–10 repetitions for one set, with 3–5 sets per treatment session.

VARIATIONS

- If only a partial effect is observed, then vary the MWM glide force or the resistance.
- If the symptoms are worse with the muscle contraction, trial resistance/muscle contraction in the opposite direction.
- The technique can be progressed through the range, with increasing resistance.
- Muscle contraction can be isometric, concentric or eccentric.
- External rotation can be managed in a similar fashion (see Fig. 5.40).

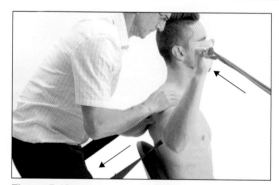

Figure 5.40
Shoulder external rotation contraction combined with MWM: end position

COMMENTS

- The therapist's hand on the scapula is important. This hand can control the scapula movement and thereby improve motor control of the shoulder.
- Rotation can be performed in scaption, if abduction in the frontal plane increases symptoms.
- Ensure the belt pulls downwards, backwards and laterally. This ensures that the humeral head does not ride up in the glenoid fossa.
- Ensure excessive glide force is not used as this could cause excessive posterior glide and potentially increase symptoms.
- Contraction combined with MWM is being developed for a wide range of clinical applications in various body regions by Yuval David.

ANNOTATIONS

sit R GH 90 degrees Ab belt Post-lat/Inf gl MWM res IR (blue stretch band)×10(5)

sit R GH 90 degrees Ab belt Post-lat/Inf gl MWM res ER (blue stretch band)×10(5)

5

References

Bisset, L., Hing, W., Vicenzino, B., 2011. A systematic review of the efficacy of MWM. In: Vicenzino, B., Hing, W., Rivett, D., Hall, T. (Eds.), Mobilisation With Movement: The Art and the Science. Churchill Livingstone Australia, Chatswood, NSW, pp. 26–64.

Boruah, L., Dutta, A., Deka, P., Roy, J., 2015. To study the effect of scapular mobilization versus mobilization with movement to reduce pain and improve gleno-humeral range of motion in adhesive capsulitis of the shoulder: a comparative study. Int. J. Physiother. 2 (5), 811–818.

Delgado-Gil, J.A., Prado-Robles, E., Rodrigues-de-Souza, D.P., Cleland, J.A., Fernandez-de-las-Penas, C., Alburquerque-Sendin, F., 2015. Effects of mobilization with movement on pain and range of motion in patients with unilateral shoulder impingement syndrome: a randomized controlled trial. J. Manipulative Physiol. Ther. 38 (4), 245–252.

DeSantis, L., Hasson, S.M., 2006. Use of mobilization with movement in the treatment of a patient with subacromial impingement: a case report. J Man Manipulative Ther. 14 (2), 77–87.

Doner, G., Guven, Z., Atalay, A., Celiker, R., 2013. Evalution of Mulligan's technique for adhesive capsulitis of the shoulder. J. Rehabil. Med. 45 (1), 87–91.

Guimarães, J.F., Salvini, T.F., Jr., Siqueira, A.L., Ribeiro, I.L., Camargo, P.R., Alburquerque-Sendín, F., 2016. Immediate effects of mobilization with movement vs sham technique on range of motion, strength, and function in patients with shoulder impingement syndrome: randomized clinical trial. J. Manipulative Physiol. Ther. 39 (9), 605–615.

Hanchard, N.C., Lenza, M., Handoll, H.H., Takwoingi, Y., 2013. Physical tests for shoulder impingements and local lesions of bursa, tendon or labrum that may accompany impingement. Cochrane Database Syst. Rev. (4), CD007427.

Howick, J., Chalmers, I., Glasziou, P., Greenhalgh, T., Heneghan, C., Liberati, A., et al., 2011. The Oxford Levels of Evidence 2. Oxford Centre for Evidence-Based Medicine, Oxford.

Kachingwe, A.F., Phillips, B., Sletten, E., Plunkett, S.W., 2008. Comparison of manual therapy techniques with therapeutic exercise in the treatment of shoulder impingement: a randomized controlled pilot clinical trial. J. Man. Manipulative Ther. 16 (4), 238–247.

Kibler, W.B., Ludewig, P.M., McClure, P.W., Michener, L.A., Bak, K., Sciascia, A.D., 2013. Clinical implications of scapular dyskinesis in shoulder injury: the 2013 consensus statement from the 'Scapular Summit'. Br. J. Sports Med. 47 (14), 877–885.

Lewis, J.S., 2009. Rotator cuff tendinopathy/subacromial impingement syndrome: is it time for a new method of assessment? Br. J. Sports Med. 43 (4), 259–264.

Mulligan, M., 2003. The painful dysfunctional shoulder. A new treatment approach using 'Mobilisation with Movement'. N. Z. J. Physiother. 31 (3), 140–142.

Ribeiro, D.C., de Castro, M.P., Sole, G., Vicenzino, B., 2016. The initial effects of a sustained glenohumeral postero-lateral glide during elevation on shoulder muscle activity: a repeated measures study on asymptomatic shoulders. Man. Ther. 22, 101–108.

Romero, C.L., Torres Lacomba, M., Montoro, Y.C., Merino, D.P., Pacheco da Costa, S., Velasco Marchante, M.J., et al., 2015. Mobilization with movement for shoulder dysfunction in older adults: a pilot trial. J. Chiropr. Med. 14 (4), 249–258.

Satpute, K.H., Bhandari, P., Hall, T., 2015. Efficacy of hand behind back mobilization with movement for acute shoulder pain and movement impairment: a randomized controlled trial. J. Manipulative Physiol. Ther. 38 (5), 324–334.

Tate, A.R., McClure, P.W., Kareha, S., Irwin, D., 2008. Effect of the Scapula Reposition Test on shoulder impingement symptoms and elevation strength in overhead athletes. J. Orthop. Sports Phys. Ther. 38 (1), 4–11.

Teys, P., Bisset, L., Collins, N., Coombes, B., Vicenzino, B., 2013. One-week time course of the effects of Mulligan's Mobilisation with Movement and taping in painful shoulders. Man. Ther. 18 (5), 372–377.

Timmons, M.K., Thigpen, C.A., Seitz, A.L., Karduna, A.R., Arnold, B.L., Michener, L.A., 2012. Scapular kinematics and subacromial-impingement syndrome: a meta-analysis. J. Sport Rehabil. 21 (4), 354–370.

Wright, A.A., Wassinger, C.A., Frank, M., Michener, L.A., Hegedus, E.J., 2013. Diagnostic accuracy of scapular physical examination tests for shoulder disorders: a systematic review. Br. J. Sports Med. 47 (14), 886–892.

Yang, J.L., Chang, C.W., Chen, S.Y., Wang, S.F., Lin, J.J., 2007. Mobilization techniques in subjects with frozen shoulder syndrome: randomized multiple-treatment trial. Phys. Ther. 87 (10), 1307–1315.

Youngjoon, S., Jaeseok, L., Dongwook, H., 2015. The effects of spinal mobilization with arm movements on shoulder muscle strengthening. J. Phys. Ther. Sci. 27 (1), 11–13.

5

Elbow region

INTRODUCTION

The elbow joint consists of the articulation between the humerus and ulna and the humerus and radius. Sharing the joint capsule with the elbow joint, but functionally distinct, is the proximal forearm articulation of the superior radioulnar joint. One of the often worrisome and sometimes difficult to treat sequelae of traumatic elbow injuries (e.g. fractures and immobilisation) is a reasonably difficult to alleviate limitation of motion. The combination of accessory glides with physiological movements along with the fundamental tenet of pain-free application and ability to self-treat are characteristics of MWM techniques that are useful in improving and maintaining motion in the elbow. A substantial part of this chapter describes MWM techniques that can be useful in improving elbow function through improved motion.

The elbow serves as one of the emblematic examples of how MWM can be used to treat conditions that are not conventionally conceived as being predominantly articular in nature. For example, tennis elbow (or lateral epicondylalgia), which is conventionally conceived as a tendinopathy, has been shown to respond favourably to MWM (see levels of evidence below). This chapter deals first with MWM techniques that, along with a graduated exercise programme, might be useful in managing tennis elbow.

Tennis elbow is characterised by pain over the lateral elbow that might extend down the forearm but not into the hand or proximal to the elbow. The patient often presents with disability related to activities that include gripping and activities involving the stabilising muscles of the wrist, of which the tendons are probably the source of the pain. There is evidence from laboratory studies that the MWM treatment techniques of Mulligan can produce immediate improvements in force generation of the involved muscles at pain threshold as well as improvements in mechanical hyperalgesia (Bisset et al., 2006). Two high-quality RCTs have shown that MWM combined with a graduated and progressive exercise programme delivered by qualified physiotherapists speeds up resolution at a similar extent to a corticosteroid injection but without the long-term delay in recovery and high recurrence rates of the latter (Bisset et al., 2006). Modelling of the recovery curves indicates that the MWM technique combined with exercise doubles the recovery rate compared with adopting a 'wait and see' policy. This section describes the MWM techniques included in the clinical trials and laboratory studies (lateral glide and posteroanterior (PA) radial glide) as well as others that have been described by Mulligan for this condition. The practitioner might wish to first try either the lateral glide MWM or the posteroanterior radial glide and in the event that the first-applied technique proves ineffective to progress to the other one. This chapter also presents some MWM techniques that might be useful for the tennis elbow analogue on the medial side (golfer's elbow).

Levels of evidence

Level 2: six RCTs, two case series

There is level 2 evidence in the form of six RCTs of efficacy of either stand-alone MWM treatment (Bagade & Verma, 2015; Kakati & Dutta, 2015; Rahman et al., 2016) or MWM combined with either exercise (Bisset et al., 2006), electrotherapy (Afzal et al., 2016) or traditional treatment (Amro et al., 2010) for lateral epicondylalgia. A number of lower-level studies in the form of two case series (González-Iglesias et al., 2011; Marcolino et al., 2016), case reports and laboratory-based studies of immediate effects also attest to MWM's efficacy in treating lateral epicondylalgia.

Overall, the outcomes of the available RCTs support the use of MWM in the treatment of lateral epicondylalgia. Kakati and Dutta (2015) compared the effectiveness of MWM and elbow orthosis on pain and grip strength in housewives with lateral epicondylitis. Although both interventions improved grip strength, the MWM group was more effective in reducing pain by 45%, measured through VAS immediately post the MWM session. Similarly, Rahman and colleagues (Rahman et al., 2016) demonstrated that MWM intervention was superior to a supervised exercise programme in improving both pain (VAS reduction from 6.76 ± 0.76 to 3.1 ± 0.75) and grip strength in patients with lateral epicondylitis. The study by Bagade and Verma (2015) supports the efficacy of MWM in pain management, as reductions of over 63% were observed on the results of a VAS questionnaire immediately post intervention. Interestingly, this same group demonstrated significant and continued reduction of pain in patients who received MWM treatment compared with hydrocortisone injection at follow-up assessment at 1 month, 3 months and 6 months.

TENNIS ELBOW: LATERAL ELBOW PAIN

Lateral elbow pain: manual lateral glide MWM with gripping

TECHNIQUE AT A GLANCE

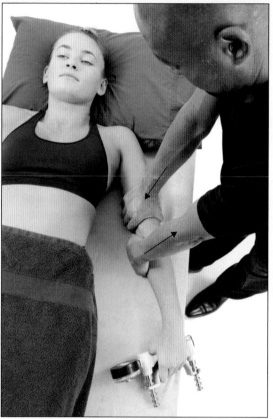

Figure 6.1
Elbow lateral glide with dynamometer

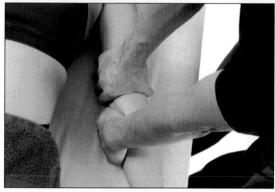

Figure 6.2
Elbow lateral glide: close view

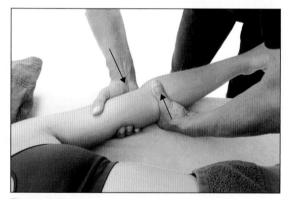

Figure 6.3
Elbow lateral glide: without dynamometer

- The patient lies supine with the elbow extended and pronated.
- The therapist stabilises the distal humerus laterally with one hand.
- The proximal ulna is glided laterally and painlessly with the other hand.
- While the glide is sustained, the patient grips a dynamometer to first onset of pain.
- Finish with the lateral glide applied and sustained during several repetitions (approximately 10) of pain-free elbow flexion/extension to prevent elbow pain on first moving after MWM.
- See Figs 6.1–6.3.

INDICATION

Pain over lateral elbow with gripping or wrist / finger extensor muscle activity.

POSITIONING

Patient:	Supine with upper limb fully supported on a treatment table.
Treated body part:	Relaxed extension of the elbow, shoulder internal rotation, with pronation of the forearm. Hands loosely around the grip dynamometer handles.
Therapist:	Adjacent to the affected elbow facing towards the head of the patient.
Hands / contact points:	Stabilising hand: entire palm of the hand with a focus through the first web-space placed on the lateral surface of the distal humerus (best achieved by pronation of the therapist's forearm).
	Gliding hand: index finger and first metacarpal or heel of the hand and web-space to spread the load, placed on the medial surface of the patient's ulna just distal to the joint line, ensuring not to exert force through the medial muscle mass (of the wrist and finger flexors).

APPLICATION GUIDELINES

- A grip dynamometer is to be used to quantify the grip force required to first onset of pain, allowing for accurate assessment of treatment effects.
- Apply a laterally directed glide across the elbow joint.
- While sustaining the lateral glide force, have the patient repeat the gripping activity to the onset of pain only.
- Note the grip strength obtained before relaxing the grip and then release the glide.
- Apply 6–10 repetitions in a set, with 3–5 sets in a treatment session, but only if there is a substantial increase in force with gripping to pain onset during the application of the technique and no latent pain responses.
- If grip force to pain onset does not change substantially then inclining the glide anterior to lateral some 5° or slightly caudad should be trialled before discarding the technique, as these directions have been shown in a study to be more effective (Abbott et al., 2001).
- There is some preliminary evidence (below in comments) as to applied manual force.
- Do not allow the patient to move out of the elbow extended position spontaneously. The therapist must apply a glide and then the patient flexes the elbow from the treatment position, repeating this 6–10 times with increasing ranges of motion each time. There is a great risk of the patient experiencing some pain if they move spontaneously (i.e. without a glide in place) into elbow flexion from the treatment position of elbow extension, the pain being sufficient to reduce the effectiveness of the lateral glide on subsequent occasions.

6

(continued next page...)

- An alternative application is with the aid of a treatment belt. This may be particularly useful when the patient's limb is large (see Fig. 6.4).

- The same application guidelines apply as for manual application, with critical points being: (a) a grip dynamometer is used to quantify grip force, (b) the belt uniformly applies a lateral force across the elbow, (c) there is a substantial increase in grip force with each repetition and immediately afterwards, and (d) remembering to do 6–10 repetitions of a lateral glide with elbow flexion and extension immediately after the sustained glides with gripping.

- In the event that a substantial increase in grip force does not occur with each repetition of the MWM then consider: (a) applying the lateral glide somewhat posteriorly by internally rotating the humerus further by approximately 5°–10°, and (b) ensuring optimal force level is applied.

- A progression from this technique is where the patient performs isometric finger and wrist extension. This may be considered a progression when gripping is no longer painful.

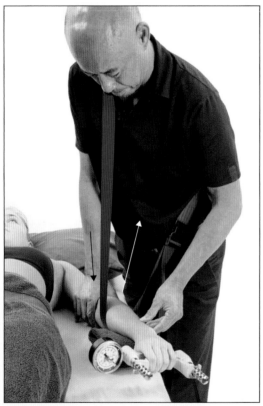

Figure 6.4A
Elbow lateral glide with a treatment belt: with dynamometer

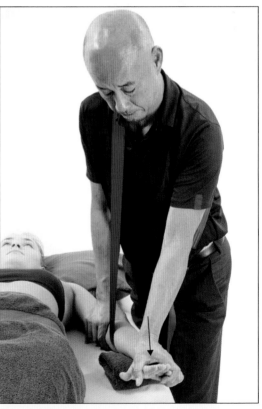

Figure 6.4B
Elbow lateral glide with a treatment belt: isometric wrist extension

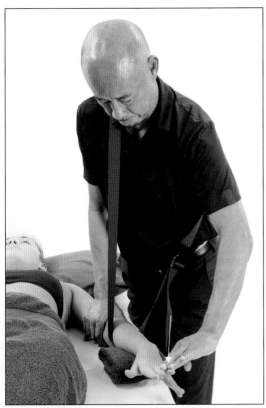

Figure 6.4C
Elbow lateral glide with a treatment belt: isometric
finger extension

COMMENTS

- Ensure that the stabilising hand has a broad contact so it does not compress the lateral epicondyle in such a way to cause pressure pain that reproduces the patient's symptoms.

- Attempt no more than four trials to elicit a positive response in any one treatment session, as failure to relieve pain over this number of trials will prove counterproductive.

- Do not release the sustained lateral glide before the patient relaxes the grip.

- The amount of force that should be applied during this treatment technique has been found to be approximately two-thirds that which the therapist was prepared to apply maximally (McLean et al., 2002). The interesting finding in that study was that there was a threshold of manual force application beyond which no additional benefit was gained in pain-free grip force and below which no benefit accrued (Vicenzino et al., 2011a). More information is available on DVD and in text in the book *Mobilisation with Movement: The Art and the Science* (Vicenzino et al., 2011b).

(continued next page...)

SELF-MANAGEMENT

- The patient can perform self-treatment (Fig. 6.5) by stabilising the humerus of the affected side against the doorframe, with a small towel as a cushion for comfort.
- The elbow is in slight flexion, with the shoulder slightly flexed (10°–15°) and rotated to align the tips of the epicondyles in the frontal plane, with supination of the forearm and a small towel or other compressible object held loosely in the hand (to squeeze and grip). At the same time, the patient reaches across their body and places their thumb posteriorly and fingers anteriorly to the affected forearm, immediately distal to the elbow joint.
- Via their first web-space, but with broad palmar contact of the forearm, the patient glides the affected forearm in a lateral direction, mimicking the lateral glide applied by the therapist.
- While sustaining the glide force, the patient repeats the gripping activity to the onset of pain only, performing 10 repetitions in a session, with 3–5 sessions in a day.
- Direct the patient to alter the glide force and glide direction if pain relief is not achieved.
- Following the sustained glides and gripping repetitions, the patient must sustain a glide while moving the elbow from the treatment position into both flexion and extension limits for 6–10 repetitions.
- An alternative is to use a wide cloth belt for stabilisation of the humerus (Fig. 6.5B) or their other hand to apply the lateral glide (see Figs 6.5C and 6.19).

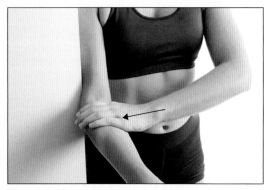

Figure 6.5A
Elbow lateral glide self-treatment with gripping: doorframe stabilisation

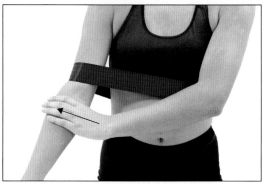

Figure 6.5B
Elbow lateral glide self-treatment with gripping: belt stabilisation

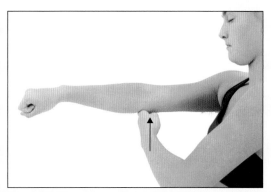

Figure 6.5C
Elbow lateral glide self-treatment with gripping: opposite arm stabilisation

TAPING

- Taping can be used to sustain the treatment effect of the lateral glide and is shown in Fig. 6.6.
- Use 30-mm non-stretch sports tape or flexible tape at greater than 50% elongation.
- Start the tape medially below the elbow joint line, spiralling in a proximal direction across the anterior aspect of the elbow. End the tape on the posterolateral aspect of the distal humerus (Fig. 6.6).
- To achieve good tension on the tape it is advisable to lay the tape on with the forearm pre-positioned in maximum supination and with the elbow flexed to 30° (see Fig. 6.6). Thus when the patient extends the elbow and pronates the arm the tape will be under maximum tension.
- Elbow extension and forearm pronation is usually the provocative position for lateral elbow pain, so maximum effect is achieved in the most important position.
- The patient may apply the tape at home, although the degree of tape tension achieved may not be as much as that obtained by the therapist.

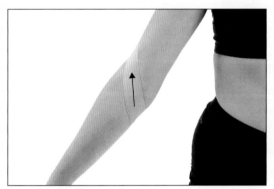

Figure 6.6A
Elbow lateral glide tape: front view

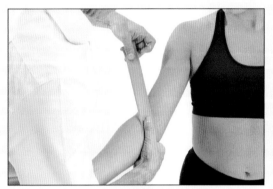

Figure 6.6B
Elbow lateral glide tape: application

ANNOTATIONS

sup ly R Elb Lat gl MWM res grip (dynamometer)×6(3)
sup ly R Elb belt Lat gl MWM res grip (dynamometer)×6(3)
sup ly R Elb belt Lat gl MWM res Wr E×6(3)
sup ly R Elb belt Lat gl MWM res Finger E×6(3)
st R Elb self Lat gl MWM grip×10
L Elb Lat gl tape

Proximal radioulnar joint posteroanterior MWM

TECHNIQUE AT A GLANCE

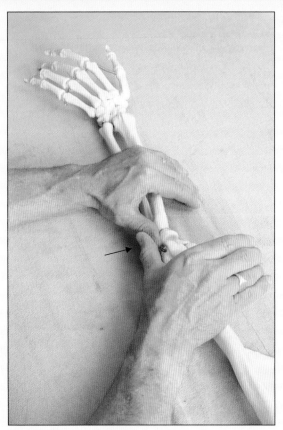

Figure 6.7
Radial head PA glide: model view

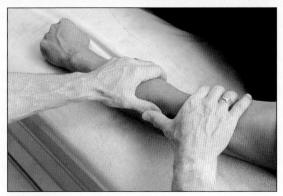

Figure 6.8
Radial head PA glide: wide view

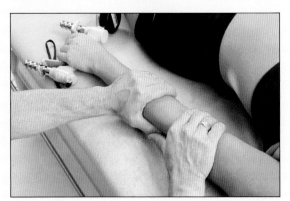

Figure 6.9
Radial head PA glide: with dynamometer

- The patient is lying supine with the arm resting by the side, shoulder internally rotated, elbow extended and forearm pronated.
- The distal humerus and proximal ulna are stabilised by the therapist's fingers.
- The radial head is glided anteriorly by thumb pressure.
- While the glide is sustained, the patient grips the dynamometer.
- See Figs 6.7–6.9.

INDICATION

Lateral elbow pain on gripping, making a fist.

POSITIONING

Patient:	Lying supine with the arm resting by side and shoulder internally rotated.
Treated body part:	The forearm is in end-range pronation and with elbow in extension and hand relaxed.
Therapist:	Adjacent to the affected elbow, facing across the patient.
Hands/contact points:	Stabilising hand: fingers of one hand wrap around the distal humerus, while the fingers of the other hand wrap around the proximal ulna to stabilise the ulna and humerus. Gliding hand: thumbs of both hands overlay each other on the posterior aspect of the head and neck of the radius.

APPLICATION GUIDELINES

- With one thumb reinforcing the other, the therapist glides the radial head anteriorly, while stabilising the ulna and humerus with their fingertips.
- While sustaining the anterior glide, ask the patient to make a fist. A grip dynamometer can be used to quantify the grip force achievable to first onset of pain, allowing for accurate assessment of treatment effects.
- Note the grip strength obtained before relaxing the grip and then release the glide.
- Apply 6–10 repetitions in a set, with 3–5 sets in a treatment session, but only if there is a substantial increase in force with gripping to pain onset during the application of the technique and no latent pain responses.

VARIATIONS

- In some individuals, the cervical spine may contribute to lateral arm pain symptoms. In this case the elbow symptoms may not be relieved by local elbow techniques. Spinal mobilisation with arm movement should be considered if there is a poor response to either an elbow lateral glide or a radial head PA glide (Chapter 3, Figs 3.28–3.31).

COMMENTS

- If pain is relieved with this technique then teach the patient an exercise to replicate the PA glide. Tape may also be helpful to maintain the treatment effect.
- This MWM can be applied in various elbow flexion or extension positions, depending on the most provocative position for making a fist or isometric finger and wrist extension.
- The radial head is commonly a sensitive contact point for mobilisation so foam should be used to minimise discomfort during mobilisation. Additionally, to minimise contact discomfort, draw the soft tissue from medial to lateral when first contacting the radial head.
- The magnitude and direction of accessory glide force may need to be altered to assure a pain-free technique. If making a fist does not provoked pain then isometric wrist and finger extension can be utilised as the pain-provocative activity.

(continued next page...)

SELF-MANAGEMENT

- The patient can perform self-treatment (Fig. 6.10) by stabilising the humerus of the affected side by their side.
- The elbow is in full extension and pronation.
- A small towel or other compressible object is held loosely in the hand (to squeeze and grip). At the same time, the patient reaches across their body and places all fingers on the posterior aspect of the radius, immediately distal to the radial head.
- Via their fingertips, the patient glides the radius anteriorly, mimicking the radial head PA glide applied by the therapist.
- While sustaining the glide force, the patient repeats the gripping activity to the onset of pain only, performing 10 repetitions in a session, with 3–5 sessions in a day.
- To be effective, the grip force to pain onset has to improve during each of the repetitions of the self-treatment technique.
- Direct the patient to alter the glide force and glide direction if pain relief is not achieved.
- Repeat 10 times in a session, with 3–5 sessions per day.

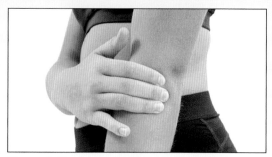

Figure 6.10
Radial head PA self-mobilisation for lateral epicondylalgia

TAPING

- Taping can be used to sustain the treatment effect of the radial head PA glide and is shown in Fig. 6.11.
- Use 30-mm non-stretch sports tape or flexible tape at greater than 50% elongation.
- With the elbow in full extension and forearm maximally pronated, the tape starts posteriorly in the midline, immediately below the radial head.
- Take up the soft tissue tension in a lateral direction and glide the radial head anteriorly while pulling the tape under tension across the anterior forearm. End the tape on the medial aspect of the ulna (see Fig. 6.11). Do not make a complete circle with the tape.
- Apply two layers of tape for maximal effect.
- The patient may apply the tape at home, although the degree of tape tension achieved may not be as much as that obtained by the therapist.

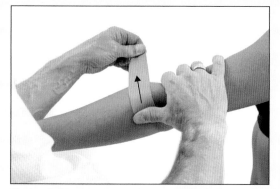

Figure 6.11
Elbow radial head PA tape

ANNOTATION

sup ly L Radial head Ant gl MWM grip×6 (3)
sup ly L Radial head Ant gl MWM res grip (dynamometer)×6 (3)
st R Radial head self Ant gl MWM grip×10
R Radial head Ant gl tape

GOLFER'S ELBOW: MEDIAL ELBOW PAIN

Olecranon medial and lateral tilt (lateral and medial rotation)

TECHNIQUE AT A GLANCE

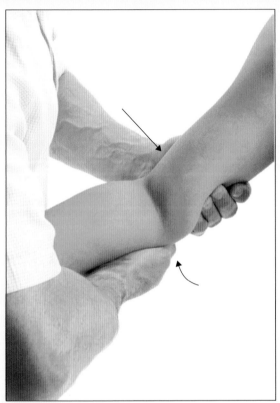

Figure 6.12
Ulna lateral tilt with gripping: hand position

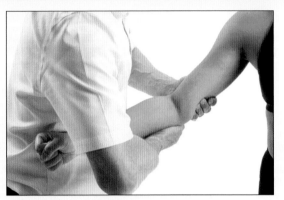

Figure 6.13
Ulna lateral tilt with gripping: wide view

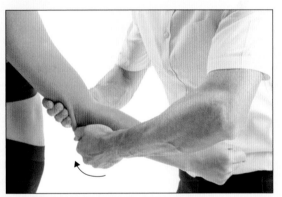

Figure 6.14
Ulna medial tilt with gripping

- The patient stands with their arm by their side.
- The therapist stabilises the distal humerus with one hand.
- The medial aspect of the olecranon is tilted laterally (Figs 6.12 and 6.13), creating painless medial rotation of the ulna. Alternatively the lateral aspect of the olecranon is tilted medially (Fig. 6.14), creating painless lateral rotation of the ulna.
- While the tilt is maintained, the patient makes a fist or flexes the wrist or finger.
- See Figs 6.12–6.14.

INDICATION

Medial elbow pain with resisted flexion of the wrist or finger(s) or with gripping.

POSITIONING

Patient:	Standing.
Treated body part:	Relaxed position with elbow and shoulder slightly flexed; patient's arm is supported by the therapist.
Therapist:	Standing facing/side on to the patient, slightly to the side of the symptoms.
Hands/contact points:	For medial tilt, contact the lateral aspect of the olecranon using the thenar eminence. The therapist's other hand stabilises the medial aspect of the distal humerus.

APPLICATION GUIDELINES

- For a medial tilt, stabilise the humerus on the medial distal aspect (Fig. 6.14).
- Apply a medial tilt of the ulna via the olecranon, using the thenar eminence on the lateral aspect of the posterior-most part of the olecranon.
- The patient performs a pain-provocative movement, which typically is making a fist or wrist flexion.
- Use of a grip dynamometer as for tennis elbow will provide a better appreciation of the amount of improvement gained with the MWM.
- While sustaining the tilt, have the patient repeat the provocative movement (CSIM), which is rendered pain-free by the mobilisation.
- Perform up to 10 repetitions in a set, with 3–5 sets per treatment session.

VARIATIONS

- For a lateral tilt, stabilise the humerus on the lateral distal aspect (Fig. 6.12).
- Apply a lateral tilt of the ulna via the olecranon, using the thenar eminence on the medial aspect of the posterior-most part of the olecranon.
- The patient performs a pain-provocative movement, which typically is making a fist or wrist flexion.
- Perform up to 10 repetitions in a set, with 3–5 sets per treatment session.

COMMENTS

- Instruct the patient to move slowly when performing the provocative activity so you are able to sustain the correct olecranon tilt throughout the motion.
- Be careful of the stabilising hand position on the medial aspect, as this region can be very sensitive in patients with medial elbow pain. Use a broad palmer contact and, if required, foam rubber to soften the contact pressure.

TAPING

- This taping technique is used when the patient has relief with the golfer's elbow medial olecranon tilt technique; it is shown in Fig. 6.15.
- Use 30-mm non-stretch sports tape or flexible tape at greater than 50% elongation in two layers, although the tape width may vary depending on the size of the patient's arm.
- The patient's elbow should be slightly flexed and supinated when applying the tape.
- Position the tape on the lateral aspect of the olecranon, slightly away from the olecranon, to allow for soft tissue slack take-up when applying tension to the tape.
- The tape is tensioned medially while spiralling up the arm from distal to proximal, ending by attaching it to the lateral humerus.
- After application, the original pain-provocative activity (e.g. gripping) should now be pain-free.

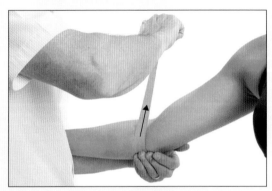

Figure 6.15A
Olecranon medial tilt tape for golfer's elbow:
application

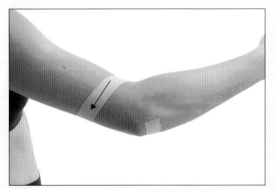

Figure 6.15B
Olecranon medial tilt tape for golfer's elbow:
complete

ANNOTATIONS

st R Olecranon Med tilt MWM grip×6
st R Olecranon Med tilt MWM res Wr F×6
st R Olecranon Lat tilt MWM res grip (dynamometer)×10(3)
st R Olecranon Med tilt MWM res Finger F×6
R Olecranon Med tilt tape

ELBOW MOVEMENT DYSFUNCTION

Elbow extension manual lateral and medial glide

TECHNIQUE AT A GLANCE

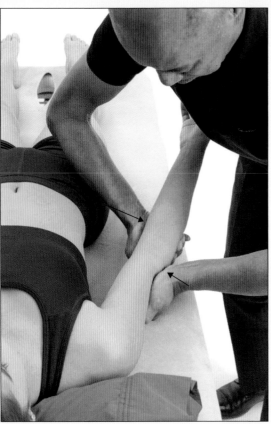

Figure 6.16
Elbow manual lateral glide: start position

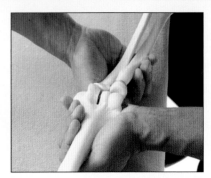

Figure 6.17
Elbow manual lateral glide: model view

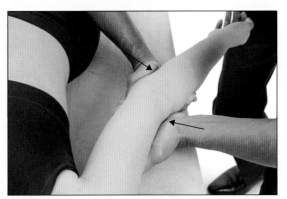

Figure 6.18
Elbow manual lateral glide: end position

- The patient lies supine, close to the edge of the treatment table with the elbow flexed.
- The therapist stabilises the distal humerus laterally with one hand.
- Glide proximal ulna laterally with the other hand.
- Maintain the glide while the patient extends their elbow.
- Use over-pressure at the end range if appropriate.
- See Figs 6.16–6.18.

INDICATION

Painful and/or restricted elbow extension movement.

POSITIONING

Patient:	Laying supine with upper limb fully supported on a treatment table, shoulder external rotation, with supination of the forearm.
Treated body part:	Elbow in a flexed position away from the limitation.
Therapist:	Standing adjacent to the affected elbow facing towards the head of the patient.
Position hands/contact points:	Stabilising hand: the entire palm of the hand stabilises the lateral surface of the distal humerus. Gliding hand: the entire palm of the hand contacts the medial surface of the proximal ulna just distal to the elbow joint line.

APPLICATION GUIDELINES

- Apply a laterally directed glide across the elbow joint.
- While sustaining the glide force, have the patient repeat the elbow extension movement to the onset of pain only.
- If movement is still restricted and no pain is being experienced then over-pressure is applied.
- Ensure to allow for the carrying angle in the terminal ranges of extension if it is present.
- Apply 6–10 repetitions in a set, with 3–5 sets in a treatment session, but only if there is a substantial increase in movement to pain onset during and after the application of the technique.
- If the technique is indicated the patient should experience a gain in movement.

VARIATIONS

- A manual therapy belt may also be used for easier application of the gliding force (Fig. 6.19).
- The distal humerus is stabilised laterally with one hand.
- The treatment belt loops around the therapist's pelvis and the upper aspect of the patient's forearm, contacting the ulna medially.
- Maintain the glide with the treatment belt while the patient extends their elbow.
- The practitioner needs to pay particular attention to the evenness of belt contact with the forearm for maximum comfort.

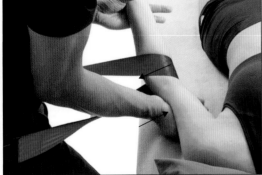

Figure 6.19A
Lateral glide using a belt for elbow extension: start position

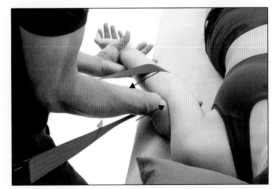

Figure 6.19B
Lateral glide using a belt for elbow extension: end position

(continued next page...)

- Elbow extension may be undertaken in any range of forearm pronation or supination, depending on the CSIM and symptomatic response to the MWM.
- If a lateral glide is not successful, try a medial glide of the ulna (Fig. 6.20). For this technique position the shoulder is in 90° abduction. The MWM can be achieved manually with the hands or with a treatment belt (Fig. 6.20).

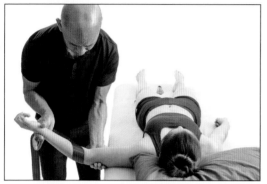

Figure 6.20A

Medial glide using a belt for elbow extension: start position

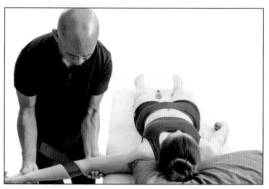

Figure 6.20B

Medial glide using a belt for elbow extension: end position

- In the presence of a sensitised median nerve, the medial glide technique can be applied in a modified position, with the patient positioned lying on their symptomatic side and shoulder flexed to 90° (Fig. 6.21). This shoulder flexion position will not stress the median nerve as much as the abduction position in Fig. 6.20.

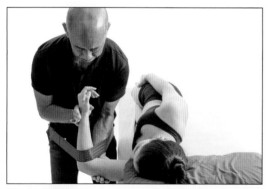

Figure 6.21A

Modified medial glide using a belt for elbow extension: start position

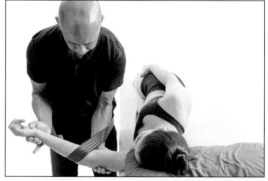

Figure 6.21B

Modified medial glide using a belt for elbow extension: end position

- If a medial glide is not successful, try a medial tilt of the olecranon; this technique was described earlier in this chapter (see Fig. 6.14).

COMMENTS

- Ensure that the stabilising hand has a broad contact so that it does not compress the lateral soft tissues in such a way as to cause pressure pain or discomfort. If the elbow extension does not change substantially then try altering the glide direction or glide force before discarding the technique.

- Ensure that you do not place strong force through the muscle mass (of the wrist and finger flexors), but rather make contact directly on the ulna, which is somewhat posterior to the muscle mass.

- Do not release the glide force until the elbow returns to the start position. The amount of force that should be applied during this treatment technique may vary, but should be sufficient for the movement to be pain-free.

ANNOTATION

sup ly R Elb Lat gl MWM E×6(3)

sup ly L Elb belt Lat gl MWM E +OP×6(3)

sup ly L Elb Med gl MWM E×6(3)

sup ly L sh 90 degrees Ab R Elb belt Med gl MWM E×6(3)

R s ly L Sh 90 degrees F R Elb belt Med gl MWM E +OP×6(3)

Elbow flexion manual lateral and medial glide

TECHNIQUE AT A GLANCE

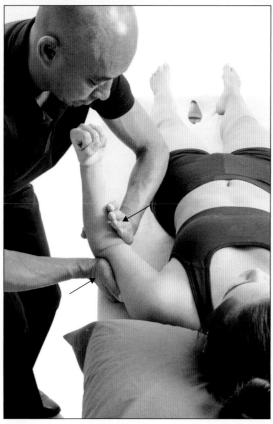

Figure 6.22
Elbow manual lateral glide for flexion: start position

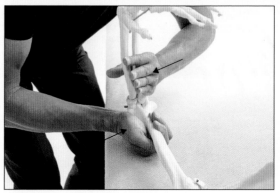

Figure 6.23
Elbow manual lateral glide for flexion: model view

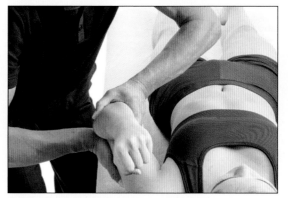

Figure 6.24
Elbow manual lateral glide for flexion: end position

- The patient lies supine close to the edge of the treatment table with the elbow in a pain-free position of flexion/extension and supinated.
- The therapist stabilises the distal humerus laterally with one hand.
- The therapist glides the proximal radius and ulna laterally with the other hand.
- The therapist maintains the glide while the patient flexes their elbow.
- Over-pressure by the patient is used at the end range into flexion if appropriate.
- See Figs 6.22–6.24.

INDICATION

Painful and/or restricted elbow flexion movement.

POSITIONING

Patient:	Supine with shoulder flexed slightly.
Treated body part:	Relaxed and pain-free mid position of flexion/extension of the elbow, with supination of the forearm.
Therapist:	Adjacent to the affected elbow facing towards the head of the patient.
Position hands/contact points:	Stabilising hand: base of index finger of the pronated hand on the lateral surface of the distal humerus. Gliding hand: base of index finger of the pronated hand placed on the medial surface of the patient's forearm just distal to the joint line.

APPLICATION GUIDELINES

- Apply a laterally directed glide across the elbow joint.
- While sustaining the lateral glide force, have the patient repeat elbow flexion to the onset of pain only.
- Apply 6–10 repetitions in a set, with 3–5 sets in a treatment session, but only if there is a substantial increase in movement to pain onset during and after the application of the technique and no latent pain responses.
- If the technique is indicated the patient should experience a gain in movement with every repetition.

VARIATIONS

- A manual therapy belt may also be used for easier application of the gliding force (Fig. 6.25).
- The distal humerus is stabilised laterally with one hand.
- The treatment belt loops around the therapist's pelvis and the upper aspect of the patient's forearm, immediately distal to the patient's medial epicondyle.
- Maintain the glide with the treatment belt while the patient flexes their elbow.
- The practitioner needs to pay particular attention to the evenness of belt contact with the forearm for maximum comfort.
- Ensure that the therapist moves their pelvis in unison with the patient's elbow movement to maintain the correct glide.

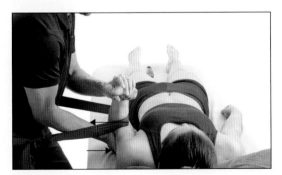

Figure 6.25A
Lateral glide using a belt for elbow flexion: start position

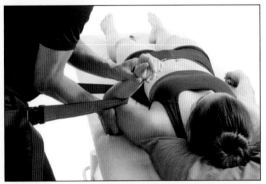

Figure 6.25B
Lateral glide using a belt for elbow flexion: end position

(continued next page...)

- Elbow flexion may be undertaken in any range of forearm pronation or supination, depending on the CSIM and symptomatic response to the MWM.
- If a lateral glide is not successful, try a medial glide of the radius and ulna using the hands for the glide or a treatment belt (Fig. 6.26).

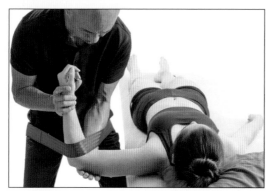

Figure 6.26A
Medial glide using a belt for elbow flexion: start position

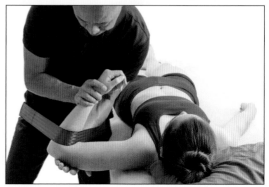

Figure 6.26B
Medial glide using a belt for elbow flexion: end position

6

- Instead of a lateral or medial glide, a manual lateral or medial rotation of the ulna may be used to gain pain-free movement into flexion (see Fig. 6.27). Note: use the olecranon to hook on for a better contact. The index finger stays in contact with the ulna/radius on the anterior part of the forearm. Always move the fingers away from the anterior elbow surface so as not to hinder attainment of full flexion.

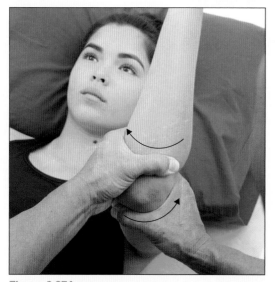

Figure 6.27A
Forearm rotation for elbow flexion: start position

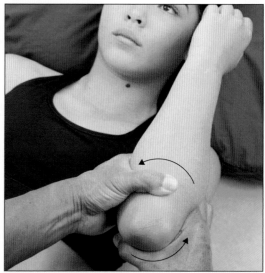

Figure 6.27B
Forearm rotation for elbow flexion: end position

COMMENTS

- Ensure that the stabilising hand has a broad contact so it does not compress the humeral epicondyle in such a way to cause pressure pain.
- If the movement to pain onset does not change substantially then inclining the glide slightly in a different direction should be trialled before discarding the technique.
- Do not release the sustained glide before the elbow returns back to the start position.
- The amount of force that should be applied during this treatment technique may vary, but should be enough to avoid pain during the movement.
- If hands are blocking elbow flexion towards end range, the therapist can move both hands away from the anterior elbow while sustaining the glide.
- Do not release the glide force until the elbow returns to the start position. The amount of force that should be applied during this treatment technique may vary, but should be sufficient for the movement to be pain-free.

ANNOTATIONS

sup ly L Elb Med gl MWM F×6(3)
sup ly L Elb belt Med gl MWM F×6(3)
sup ly L Fra IR MWM F×6(3)
sup ly L Fra ER MWM F×6(3)
sup ly L Sh 90 degrees Ab L Elb belt Lat gl MWM F×6(3)

6

Elbow flexion and extension manual olecranon lateral tilt/medial rotation

TECHNIQUE AT A GLANCE

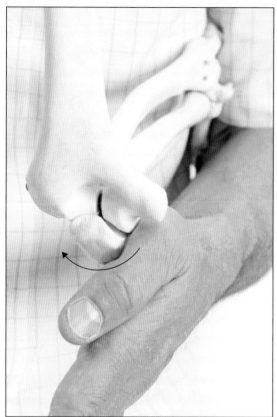

Figure 6.28
Olecranon lateral tilt for extension: model view showing hand placement

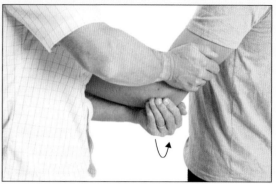

Figure 6.29
Olecranon lateral tilt for extension: start position

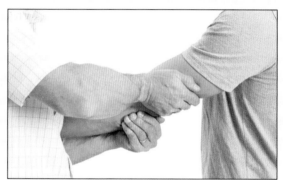

Figure 6.30
Olecranon lateral tilt for extension: end position

- The patient stands with the arm supported by the therapist.
- The therapist stabilises the distal humerus laterally with one hand.
- The medial aspect of the posterior olecranon is tilted laterally, creating medial rotation of the ulna with the other hand.
- While the tilt is maintained the patient moves the elbow towards the limited range (in this case extension).
- See Figs 6.28–6.30.

6

INDICATION

Limitation of elbow flexion or extension due to pain or stiffness.

POSITIONING

Patient:	Standing with arm supported by the therapist. (Note: it can also be performed with patient sitting.)
Treated body part:	Shoulder slightly flexed with the elbow in a pain-free position close to the point of limitation or pain.
Therapist:	Adjacent to the affected elbow facing towards the patient.
Hands/contact points:	The thenar eminence of the mobilising hand contacts the medial aspect of the olecranon posteriorly distal to the elbow joint line. The fingers of this hand wrap around the back of the olecranon. The stabilising hand contacts the lateral aspect of the distal humerus just above the joint line.

APPLICATION GUIDELINES

- Support the patient's arm, resting the forearm against the side of the therapist's body closest to the patient.
- Prior to commencing the glide, move the elbow close to the point in range of symptom onset.
- Stabilise the lateral aspect of the distal humerus.
- The thenar eminence of the therapist's medial hand applies a lateral tilt creating medial rotation of the ulna.
- The patient moves actively into flexion or extension.
- If full range is achieved, the patient will apply over-pressure to their forearm with their free hand.
- Apply 6–10 repetitions in a set, with 3–5 sets in a treatment session, but only if there is a substantial increase in pain-free ROM.

COMMENTS

- This technique is frequently effective when used in isolation.
- The hand position for this technique when addressing elbow flexion versus extension is critical as the end positions are quite different (see Fig. 6.31).

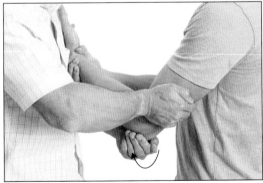

Figure 6.31A
Olecranon lateral tilt for flexion: hand position in start position

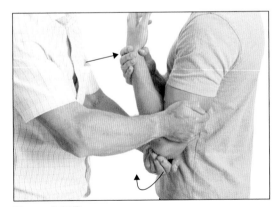

Figure 6.31B
Olecranon lateral tilt for flexion: end position

(continued next page...)

TAPING

- The taping technique is used when the patient has relief with the olecranon tilt technique (Figs 6.28–6.31) and it is shown in Fig. 6.32.

- Use 30-mm non-stretch sports tape or flexible tape at greater than 50% elongation in two layers, although the tape width may vary depending on the size of the patient's arm.

- The elbow should be flexed to 30° and fully supinated when applying the tape. It is usually possible to tilt the olecranon at the same time as the tape is applied, thus increasing tape tension and tape efficacy.

- Position the tape on the medial aspect of the olecranon, slightly away from the olecranon, to allow for soft tissue slack take-up when applying tension to the tape.

- The tape is tensioned laterally while spiralling up the arm from distal to proximal, ending by attaching to the medial humerus.

- After application, the original pain-provocative activity (e.g. elbow flexion or extension) should now be pain-free.

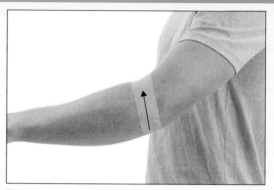

Figure 6.32
Olecranon lateral tilt taping technique

ANNOTATIONS

st L Olecranon Lat tilt MWM E×6
st L Olecranon Lat tilt MWM F +OP×10(3)
R Olecranon Lat tilt tape

Elbow flexion and extension manual olecranon medial tilt/lateral rotation

TECHNIQUE AT A GLANCE

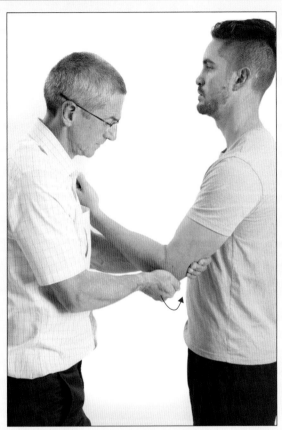

Figure 6.33
Olecranon medial tilt for flexion: overview

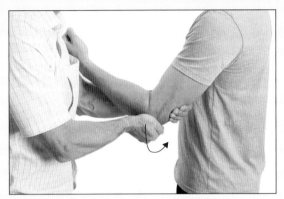

Figure 6.34
Olecranon medial tilt for flexion: start position

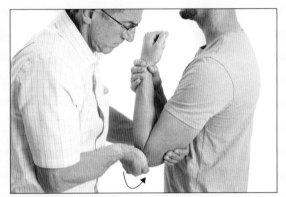

Figure 6.35
Olecranon medial tilt for flexion: end position

- The patient stands with their arm by their side.
- The therapist stabilises the distal humerus medially with one hand.
- The lateral aspect of the olecranon is medially tilted, creating painless lateral rotation of the ulna with the other hand.
- While the tilt is maintained the patient moves the elbow towards the limited range.
- See Figs 6.33–6.35.

INDICATION

Limitation of elbow flexion or extension due to pain or stiffness.

POSITIONING

Patient:	Standing with arm supported by the therapist (can be performed with patient sitting).
Treated body part:	Shoulder slightly flexed, with the elbow in a pain-free position close to the point of limitation or pain.
Therapist:	Adjacent and medial to the affected elbow facing towards the patient.
Hands/contact points:	The thenar eminence of the mobilising hand contacts the lateral aspect of the olecranon. The fingers of this hand wrap around the back of the olecranon. The stabilising hand contacts the medial aspect of the distal humerus just above the joint line.

APPLICATION GUIDELINES

- Support the patient's arm, resting the forearm against the lateral side of the therapist's body.
- Move the elbow close to the point in range of symptom onset.
- Stabilise the medial aspect of the distal humerus.
- The thenar eminence of the therapist's lateral hand applies a medial tilt to the olecranon on its most posterior lateral aspect. As the olecranon is more posterior and inferior to the elbow joint plane, the resultant force will be more of a tilt than a true glide.
- The patient moves actively into flexion (Fig. 6.35) or extension (Fig. 6.36).
- If full range is achieved, the patient will apply over-pressure to their forearm with their free hand.
- Apply 6–10 repetitions in a set, with 3–5 sets in a treatment session, but only if there is a substantial increase in pain-free ROM.

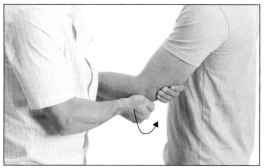

Figure 6.36A
Olecranon medial tilt for elbow extension: start position

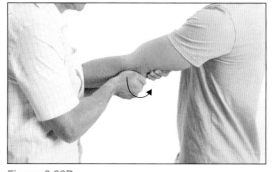

Figure 6.36B
Olecranon medial tilt for elbow extension: end position

COMMENTS

- There is only a very small contact area on the lateral olecranon for application of force.
- Ensure that you take up the soft tissue slack to obtain a good contact of the bone surface.

TAPING

- This taping technique is used when the patient has relief with the olecranon tilt technique (Fig. 6.33) and is shown in Fig. 6.37.
- Use 30-mm non-stretch sports tape or flexible tape at greater than 50% elongation in two layers, although the tape width may vary depending on the size of the patient's arm.
- The patient's elbow should be flexed to 30° and fully supinated when applying the tape. It is usually possible to tilt the olecranon at the same time as the tape is applied, thus increasing tape tension and tape efficacy.
- For a medial tilt, position the tape on the medial aspect of the olecranon, slightly away from the olecranon, to allow for soft tissue slack take-up when applying tension to the tape.
- The tape is tensioned medially while spiralling up the arm from distal to proximal, ending by attaching to the lateral humerus.
- After application, the original pain-provocative activity (e.g. elbow flexion or extension) should now be pain-free.

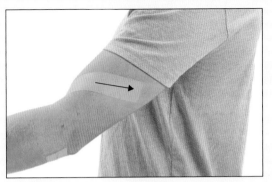

Figure 6.37
Olecranon medial tilt taping technique

ANNOTATIONS

st L Olecranon Med tilt MWM F +OP×6
st L Olecranon Med tilt MWM E +OP×10(3)
R Olecranon Med tilt tape

FOREARM: TREATED PROXIMALLY

Proximal radioulnar joint posteroanterior MWM to improve supination and pronation

TECHNIQUE AT A GLANCE

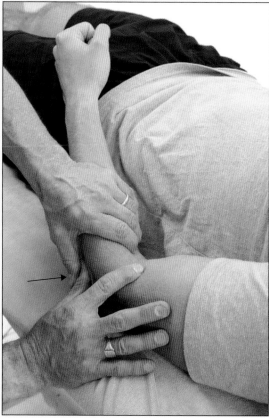

Figure 6.38
Radial head PA glide during supination: start position

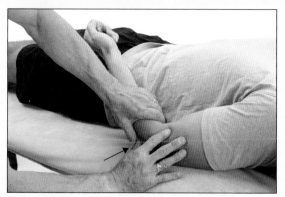

Figure 6.39
PA glide of the radial head: supination

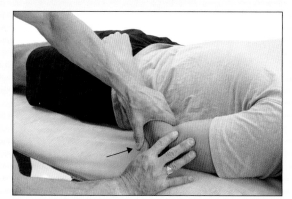

Figure 6.40
PA glide of the radial head: pronation

- The patient is supine with the elbow flexed between 30° and 90°.
- The therapist stabilises the proximal ulna with their fingers.
- The radial head is glided anteriorly by thumb pressure.
- While the glide is sustained, the patient actively supinates or pronates the forearm.
- Over-pressure is applied at end range with the hand of the uninvolved upper extremity.
- See Figs 6.38–6.40.

INDICATION

Limitation of forearm pronation or supination movement due to pain or stiffness of the proximal radioulnar joint.

POSITIONING

Patient:	Supine with the elbow flexed between 30° and 90°.
Treated body part:	The forearm is in mid-range pronation and supination with the fingers pointing up.
Therapist:	Adjacent to the affected elbow facing towards the patient's head.
Hands/contact points:	Stabilising hands: fingers of the caudal hand wrap around the proximal forearm to stabilise the ulna. Gliding hand: thumbs of both hands overlay each other on the posterior aspect of the head and neck of the radius.

APPLICATION GUIDELINES

- With one thumb reinforcing the other, the therapist glides the radial head anteriorly, while stabilising the ulna with their fingertips.
- While sustaining the anterior glide, ask the patient to actively supinate or pronate their forearm.
- Apply 6–10 repetitions in a set, with 3–5 sets in a treatment session.
- The patient may apply pain-free passive over-pressure with their other hand through pressure applied using their distal forearm on the symptomatic side.

COMMENTS

- The MWM can be applied in various elbow flexion or extension positions, depending on the most provocative or limited point in elbow range at which supination or pronation movement is painful.
- The radial head is commonly a sensitive contact point for mobilisation so foam should be used to minimise discomfort during mobilisation. Additionally, to minimise contact discomfort, draw the soft tissue from medial to lateral when first contacting the radial head.
- The magnitude and direction of accessory glide force may need to be altered to assure a pain-free technique. If gliding the radial head anteriorly does not result in pain-free supination or pronation, consider anteroposterior (AP) radial head mobilisation. The anterior aspect of the head of radius is quite sensitive, so be careful to ensure maximum comfort by pushing the soft tissue laterally before applying AP pressure.

ANNOTATIONS

sup R Elb 30 degrees F R Radial head Ant gl MWM Supin×6
sup R Elb 90 degrees F R Radial head Ant gl MWM Pron×6(3)

References

Abbott, J.H., Patla, C.E., Jensen, R.H., 2001. The initial effects of an elbow mobilisation with movement technique on grip strength in subjects with lateral epicondylalgia. Man. Ther. 6 (3), 163–169.

Afzal, M.W., Ahmad, A., Waqas, M.S., Ahmad, U., 2016. Effectiveness of therapeutic ultrasound with and without Mulligan mobilization in lateral epicondylitis. Ann. King Edward Med. Uni. 22 (1), 47–59.

Amro, A., Diener, I., Bdair, W.O., Hameda, I.M., Shalabi, A.I., Ilyyan, D.I., 2010. The effects of Mulligan mobilisation with movement and taping techniques on pain, grip strength, and function in patients with lateral epicondylitis. Hong Kong Physiother. J. 28 (1), 19–23.

Bagade, V.K., Verma, C., 2015. Effect of Mulligan mobilization with movement (MWM) in the treatment of chronic lateral epicondylitis: 24 weeks follow-up study. Indian J. Physiother. Occup. Ther. 9 (4), 199–204.

Bisset, L., Beller, E., Jull, G., Brooks, P., Darnell, R., Vicenzino, B., 2006. Mobilisation with movement and exercise, corticosteroid injection, or wait and see for tennis elbow: randomised trial. BMJ 333 (7575), 939.

González-Iglesias, J., Cleland, J.A., del Rosario Gutierrez-Vega, M., Fernández-de-las-Peñas, C., 2011. Multimodal management of lateral epicondylalgia in rock climbers: a prospective case series. J. Manipulative PhysiolTher. 34 (9), 635–642.

Kakati, T., Dutta, A., 2015. Comparative study to find out immediate effectiveness of movement with mobilization versus elbow orthosis on pain and grip strength in lateral epicondylitis in housewives. Int. J. Physiother. 2 (61), 1085–1090.

McLean, S., Naish, R., Reed, L., Urry, S., Vicenzino, B., 2002. A pilot study of the manual force levels required to produce manipulation induced hypoalgesia. Clin. Biomech. (Bristol, Avon) 17 (4), 304–308.

Marcolino, A.M., das Neves, L.M.S., Oliveira, B.G., Alexandre, A.A., Corsatto, G., Barbosa, R.I., et al., 2016. Multimodal approach to rehabilitation of the patients with lateral epicondylosis: a case series. Springerplus 5 (1), 1718.

Rahman, H., Chaturvedi, P.A., Apparao, P., Srithulasi, P.R., 2016. Effectiveness of Mulligan mobilisation with movement compared to supervised exercise program in subjects with lateral epicondylitis. Int. J. Physiother. Res. 4 (2), 1394–1400.

Vicenzino, B., Hing, W., Hall, T., Rivett, D., 2011a. Efficacy. In: Vicenzino, B., Hing, W., Rivett, D., Hall, T. (Eds.), Mobilisation With Movement: The Art and the Science. Churchill Livingstone Australia, Chatswood, NSW, pp. 26–63.

Vicenzino, B., Hing, W., Hall, T., Rivett, D., 2011b. Mobilisation with Movement: the art and science of its application. In: Vicenzino, B., Hing, W., Rivett, D., Hall, T. (Eds.), Mobilisation With Movement: The Art and the Science. Churchill Livingstone Australia, Chatswood, NSW, pp. 9–23.

6

Wrist and hand

TECHNIQUES FOR THE WRIST AND HAND

DISTAL FOREARM / WRIST TECHNIQUES

Inferior radioulnar joint: pain or limitation of movement during pronation or supination

Carpal lateral glide for non-weight-bearing wrist flexion and extension
  Wrist self-treatment: lateral glide for wrist flexion and extension
  Taping for lateral carpal glide for wrist flexion and extension

Carpal medial glide for non-weight-bearing wrist flexion and extension
  Wrist self-treatment: medial glide for flexion and extension
  Taping for medial carpal glide for wrist flexion and extension

Carpal lateral glide for weight-bearing wrist extension
  Wrist self-treatment for weight -bearing wrist extension – lateral and medial glide

Carpal rotation for wrist flexion and extension
  Carpal rotation for wrist flexion or extension: self-management
  Taping for carpal rotation for wrist flexion and extension

Scaphoid PA or AP glide non-weight-bearing
  Scaphoid PA in weight-bearing wrist extension

HAND

Metacarpal PA and AP glide with fist clenching

FINGER – PROXIMAL INTERPHALANGEAL (PIP) JOINT PAIN AND / OR RESTRICTION

Finger PIP joint pain / restriction with flexion manual lateral / medial glide
  Manual internal / external rotation with flexion
  Finger self-management: rotation and glide
  Taping fingers: rotation and lateral glide

INTRODUCTION

The wrist is a complex of articulations involving the distal radioulnar, radiocarpal, ulnocarpal, intercarpal and carpometacarpal joints. Understanding the anatomy of the wrist complex is important, particularly when applying MWM, to ensure the correct direction of glide. The radius forms the major part of the articulation with the carpal bones, being much wider at the wrist than the ulna. The articular surface of the radius has two concave facets, which articulate with the scaphoid and the lunate directly, while the ulna articulates with the articular disc and not directly with the carpal bones. The radius has a long styloid process typically projecting 1 cm further distally than the ulnar styloid process. Hence, the treatment plane for MWM at the ulnoradiocarpal joint is oblique, lying from proximal/medial to distal/lateral with the arm in the anatomical position.

Wrist pain can be generalised, requiring a general MWM technique, or it can be more localised, involving a specific articulation of the radiocarpal or intercarpal joints, and requiring a localised MWM technique.

The proximal row of the carpal bones consists of the scaphoid, lunate, triquetrum and the pisiform, while the distal row consists of the trapezium, trapezoid, capitate and hamate. Movement of an individual bone relative to its joint partner can be applied to restore pain-free ROM. If uncertain, it would be advisable to trial a generalised carpal row MWM, and if unsuccessful then move to a specific localised MWM, usually of the bones underlying the pain.

Movement at the wrist can occur in a number of different directions including pronation/supination (predominantly occurring at the distal radioulnar joint), as well as flexion/extension and deviation at the ulnoradiocarpal and intercarpal joints. There is a small amount of movement of horizontal flexion and extension in the intermetacarpal region of the hand. In addition, there is a large range of flexion/extension motion at the metacarpophalangeal and interphalangeal joints. MWM can be applied to manage the appropriate CSIM, which may consist of any of these movements.

Interestingly, the first patient that Brian Mulligan treated using the MWM approach was a patient with a painful proximal interphalangeal joint following a traumatic event. Brian Mulligan hypothesised that the cause of pain was a positional fault. There is evidence from magnetic resonance imaging (MRI) of a similar positional fault in the thumb, also caused by a traumatic event (Hsieh et al., 2002). As well as resolving the patient's thumb problem, MWM improved the positional fault during the course of management, but this improvement was not maintained at long-term follow-up, despite sustained improvement in pain.

In addition to pain arising from the wrist and finger joints, soft tissue disorders around the forearm and wrist can also be managed using the Mulligan Concept. Intersection syndrome is a soft tissue disorder involving inflammation and swelling; it is due to friction between the abductor pollicis longus and extensor pollicis brevis and the underlying extensor carpi radialis longus and brevis. Symptoms include crepitus, tenderness, swelling and pain. In the Mulligan Concept, symptoms can be managed by unloading the soft tissues using tape. A recent case series of five patients with this syndrome found they were successfully managed using self-applied daily Mulligan Concept unloading tape (Kaneko & Takasaki, 2011). All patients were symptom-free and maintained that status in long-term follow-up.

Levels of evidence

Level 4: three case series, three case studies

There are two case studies of successful application of a phalangeal MWM of the metacarpophalangeal joint in patients who had pain and disability of long duration (4.5 and 28 weeks) (Folk, 2001; Hsieh et al., 2002). Both cases responded well to rotational glide MWMs, rather than transverse glides, which is perhaps an indication that rotation glides ought to be the first tried. Villafañe and colleagues (Villafañe et al., 2013) reported successful management of advanced trapeziometacarpal osteoarthritis with combined use of MWM and kinesiotape in a 53-year-old female patient. The 12-week intervention promoted a decrease in pain and an increase of thumb ROM and pressure pain threshold, which were maintained at the 4-month follow-up. MWM, in particular radial glide of the carpal bones, has also been shown to reduce pain and improve wrist ROM in a case series ($n=4$; Rabin et al., 2015) and a case report (Backstrom, 2002) of patients with de Quervain's tenosynovitis. Similarly, in a series of cases ($n=5$) the MWM-like tape for intersection syndrome applied daily for 3 weeks was shown to eliminate crepitus and swelling (Kaneko & Takasaki, 2011).

7

Although these reports represent a low level of evidence (level 4 on Oxford Centre for Evidence-Based Medicine Levels of Evidence (Howick et al., 2011)) these case descriptions provide some guidance for the clinician in the clinical reasoning processes used to manage pain and disability of the thumb and fingers. There is a need for higher-level evidence to substantiate these clinical observations.

7

DISTAL FOREARM / WRIST

Inferior radioulnar joint: pain or limitation of movement during pronation or supination

TECHNIQUE AT A GLANCE

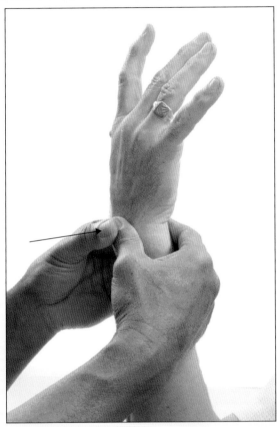

Figure 7.1
PA glide of the distal ulna with supination

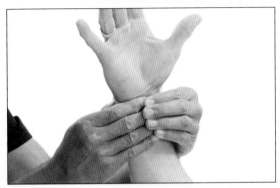

Figure 7.2
PA glide of the distal ulna: finger placement

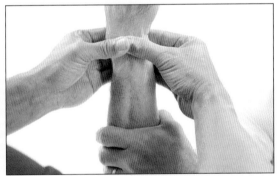

Figure 7.3
PA glide of the distal ulna with over-pressure into supination

- Stabilise the radius with fingertips on the anterior aspect of the distal aspect of the radius.
- Overlay the thumbs on the dorsal aspect of the distal end of the ulna.
- Glide the distal end of the ulna in a posteroanterior (PA) direction, with counterforce against the radius.
- Sustain the glide, while the patient performs slow repeated pronation or supination movement. The active movement must be performed slowly and also be pain-free.
- Over-pressure can be applied by the patient with their unaffected hand grasping the forearm proximal to the wrist.
- See Figs 7.1–7.3.

INDICATION

Pain or limitation of movement in the distal forearm/wrist during supination or pronation movement.

POSITIONING

Patient:	Sitting with the arm by the side, elbow flexed to 110°–130°, and hand relaxed.
Treated body part:	Forearm in mid pronation/supination position.
Therapist:	Standing at the side of patient.
Hands/contact points:	Stabilising hand: fingertips of the second to fifth fingers of each hand overlay on the anterior distal aspect of the radius.
	Gliding hand: thumbs of both hands overlay on the posterior (dorsal) aspect of the ulna (see Fig. 7.1).

APPLICATION GUIDELINES

- Stabilise the radius with fingertips on the anterior (volar) aspect of the distal aspect of the radius.
- Overlay the thumbs on the dorsal aspect of the distal end of the ulna.
- Glide the distal end of the ulna in a PA direction, with counterforce against the radius. The mobilisation must be pain-free.
- Sustain the glide, while the patient performs slow repeated pronation or supination movement. The active movement must be performed slowly and also be pain-free.
- Over-pressure can be applied by the patient with their unaffected hand grasping the forearm proximal to the wrist.
- Apply 6–10 repetitions in a set, with 3–5 sets in a treatment session, but only if there is a substantial increase in range or pain-free movement.

VARIATIONS

- In the event that a PA glide on the ulna is not effective, try a similar technique but with PA glide applied to the radius with relative fixation on the ulna (Fig. 7.4).

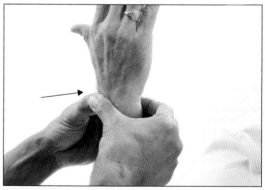

Figure 7.4
PA of the radius with pronation

COMMENTS

- The distal end of the ulna occupies one-third of the width of the distal forearm. Hence the thumbs must be on the lateral one-third of the ulnar side of the forearm.
- Use sponge rubber to reduce contact tenderness.
- The distal radioulnar joint is frequently injured within a Colles fracture (Colles, 2006), which is classically described as a fracture of the distal end of the radius. However, now the term tends to be used to describe any fracture of the distal portion of the radius with or without involvement of the ulna. Following a period of fixation for fractures, malalignment of the distal end of the radius frequently occurs. Sprains and strains of the distal forearm also result in painful loss of pronation, supination and loss of movement of the wrist.

7

SELF-MANAGEMENT

- The patient may be taught how to perform the PA glide on the ulna or the radius as an MWM home exercise.
- Glide the distal aspect of the ulna or radius in a PA direction using the fingertips of the patient's unaffected hand, while gliding the adjacent bone AP with their thumb. Sustain the glide while the movement is performed. The exercise and glide must be completely pain-free at all times.

TAPING

- Taping can be used to mimic the treatment and exercise technique, but be careful to avoid compressing the radius and ulna.
- Use 30-mm non-stretch sports tape or flexible tape at greater than 50% elongation. See the Introduction for the application of strapping tape.
- To achieve good tension on the tape it is advisable to lay the tape on with the forearm in mid-pronation / supination position, with maximum glide of the ulna maintained (Fig. 7.5).
- For a PA ulnar glide, start medially on the posterior aspect of the distal ulna, immediately proximal to the styloid process. Wrap the tape around the anterior aspect of the distal forearm while gliding the ulna in a PA direction. End the tape on the posterolateral aspect of the distal radius
- Reverse the tape direction for a PA radial glide.

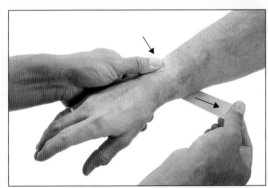

Figure 7.5A
Taping the inferior radioulnar joint for PA glide on the ulna: tape application

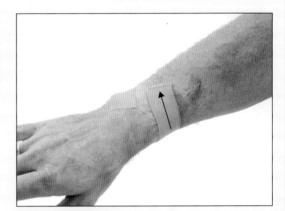

Figure 7.5B
Taping the inferior radioulnar joint for PA glide on the ulna: complete

ANNOTATIONS

sit R Inf RUJ Ulna Ant gl MWM Supin×6
sit R Inf RUJ Ulna Ant gl MWM Pron +OP×10(3)
sit R Inf RUJ Radius Ant gl MWM Supin×6
sit R inf RUJ Ulna self Ant gl MWM Supin×10
R Inf RUJ Ulna Ant gl tape

Carpal lateral glide for non-weight-bearing wrist flexion and extension

TECHNIQUE AT A GLANCE

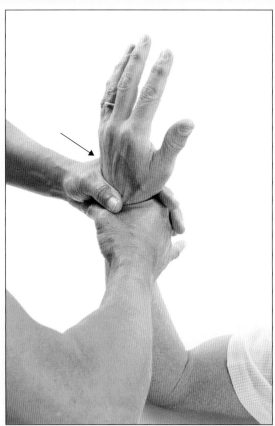

Figure 7.6
Carpal lateral glide with active non-weight-bearing wrist extension: start position

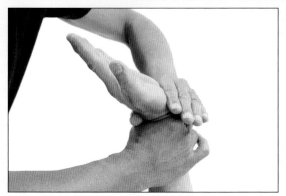

Figure 7.7
Carpal lateral glide with active non-weight-bearing wrist extension: end position

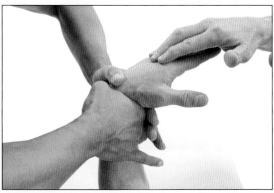

Figure 7.8
Carpal lateral glide with active non-weight-bearing wrist flexion: end position over-pressure

- Position the forearm in neutral pronation/supination.
- The therapist stabilises the lateral aspect of the distal radius using the first web-space.
- Glide the proximal row of carpal bones laterally (towards the thumb) using the first web-space of the other hand, following the joint line.
- Maintain the glide while the patient actively moves the wrist into flexion or extension.
- The patient applies over-pressure as required.
- See Figs 7.6–7.8.

INDICATION

Painful and/or restricted wrist joint flexion or extension; symptoms associated with wrist movement.

POSITIONING

Patient:	Sitting with elbow supported and flexed to 90°, forearm in mid pronation.
Treated body part:	Wrist in neutral flexion/extension position.
Therapist:	Standing facing the patient's forearm.
Hand/contact points:	Stabilising hand: first web-space contacts the lateral aspect of the radius. Mobilising hand: first web-space contacts the medial aspect of the proximal row of carpal bones.

APPLICATION GUIDELINES

- Stabilise the distal end of the radius on the lateral side.
- Apply the lateral glide on the proximal row of the carpal bones.
- Keep your hands as open as possible to avoid limiting the range of the aggravating movement.
- While sustaining the glide ask the patient to do the aggravating movement.
- It may be necessary to make slight adjustments to the direction and force of the glide to ensure a pain-free movement.
- Apply 6–10 repetitions in a set and 3–5 sets in a treatment session.
- Over-pressure may be applied to the movement; this is applied by the patient. Ensure the pressure is applied through the hand and not the fingers.

COMMENTS

- It is important that when performing MWMs on the smaller joints (i.e. forearm/wrist/fingers) the patient needs to move slowly to enable the therapist to maintain the translation/accessory glide. If the aforementioned is lost with too-rapid movement, pain may be felt and the therapist may discard the treatment though it is really the treatment of choice.
- If pain and movement are not improved with a lateral glide, then modify with subtle changes of direction.
- The patient's forearm supination/pronation position may be varied according to the clinical presentation.
- Alternative start positions can be used. Place the patient's forearm on the treatment table with the hand extending over the edge of the table. Apply the glide as before and ask the patient to repeat the limited movement.
- If pain increases with a lateral glide, change to medial glide. If it is still painful reposition the inferior radioulnar joint as above, (ulnar ventral on radius) and check active wrist movement again.
- These techniques may also be useful when managing patients with carpal tunnel syndrome, wrist tendonitis and when rehabilitating patients following immobilisation for wrist fracture.

(continued next page...)

SELF-MANAGEMENT

- If a carpal gliding technique was successful in improving wrist flexion or extension then trial a self-glide technique.
- The patient fixes their arm by their side and applies a lateral glide of the carpal bones with the fingertips or web-space of the opposite hand.
- While sustaining the glide force the patient repeats wrist movement to the onset of pain only, performing 10 repetitions in a session, with 3–5 sessions in a day (Fig. 7.9).

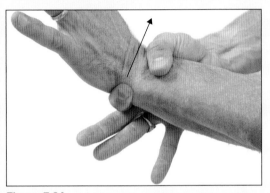

Figure 7.9A
Wrist self-treatment: lateral glide for wrist flexion and extension – extension

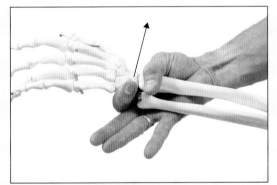

Figure 7.9B
Wrist self-treatment: lateral glide for wrist flexion and extension – model view

TAPING

- If a carpal gliding technique was successful in improving wrist movement then trial taping.
- Depending on the size of the wrist, use 20-mm non-stretch sports tape or flexible tape at greater than 50% elongation. See the Introduction for the application of strapping tape.
- Start the tape on the medial aspect of the proximal row of the carpal bones. While applying tension to the tape, spiral around the ventral and dorsal aspect of the distal forearm; end the tape over the distal aspect of the radius (Fig. 7.10).

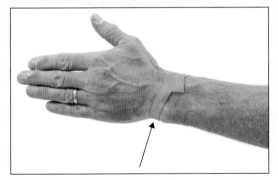

Figure 7.10
Taping for lateral carpal glide for wrist flexion and extension

ANNOTATIONS

sit R Wr Lat gl MWM E×3
sit R Wr Lat gl MWM F +OP×6(3)
st L Wr self Lat gl MWM E×6
L Wr Lat gl tape

Carpal medial glide for non-weight-bearing wrist flexion and extension

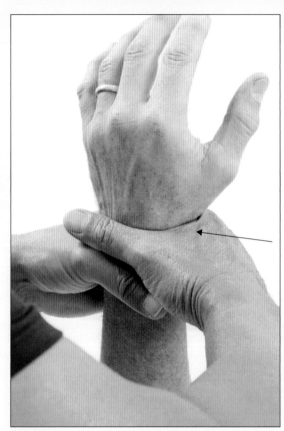

Figure 7.11
Carpal medial glide with wrist extension: start position

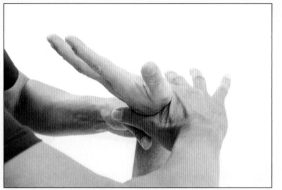

Figure 7.12
Carpal medial glide with wrist extension: end position

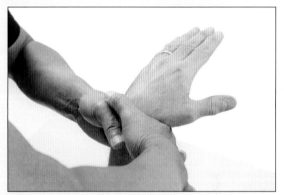

Figure 7.13
Carpal medial glide with wrist flexion: end position

- The patient positions the forearm in neutral pronation/supination.
- The therapist stabilises the medial aspect of the distal ulna using the first web-space.
- Glide the proximal row of carpal bones medially (away from the thumb) using the first web-space of the other hand, following the joint line.
- Maintain the glide while the patient actively moves the wrist into flexion or extension.
- Patient applies over-pressure as required.
- See Figs 7.11–7.13.

INDICATION

Painful and/or restricted wrist joint flexion or extension.

POSITIONING

Patient:	Sitting with elbow supported and flexed to 90°, forearm in mid pronation.
Treated body part:	Wrist neutral flexion/extension position.
Therapist:	Standing facing the patient's forearm.
Hand/contact points:	Stabilising hand: first web-space contacts the medial aspect of the distal ulna.
	Mobilising hand: first web-space contacts the lateral aspect of the proximal row of carpal bones.

APPLICATION GUIDELINES

- Stabilise the distal end of the ulna on the medial side.
- Apply the medial glide on the proximal row of the carpal bones.
- Keep your hands as open as possible to avoid limiting the range of the aggravating movement.
- While sustaining the glide ask the patient to do the aggravating movement.
- It may be necessary to make slight adjustments to the direction and force of the glide to ensure a pain-free movement.
- Apply 6–10 repetitions in a set and 3–5 sets in a treatment session.
- Over-pressure may be applied to the movement; this is applied by the patient. Ensure the pressure is applied through the hand and not the fingers.

COMMENTS

- If pain and movement is not improved with a medial glide, then modify with subtle changes of direction.
- The patient's forearm supination/pronation position may be varied according to the clinical presentation.
- Alternative start positions can be used. Place the patient's forearm on the treatment table with their hand extending over the edge of the table. Apply the glide as before and ask the patient to repeat the limited movement.
- If pain increases with a medial glide, change to a lateral glide. If it is still painful, reposition the inferior radioulnar joint as above (ulnar ventral on radius) and check active wrist movement again.
- These techniques may also be useful when managing patients with carpal tunnel syndrome or wrist tendonitis and when rehabilitating patients following immobilisation for wrist fracture.

7

SELF-MANAGEMENT

- If a carpal gliding technique is successful to improve wrist flexion or extension then trial a self-glide technique.
- The patient fixes their arm by their side, resting their pronated forearm on a table, and applies a medial glide of the carpal bones with the fingertips or web-space of the opposite hand.
- While sustaining the glide force the patient repeats wrist movement to the onset of pain only, performing 10 repetitions in a session, with 3–5 sessions in a day (Fig. 7.14).

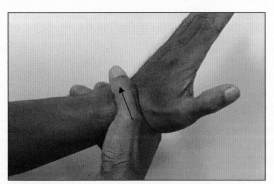

Figure 7.14A
Wrist self-treatment: medial glide for flexion and extension – extension

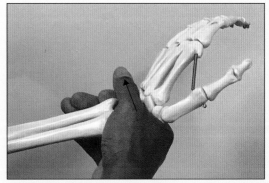

Figure 7.14B
Wrist self-treatment: medial glide for flexion and extension – extension model view

TAPING

- If a carpal gliding technique was successful in improving wrist movement then trial taping (Fig. 7.15).
- Depending on the size of the wrist, use 20-mm non-stretch sports tape or flexible tape at greater than 50% elongation. See the Introduction for general guidelines when applying strapping tape.
- Start the tape on the lateral aspect of the proximal row of the carpal bones. While applying tension to the tape, spiral around the ventral and dorsal aspects of the distal forearm; end the tape over the distal aspect of the ulna.

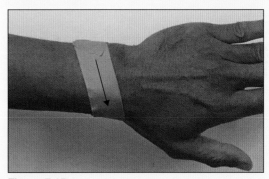

Figure 7.15
Taping for medial carpal glide for wrist flexion and extension

ANNOTATIONS

sit L Wr Med gl MWM F×3
sit L Wr Med gl MWM E +OP×6(3)
sit R Wr self Med gl MWM E×10(3)
R Wr Med gl tape

Carpal lateral glide for weight-bearing wrist extension

TECHNIQUE AT A GLANCE

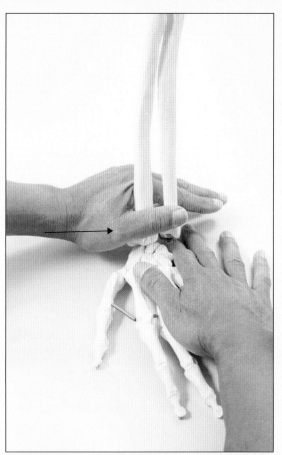

Figure 7.16
Carpal lateral glide for weight-bearing wrist extension:
model view

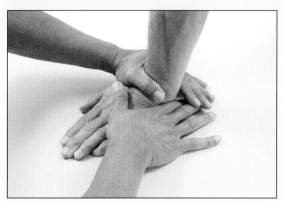

Figure 7.17
Carpal lateral glide for weight-bearing wrist extension:
end position

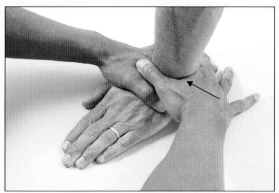

Figure 7.18
Carpal medial glide for weight-bearing wrist
extension: end position

- The patient stands with their palm on a treatment table, fingers pointing towards the therapist, and forearm in pronation (in this case the patient's left hand).
- The therapist contacts the radius or ulna with one hand.
- Stabilise the carpal bones with the opposite hand by applying stabilisation towards the thumb or conversely the little finger, using the first web-space of the other hand and following the joint line.
- Apply a glide of the radius and ulna (relative glide of the carpal bones) while the patient leans on their hand, extending the wrist.
- Patient is applying over-pressure by leaning into extension.
- See Fig. 7.16–7.18.

INDICATION

Painful and/or restricted wrist joint extension in weight-bearing.

POSITIONING

Patient:	Standing.
Treated body part:	Hand resting on the table and wrist extended.
Therapist:	Standing facing the patient's hand.
Hand/contact points:	Stabilising hand: the first web-space of the therapist's hand contacts the carpal row on the medial/ulnar side or lateral/radial side. Mobilising hand: glides the radius and ulna (creating a relative glide of the carpal bones).

APPLICATION GUIDELINES

- Stabilise the hand on the table.
- Apply the medial or lateral glide on the radius and ulna (relative lateral or medial glide of the carpal bones).
- While sustaining the glide ask the therapist to lean on their hand and extend their wrist.
- It may be necessary to make slight adjustments to the direction and force of the glide to ensure a pain-free movement.
- Apply 6–10 repetitions in a set and 3–5 sets in a treatment session.
- Over-pressure is applied by the patient leaning onto their hand.

COMMENTS

- If pain and movement are not improved with a lateral carpal glide, modify with subtle changes of direction.
- The patient's forearm supination/pronation position may be varied according to the clinical presentation.
- If pain increases with a lateral carpal glide, change to a medial carpal glide. If it is still painful, reposition the inferior radioulnar joint as above (ulnar ventral on radius) and check active wrist movement again.

7

(continued next page...)

SELF-MANAGEMENT

- If a carpal gliding technique was successful in improving weight-bearing wrist extension then trial a self-glide technique.
- The patient applies a relative lateral or medial glide of the carpal bones by gliding the radius and ulna medially or laterally using their hand or a thin strap (Fig. 7.19).
- While sustaining the glide the patient leans onto their hand resting on a folded towel, extending their wrist, and keeping the fingers flexed.
- To be effective the movement has to be pain-free during the exercise.
- Repeat 10 times in a session, with 3–5 sessions a day provided there is no pain.

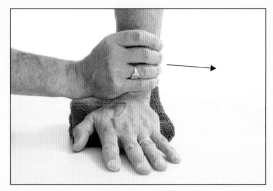

Figure 7.19A
Wrist self-treatment for weight-bearing wrist extension: lateral glide

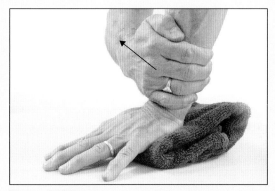

Figure 7.19B
Wrist self-treatment for weight-bearing wrist extension: medial glide

ANNOTATION

st WB L Hand L Wr Lat gl MWM E×6(3)
st WB L Hand L Wr self Lat gl MWM E×6(3)
st WB L Hand L Wr self Med gl MWM E×6(3)

Carpal rotation for wrist flexion and extension

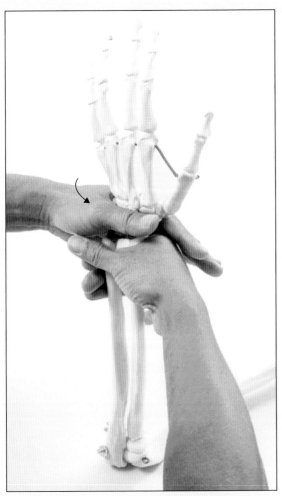

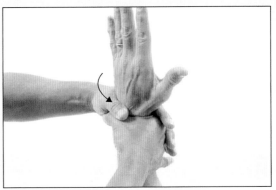

Figure 7.21
Carpal internal rotation for extension or flexion

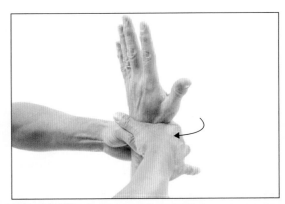

Figure 7.20
Carpal internal rotation for flexion: model view

Figure 7.22
Carpal external rotation for extension or flexion

- The patient is seated with the elbow resting on a treatment table.
- The therapist stabilises the distal radius and ulna from the lateral/radial side using the web-space between the thumb and index finger.
- The other hand grasps the medial aspect of the proximal carpal row using the web-space between the thumb and index finger.
- The proximal carpal row is internally rotated (pronated) or externally rotated (supinated).
- While the glide is sustained the patient flexes or extends the wrist.
- See Figs 7.20–7.22.

INDICATION

Limitation of wrist flexion or extension movement due to pain or stiffness of the carpal joints.

POSITIONING

Patient:	Sitting.
Treated body part:	Elbow flexed and resting on a treatment table.
Therapist:	Standing facing the patient's forearm.
Hand / contact points:	Stabilising hand: the web-space between thumb and index finger on the distal radius from the lateral / radial side.
	Gliding hand: grasp the medial aspect / ulnar side of the proximal carpal row with the web-space between the thumb and index finger.

APPLICATION GUIDELINES

- Stabilise the distal end of the radius and ulna.
- Apply the internal carpal rotation (pronation) or external carpal rotation (supination).
- Keep your hands as open as possible to avoid limiting the range of the aggravating movement.
- While sustaining the glide ask the patient to do the aggravating movement.
- It may be necessary to make slight adjustments to the direction and force of the glide to ensure a pain-free movement.
- Provided the movement is pain-free, ask the patient to repeat it.
- Apply 6–10 repetitions in a set and 3–5 sets in a treatment session.
- Over-pressure may be applied to the movement; this is applied by the patient. Ensure the pressure is applied through the hand and not the fingers.
- If one carpal rotation is not effective then try the opposite rotation.

VARIATIONS

- An alternative position to apply carpal rotation for wrist extension is shown in Fig. 7.23.

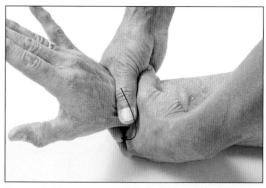

Figure 7.23
Alternative position to apply carpal rotation for wrist extension

COMMENTS

- Ensure that the stabilising hand and gliding hand are as close to the joint line as possible. If the therapist's hand position is correct, their hands should be touching.
- Ensure that only the web-spaces, thumbs and index fingers are in contact with the patient's wrist. This is to avoid limiting the ROM.

SELF-MANAGEMENT

- If a carpal rotation technique was successful in improving wrist extension or flexion then trial a self-rotation glide technique.
- For internal rotation, with the elbow flexed to 90° and the forearm pronated, the patient grasps the distal end of the radius with the thumb, and the carpal bones with the index finger applying an internal rotation glide.
- While sustaining the glide the patient repeats the restricted movement (wrist flexion or extension) (Fig. 7.24A).
- For external rotation, with the elbow flexed to 90° and the forearm supinated, the patient grasps the distal end of the ulna with the index finger, and the carpal bones with the thumb, applying an external rotation glide.
- While sustaining the glide the patient repeats the restricted movement (wrist flexion or extension) (Fig. 7.24B).
- Repeat 10 times in a session, with 3–5 sessions a day provided there is no pain.

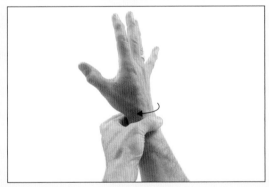

Figure 7.24A
Carpal rotation for wrist flexion or extension: internal rotation

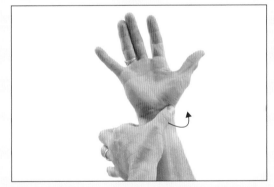

Figure 7.24B
Carpal rotation for wrist flexion or extension: external rotation

(continued next page...)

TAPING

- If a carpal rotation technique was successful in improving wrist movement then trial taping.
- Depending on the size of the wrist, use 20-mm non-stretch sports tape or flexible tape at greater than 50% elongation.
- Start the tape on the posterior aspect of the wrist over the proximal carpal row. Then apply the external rotation glide. Spiral the tape around the medial aspect of the wrist; end the tape over the distal anterior aspect of the forearm (Fig. 7.25A). Reverse the direction for the internal rotation (Fig. 7.25B).
- To achieve good tension on the tape it is advisable to lay the tape on the proximal row of the carpal bones. While applying the rotation, have the patient spiral the tape around the wrist.

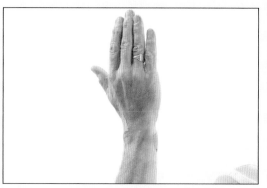

Figure 7.25A
Taping for carpal rotation for wrist flexion and extension: internal carpal rotation posterior view

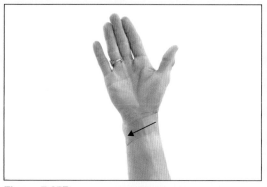

Figure 7.25B
Taping for carpal rotation for wrist flexion and extension: internal carpal rotation anterior view

ANNOTATIONS

sit L Wr IR MWM F×6
sit L Wr ER MWM E +OP×10(3)
sit R Wr self IR MWM F×10
sit R Wr self IR MWM E×10
sit R Wr self ER MWM F×10
sit R Wr self ER MWM E×10
R Wr IR tape
R Wr ER tape

Scaphoid PA or AP glide non-weight-bearing

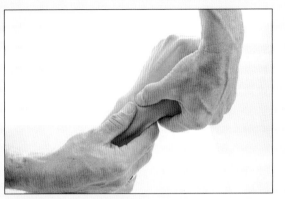

Figure 7.27
Scaphoid PA glide: start position

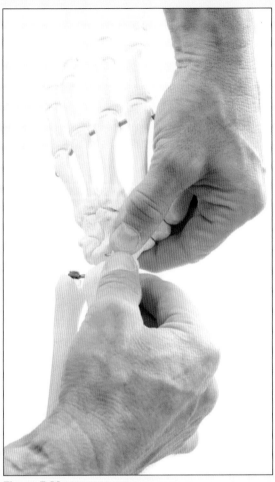

Figure 7.26
Scaphoid PA glide: model view

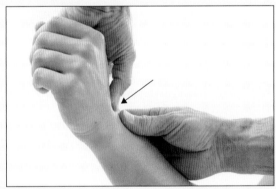

Figure 7.28
Scaphoid PA glide: mid-range extension

- The patient is sitting with the forearm resting on a treatment table.
- The therapist stabilises the distal end of the radius with the fingertips of the index finger and thumb of one hand.
- The scaphoid is mobilised by the thumb and tip of the index finger of the opposite hand.
- The scaphoid glide is in a posteroanterior (PA) or anteroposterior (AP) direction.
- While the glide is sustained the patient does the symptomatic movement (usually wrist extension).
- See Figs 7.26–7.28.

INDICATION

Limitation of wrist extension movement due to local pain over the scaphoid.

POSITIONING

Patient:	Sitting with the forearm pronated and fully supported on a treatment table.
Therapist:	Standing adjacent to the affected wrist.
Hand/contact points:	Stabilising hand: index finger and thumb of one hand stabilise the distal ventral and dorsal aspect of the radius.
	Gliding hand: index finger and thumb of the opposite hand contact the proximal end of the scaphoid.

APPLICATION GUIDELINES

- Apply a PA or an AP glide of the scaphoid relative to the radius.
- Sustain this glide and have the patient repeat the wrist extension movement.
- It may be necessary to make slight adjustments to the direction and force of the glide to ensure a pain-free movement.
- Apply 6–10 repetitions in a set and 3–5 sets in a treatment session.
- If the pain remains unchanged or increases with one glide, apply the opposite glide.

VARIATIONS

- If these scaphoid techniques are not effective the therapist should also consider performing the technique to the trapezium in a similar fashion.
- The scaphoid PA or AP glide can be applied in a weight-bearing position (Fig. 7.29).
- While the glide is sustained the patient weight-bears through the hand, taking the wrist into extension.

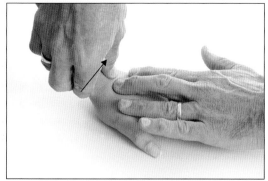

Figure 7.29
Scaphoid PA in weight-bearing wrist extension

COMMENTS

- Ensure that the glide is sustained throughout the movement and on return to the start position.

ANNOTATIONS

sit L Scaphoid Ant gl MWM Wr E×6
sit L Scaphoid Ant gl MWM Wr F +OP×10(3)
st WB L Hand L Scaphoid Ant gl MWM Wr E×6
st WB L Hand L Scaphoid Post gl MWM Wr E×10(3)

7

HAND

Metacarpal PA and AP glide with fist clenching

TECHNIQUE AT A GLANCE

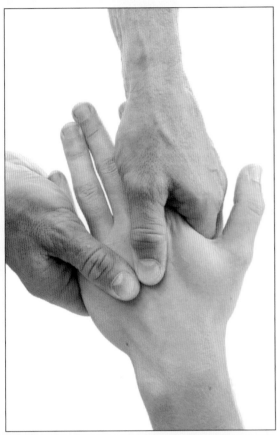

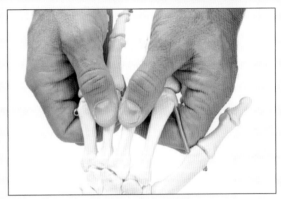

Figure 7.31
PA glide of the metacarpals with fist clenching: model view

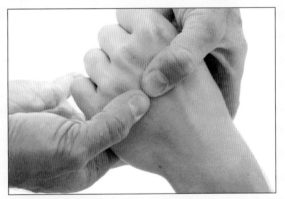

Figure 7.32
PA glide of the metacarpals with fist clenching: end position

Figure 7.30
PA glide of the metacarpals with fist clenching: start position

- The patient sits comfortably with forearm pronated, hand relaxed.
- The therapist faces the patient and supports their hand.
- The therapist stabilises the third or fourth metacarpal between the index finger and thumb of one hand while gliding the fourth or fifth metacarpal with the index finger and thumb of the other hand.
- Glide in an AP or PA direction.
- Maintain the glide while the patient makes a fist.
- See Figs 7.30–7.32.

INDICATION

Pain in the metacarpal region during gripping activities or making a fist.

POSITIONING

Patient:	Sitting with the elbow flexed to 90° and forearm pronated.
Treated body part:	Hand relaxed.
Therapist:	Facing towards the patient.
Hands/contact points:	Stabilising hand: index and thumb fix the proximal aspect of the adjacent metacarpal.
	Gliding hand: index finger and thumb glide the proximal aspect of the affected metacarpal (usually the fourth or fifth) in an AP or PA direction.

APPLICATION GUIDELINES

- Grasp the proximal third of the affected metacarpal between the thumb and index finger (e.g. fourth or fifth) while the adjacent metacarpal is stabilised between the thumb and index finger of the other hand.
- Glide the affected metacarpal in an AP or PA pain-free direction.
- Sustain the glide, while the patient performs repeated gripping movements. The active movement must also be pain-free.
- Apply 6–10 repetitions in a set, with 3–5 sets in a treatment session, but only if there is a substantial increase in range or gripping force.

COMMENTS

- Ensure that the stabilising and mobilising hand has a broad contact point to reduce local tenderness. Additionally the contact can be adjusted more proximally or distally as needed.
- Use sponge rubber to reduce contact tenderness.

SELF-MANAGEMENT

- The patient may be taught how to perform the MWM as a home exercise by gliding the proximal aspect of the affected metacarpal in an AP or PA direction using the index finger and thumb of their unaffected hand.
- Glide direction is dependent on the direction found to be effective in the therapist technique.
- If the AP is not effective then a PA glide can be trialled.

ANNOTATIONS

sit L 5th on 4th MC Ant gl MWM fist×6
sit L 4th on 3rd MC Ant gl MWM fist×6(3)
sit L 5th on 4th MC Post gl MWM fist×10(3)
sit L 4th on 3rd MC Post gl MWM fist×6(3)

FINGER – PROXIMAL INTERPHALANGEAL (PIP) JOINT PAIN AND / OR RESTRICTION

Finger PIP joint pain / restriction with flexion manual lateral / medial glide

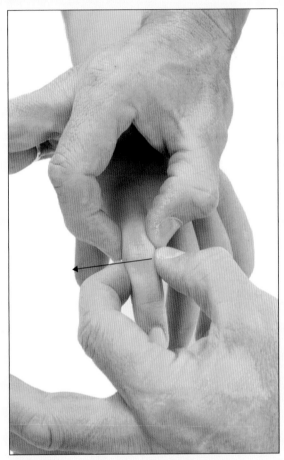

Figure 7.33
Proximal interphalangeal (PIP) joint lateral glide with flexion: start position

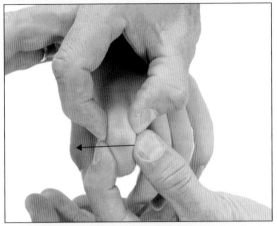

Figure 7.34
Proximal interphalangeal joint lateral glide with flexion: end position

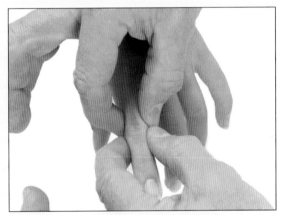

Figure 7.35
Proximal interphalangeal joint lateral glide with extension: end position

- The distal end of the proximal phalanx is stabilised with thumb and finger.
- A glide of the proximal end of the middle phalanx is applied laterally or medially and painlessly with the therapist's other hand.
- While the glide is sustained, the patient slowly flexes or extends the joint.
- When the end of active range is reached, the patient applies pain-free over-pressure on the middle phalanx.
- See Figs 7.33–7.35.

INDICATION

Painful and/or restricted PIP or distal interphalangeal (DIP) joint flexion or extension.

POSITIONING

Patient:	Sitting.
Treated body part:	Relaxed resting position; elbow or forearm may be resting on a treatment table.
Therapist:	May sit or stand as is comfortable.
Hands/contact points:	Stabilising hand: thumb and index finger contacting the medial and lateral aspects of the distal end of the phalanx.
	Gliding hand: thumb and index finger contacting the medial and lateral aspects of the proximal end of the adjacent phalanx.

APPLICATION GUIDELINES

- Apply a lateral or medial glide across the PIP or DIP joint parallel to the treatment plane.
- While sustaining the glide, have the patient repeat the provocative movement, which should now be pain-free.
- Have the patient apply over-pressure on the adjacent phalanx when pain-free end range is reached.
- Apply 6–10 repetitions in a set, with 3–5 sets in a treatment session.

VARIATIONS

- Medial and lateral glides can also be combined with rotation if required.
- Apply an internal rotation of the middle phalanx relative to the proximal phalanx before applying a medial or lateral glide.
- While sustaining the internal rotation and glide, have the patient repeat the provocative movement, which should now be pain-free (Fig. 7.36).

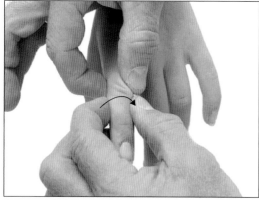

Figure 7.36A
Proximal interphalangeal joint manual internal/external rotation with flexion: external

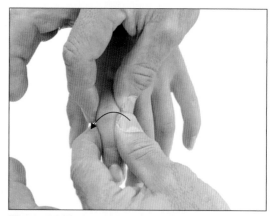

Figure 7.36B
Proximal interphalangeal joint manual internal/external rotation with flexion: internal

COMMENTS

- Instruct the patient to move slowly when actively flexing the finger so you are able to sustain the correct glide effectively throughout the motion, including over-pressure, until the patient returns the joint out of the previously provocative range.
- If a lateral glide increases the symptoms, change to a medial glide.
- If a lateral glide decreases but does not clear symptoms, vary the direction (include rotation) and force subtly until the pain-free mobilisation is found that clears the pain and restores full motion with over-pressure.

SELF-MANAGEMENT

- The patient applies the glide or rotation mobilisation that the therapist has found to be pain-free
- Rotation is achieved by mobilising the middle phalanx relative to the proximal phalanx with the first three digits of their free hand rotating the phalanx internally or externally while concurrently flexing or extending the joint.
- Glide is achieved through the thumb and index finger on adjacent phalanx.
- While sustaining the mobilisation, the patient repeats the now pain-free provocative movement.
- The patient applies over-pressure on the middle phalanx when pain-free end range is reached.
- Apply 6–10 repetitions in a set, with 3–5 sets in a treatment session (see Fig. 7.37).

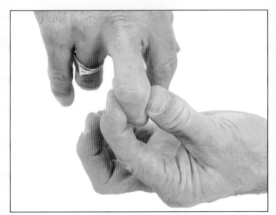

Figure 7.37A
Finger self-management: rotation

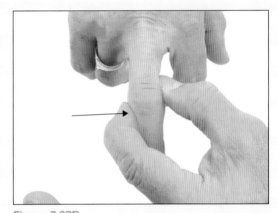

Figure 7.37B
Finger self-management: glide

(continued next page...)

TAPING

- Apply a 1-cm width strip of tape to the dorsal mid shaft of the middle phalanx at an angle from distal to proximal.
- Grip, over the tape, the medial and lateral sides of the shaft of the middle phalanx and apply the medial rotation.
- With the other hand, pull the tape obliquely around the ventral shaft of the proximal phalanx and affix to the skin.
- Re-test the provocative movement, which should now be less painful and have improved ROM.
- For lateral rotation apply the tape in the opposite direction.
- A medial or lateral glide can be achieved by applying both internal and external rotation (Fig. 7.38).

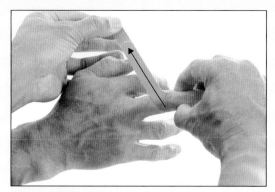

Figure 7.38A
Taping fingers: rotation application

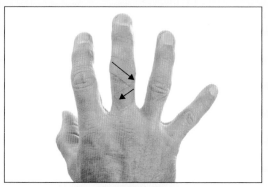

Figure 7.38B
Taping fingers: lateral glide completed

ANNOTATIONS

sit L Index PIP Lat gl MWM F×6
sit L Index PIP Lat gl MWM E +OP×6
sit R Index PIP Med gl MWM F +OP×10(5)
sit R Index PIP self IR MWM F×6
sit R Index PIP self Lat gl MWM F +OP×10(5)
R Index PIP ER tape
R Index PIP Lat gl tape

References

Backstrom, K.M., 2002. Mobilization with movement as an adjunct intervention in a patient with complicated de Quervain's tenosynovitis: a case report. J. Orthop. Sports Phys. Ther. 32 (3), 86–94, discussion -7.

Colles, A., 2006. On fracture of the carpal extremity of the radius. Clin. Orthop. Relat. Res. 445, 5–7. (Orig. pub. 1814 Edinburg. Med. Surg. J. 10, 181.)

Folk, B., 2001. Traumatic thumb injury management using mobilization with movement. Man. Ther. 6 (3), 178–182.

Howick, J., Chalmers, I., Glasziou, P., Greenhalgh, T., Heneghan, C., Liberati, A., et al., 2011. The Oxford Levels of Evidence 2. Oxford Centre for Evidence-Based Medicine, Oxford.

Hsieh, C.Y., Vicenzino, B., Yang, C.H., Hu, M.H., Yang, C., 2002. Mulligan's mobilization with movement for the thumb: a single case report using magnetic resonance imaging to evaluate the positional fault hypothesis. Man. Ther. 7 (1), 44–49.

Kaneko, S., Takasaki, H., 2011. Forearm pain, diagnosed as intersection syndrome, managed by taping: a case series. J. Orthop. Sports Phys. Ther. 41 (7), 514–519.

Rabin, A., Israeli, T., Kozol, Z., 2015. Physiotherapy management of people diagnosed with de Quervain's disease: a case series. Physiother. Can. 67 (3), 263–267.

Villafañe, J.H., Langford, D., Alguacil-Diego, I.M., Fernández-Carnero, J., 2013. Management of trapeziometacarpal osteoarthritis pain and dysfunction using mobilization with movement technique in combination with kinesiology tape: a case report. J. Chiropr. Med. 12 (2), 79–86.

Thoracic spine and rib cage

TECHNIQUES FOR THORACIC SPINE AND RIB CAGE

THORACIC SPINE
Thoracic traction with a belt
   Thoracic spine self-traction
Thoracic SNAG central (and unilateral) for flexion, extension, lateral flexion or rotation
   Thoracic SNAG – central for flexion
   Unilateral thoracic SNAG
   Unilateral thoracic SNAG for extension, lateral flexion and rotation
   Thoracic self-SNAG for extension, rotation and lateral flexion
   Taping in acute thoracic pain scenarios

THORAX – RIB AND SPINE
Upper and lower rib MWM
   Unilateral
   Bilateral
   Rib MWM using thumbs combined with shoulder elevation
Costovertebral MWM for first or second rib

INTRODUCTION

The thoracic spine is rendered relatively stiff when compared with the rest of the spine because of the rib cage, associated ligaments and relatively thin, rigid intervertebral disc. The ribs attach to the spine through the strong radiate ligament, binding each rib to adjacent vertebral bodies and the intervertebral disc. Each rib articulates at the costovertebral, the costotransverse and in the case of some ribs the costosternal joints. Hence movement of the spine cannot be considered without movement of the ribs and sternum. Despite this complexity, the thoracic cage is still capable of substantial movement, with key movements of rotation, extension and respiration (Edmondston & Singer, 1997).

The precise incidence of thoracic spine pain is poorly understood (Edmondston et al., 2007), but is believed to account for approximately 10% of spinal pain disorders in the general population (Briggs et al., 2009). In contrast, rib pain is less common, accounting for less than 2% of patients seen in clinical practice (Hinkley & Drysdale, 1995). Despite the lower prevalence of thoracic spine pain compared with other regions of the spine, disability associated with thoracic spine disorders is at least comparable with pain disorders of the lumbar spine (Occhipinti et al., 1993).

The thoracic spine is a relatively forgotten region of the spine, particularly with respect to research evidence regarding the efficacy of manual therapy for thoracic pain disorders. In contrast there is a growing body of knowledge confirming the importance of the thoracic spine in regard to shoulder pain disorders (Mintken et al., 2010; Norlander & Nordgren, 1998; Sobel et al., 1996) and mechanical neck pain (Cross et al., 2011).

One explanation for this is that the thoracic spine is a region of interdependence (Strunce et al., 2009) contributing to movement of the shoulder and the neck. Indeed, Crosbie and colleagues (Crosbie et al., 2008) reported a strong contribution of movement from the thoracic spine during arm elevation. Hence lack of movement in the thoracic spine may perpetuate a pain disorder in the shoulder and neck and vice versa. Mulligan Concept techniques are well suited to address movement impairment in the thorax as they can be directed to an individual segment in the spine or to any rib.

In the Mulligan Concept there is the potential to explore the contribution that thoracic spine movement impairment contributes to a range of thoracic and cervical spine, shoulder and arm pain disorders as the effects can be immediately evaluated. An example of this is the spinal mobilisation with arm movement (SMWAM) technique. As just stated, shoulder movement in all directions induces movement of the thoracic spine (Crosbie et al., 2008) and neck (Takasaki et al., 2009). Improvement in shoulder or neck movement as a result of a SMWAM technique can be immediately judged and the technique modified accordingly. There is evidence that segmentally directed mobilisation of the spine improves shoulder pain and movement impairment (McClatchie et al., 2009). The value of this technique is that the impact of the technique can be judged immediately and painlessly.

From a pragmatic perspective in the application of Mulligan Concept techniques in the thoracic spine and ribs, the placement and direction of the manual force will vary according to the region of the thoracic spine being treated. The relationship of spinous and transverse processes varies slightly across the thoracic spine, but one study indicated that for the vertebral levels T1–10 the transverse process was approximately level with the spinous process of the vertebral level above (Geelhoed et al., 2006). Knowledge of the orientation of the facet joints will help the practitioner's initial decision of the direction of the applied manual glide. The orientation of the facet in the sagittal plane increases in pitch from approximately 60° upwards from the transverse plane at the upper thoracic spine to 70° in the low thoracic spine (Williams et al., 1989).

Although the following describe specific start positions of the patient, thorax and therapist, there will be many times when there needs to be variations to these in order to match the patient's presentation.

Levels of evidence

Level 4: one case series and one case report

A recent case series (*n*=7) demonstrated the efficacy of thoracic SNAG in reducing pain during active shoulder abduction in subjects classified with secondary impingement syndrome (Andrews et al., 2018). Further, this group demonstrated significant decrease in pain (measured by NRS) during resisted external rotation of the shoulder and active abduction both immediately and 48 hours post-intervention (Andrews et al., 2018).

A single case report describes the favourable response of a 20-year-old male university student who presented with an unusual case of acute left-side thoracic pain with a list of the spine (Horton, 2002). At the first session a

SNAG (T8) was applied several times to alleviate the spinal list, which it did. The first session was completed after some tape was applied to maintain the improvement in spinal posture. The patient reported a 95% improvement in his condition at the second visit 24 hours later. This is an example of the degree of improvement expected initially and afterwards. Though this constitutes level 4 evidence, it does provide a description of an actual case that will assist practitioners in the application of the MWM concept. There is no other higher-level evidence on MWM at the thoracic spine.

8

THORACIC SPINE

Thoracic traction with a belt

TECHNIQUE AT A GLANCE

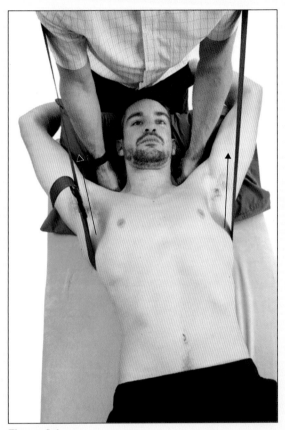

Figure 8.1
Thoracic traction using a belt with hands above head

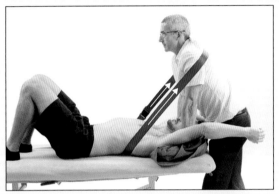

Figure 8.2
Thoracic traction using a belt with hands above head: side view

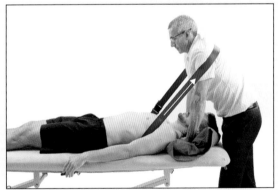

Figure 8.3
Thoracic traction variation

- The patient is supine on a treatment couch.
- A manual therapy belt is positioned under the patient's thoracic spine to align at the level of the spinous process of the superior vertebra of the offending motion segment. The belt is then looped around the therapist's shoulders.
- The patient elevates the shoulders to place them in a relaxed position above the head.
- The therapist, with fists that are clenched and placed to the side of the patient's head, gently pivots on his arms and leans backwards to generate a traction effect with the belt around the patient's thorax.
- This traction effect can be sustained for several seconds and should create pain relief for the patient.
- See Figs 8.1–8.3.

INDICATION

Thoracic pain at rest, in single or multiple directions of movement and/or upon deep breathing.

POSITIONING

Patient:	Lying supine, shoulders level with the end of the couch.
Treated body part:	Thoracic spine relaxed with arms elevated and resting to move the scapulae laterally away from the spine.
Therapist:	Standing at the head of the treatment couch.
Hands/contact points:	A manual therapy belt is positioned under the patient's thoracic spine, looped around the spinous process of the superior vertebra of the symptomatic motion segment. The manual therapy belt is then looped around the upper thorax of the therapist. The therapist positions their clenched hands on the treatment couch maintaining slightly flexed elbows. Here the hands can be placed beside the patient's head or beside their armpits. The therapist now gently leans backwards creating a traction effect through to the patient's thoracic spine. The therapist uses their clenched hands on the couch to provide a fulcrum effect to generate the traction force.

APPLICATION GUIDELINES

- Apply sustained traction with the belt, which can be maintained for more than 10 seconds.
- While sustaining the traction force, the patient should experience relief of their symptoms.
- Apply several repetitions in a treatment session, but only if there is a substantial increase in pain-free movement or breathing following the application of the technique and no latent pain responses.

COMMENTS

- The duration and degree of traction force can be altered according to the patient's response.
- This technique may be applied for vertebral levels from T4 to T12.

VARIATIONS

- For some patients, positioning the knees and hips in flexion makes the technique more comfortable.
- Placing the patient's arms by their side may reduce the degree of thoracic extension, which may be preferable for some.

SELF-MANAGEMENT

- The patient stands at the edge of a kitchen bench or a table.
- The patient places each hand on the bench edge.
- The patient slowly takes their body weight by flexing the knees so that the body weight is taken through the arms with extended elbows.
- The shoulder girdle is relaxed also so that the thoracic spine musculature is relaxed and the traction effect will be translated through the thoracic area.
- See Fig. 8.4.

8

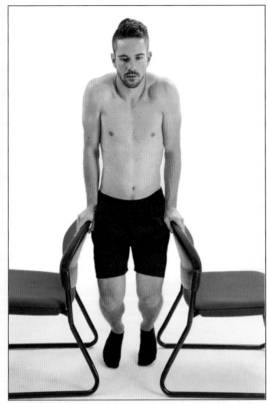

Figure 8.4A
Thoracic spine self-traction: using two chairs

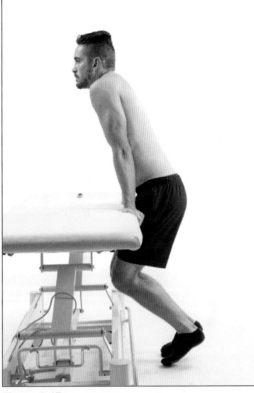

Figure 8.4B
Thoracic spine self-traction: using a bench or table

- This technique is particularly helpful for the patient as it can be performed away from the clinic (at home or at work). It is helpful for the patient with a unidirectional or a multidirectional pain disorder (i.e. any physiological thoracic movement or deep breathing).
- While sustaining the traction effect, the patient should experience relief of their symptoms.
- Apply the self-traction for approximately 10 seconds. Apply 6–10 repetitions in a session, but only if there is a substantial increase in pain-free movement or breathing after the application of the technique and no latent pain responses occur.
- Ensure that the feet are positioned so that when the weight is taken through the upper extremities the thoracic spine is not forced into an extended position. If extension occurs, the pain may be aggravated and the effect of the self-traction may be negated.
- If pain relief is not achieved on the first attempt, the patient should position the feet slightly further forwards until the thoracic spine pain is relieved.

ANNOTATIONS

sup ly T9 belt Tr×10 sec(6)
st self chair Tr×10 sec(3)

Thoracic SNAG central (and unilateral) for flexion, extension, lateral flexion or rotation

Thoracic SNAG – central for flexion

TECHNIQUE AT A GLANCE

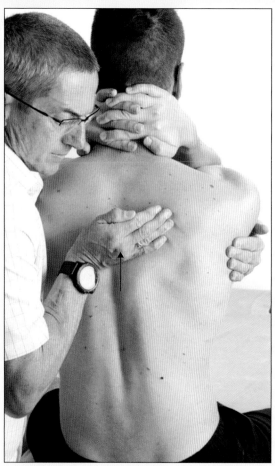

Figure 8.5
Thoracic SNAG central contact

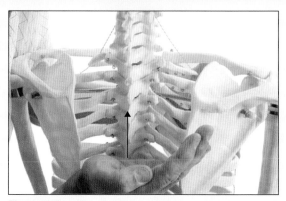

Figure 8.6
Thoracic SNAG: start point model view

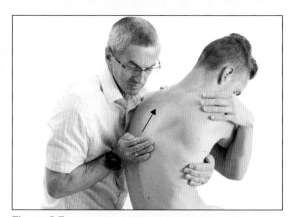

Figure 8.7
Thoracic SNAG: end point into flexion

- The patient sits astride or across the end of the plinth in order to stabilise the pelvis and the therapist stands on the side towards which movement will occur (i.e. in the direction of limitation).

- The patient's hands are placed behind the neck to protract the scapulae and allow the therapist to make hand contact with the mid-thoracic spine.

- The therapist's mobilising hand (ulnar border) will be either central or on one side over the facet joint/transverse process (ipsilateral – usually to the side of pain or limitation – see variation outlined below) and the other arm holds anteriorly over the chest wall above the level to be mobilised.

- The cephalad glide is applied parallel to the facet joint plane.
- Traction is also applied prior to glide and movement, which is achieved by therapist's knee extension.
- See Figs 8.5–8.7.

INDICATION

Midline and/or bilateral thoracic pain occurring with a loss of thoracic (trunk) movement. This could be extension, flexion, lateral flexion or rotation.

POSITIONING

Patient:	Sitting on edge of treatment plinth.
Treated body part:	Sitting astride one end of the treatment plinth facing the other end with hands placed behind the neck to protract the scapulae and allow the therapist to make hand contact with the mid-thoracic spine.
	The pelvis is stabilised by the patient's abducted hips with lower limbs over each side or across the corner of the plinth.
	The thoracic spine is in neutral upright position.
Therapist:	Standing slightly behind the patient on the side of symptoms for a unilateral technique, or on either side, in the case of central or bilateral pain.
Hands/contact points:	One arm is placed around the patient's chest anteriorly above the level to be mobilised.
	The ulnar border of the therapist's mobilising hand is placed over the thoracic spinous process (central) in such a way that a cephalad glide can be applied parallel to the facet joint plane.

APPLICATION GUIDELINES

- It is possible to use thoracic SNAGs from T3/T4 down to T12.
- Ensure that the treatment plinth is adjusted to a height that allows the therapist to use knee extension to perform the traction component of the technique.
- The therapist must maintain the traction and glide until the patient returns to the start position.
- A cephalad glide is applied to the involved spinal level and sustained as the patient actively moves the trunk.
- End-of-range over-pressure is applied by the hand around the anterior chest for the rotation or lateral flexion technique.

(continued next page...)

- A unilateral SNAG may be trialled in the event that a central SNAG is not effective. The ulnar border of the hand is placed immediately lateral to the spinous process, contacting the transverse process of the same vertebral level.
- Unilateral thoracic SNAGs are suggested to be required more often than central thoracic SNAGs and rotation is the most commonly used technique (Fig. 8.8A and B).
- If a unilateral thoracic SNAG is used, it will most likely be applied on the symptomatic side to be effective.
- If the thoracic technique is applied unilaterally, where possible and if indicated, try to include the rib of the involved level by aligning the ulnar border of the hand along the rib line. A better outcome may often be achieved if the rib is included.
- Thoracic SNAGs can be used for all thoracic movements.

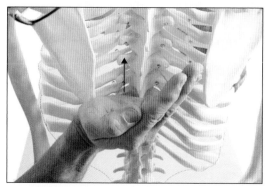

Figure 8.8A
Unilateral thoracic SNAG: model view

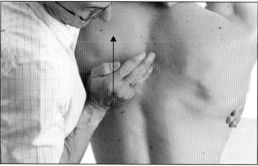

Figure 8.8B
Unilateral thoracic SNAG: hand position

- If indicated, the rotation SNAG can be applied with a combination of movements. For example, the best response may be achieved if the involved segment is placed in flexion or side flexion before the rotation SNAG is applied (Fig. 8.9).
- Respiration can be combined with the SNAG in any direction, but is particularly effective for rotation. Breathing out as approaching the outer ROM allows over-pressure to move the trunk further into the end of range.
- If the patient cannot comfortably straddle the treatment plinth (often due to limited hip or general flexibility), the patient can straddle a corner of the treatment plinth. The therapist should stand to the side of the plinth and rotate the patient towards them. This technique is more physically challenging for the therapist owing to the reach distance caused by the edge of the plinth.

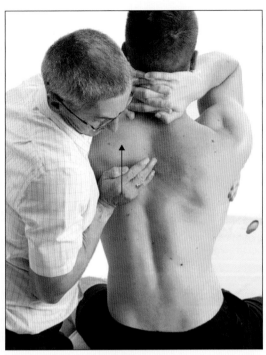

Figure 8.9A
Unilateral thoracic SNAG for extension

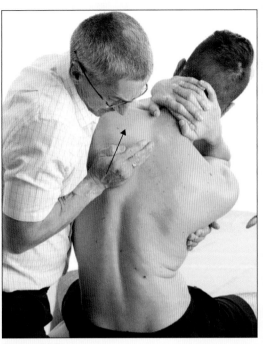

Figure 8.9B
Unilateral thoracic SNAG for lateral flexion

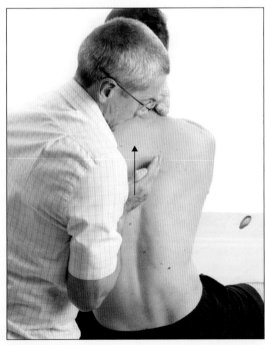

Figure 8.9C
Unilateral thoracic SNAG for rotation

(continued next page...)

COMMENTS

- If the pain is acute or severe, use minimal force to apply the cephalad glide then increase the amount of applied force as indicated by the response. Often, more force is required if the movement is limited by stiffness more than pain.

- Slightly vary the angle of applied mobilising force (Mulligan expresses this as 'constructive fiddling') to fine-tune the technique and optimise the response.

- If the desired response is not achieved at that spinal level, try applying the technique at segments above or below it.

- It is often not necessary to perform the technique from the neutral position to end range. If the restriction or pain is at or near end range, the patient may be rotated to a range short of symptoms and the technique applied from that point to end range. This is often easier for the therapist to control.

- If the point of application for the mobilisation is tender, use a foam pad.

- If the therapist's or the patient's skin is moist and slippery, use a paper tissue between the mobilising hand and the skin.

- Some smaller therapists may be unable to perform this technique on a significantly larger patient.

- The SNAG technique for flexion differs from the others in that the therapist's forearm is used as a fulcrum over which the trunk is flexed. As such, the forearm is placed directly anterior of the involved level to provide a pivot point.

- If rotation is limited in both directions, the SNAG may be performed to the left and right in the same treatment session. Movement in both directions should be cleared. However, do not over-treat, particularly on the first visit. As soon as a significant improvement has been achieved, stop.

SELF-MANAGEMENT

- The patient replicates the technique as a home exercise by using a self-SNAG strap in contact with the spinous process at the involved level.

- A cranially inclined glide is achieved by pulling upwards with both arms. The glide is sustained as the patient actively moves their thoracic spine according to their individual complaint (Fig. 8.10). The motion must be symptom-free or not carried out.

- The angle and / or amplitude of the glide are adjusted to ensure symptom-free active movement.

- Up to 10 repetitions are performed and the symptoms are then reassessed. This process is repeated 3–5 times per day until all symptoms have resolved.

- A small piece of tape can be used to assist the patient in finding the spinous process of the involved vertebral level.

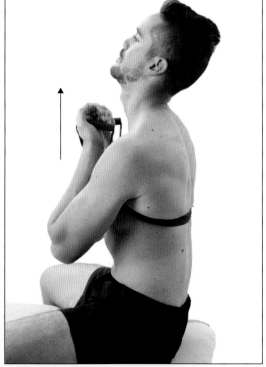

Figure 8.10A
Thoracic self-SNAG: extension

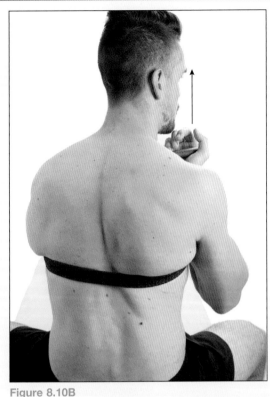

Figure 8.10B
Thoracic self-SNAG: rotation

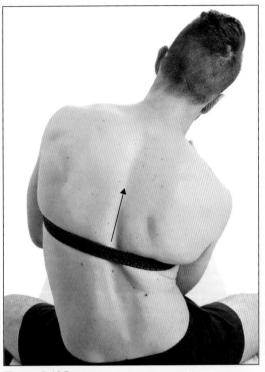

Figure 8.10C
Thoracic self-SNAG: lateral flexion

8

TAPING

- In more acute cases, two pieces of sports tape may be applied over the involved level for support. This is left in place for 48 hours (Fig. 8.11).

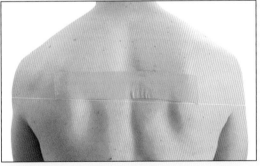

Figure 8.11
Taping in acute thoracic pain scenarios

ANNOTATIONS

sit T5 SNAG F×3
sit L T7 SNAG E×6(3)
sit L T7 SNAG LF R×3
sit L T7 SNAG Rot R×6(3)
sit T7 self strap SNAG E×3
sit T7 self strap SNAG Rot R×3
sit R T7 self strap SNAG LF R×6(3)
T4 Horiz tape

THORAX – RIB AND SPINE

Upper and lower rib MWM

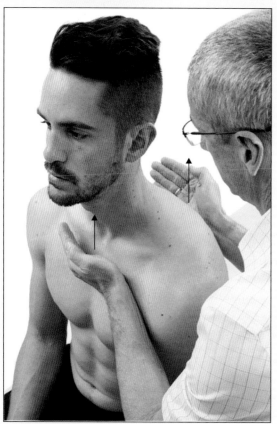

Figure 8.12
Upper rib MWM: unilateral hand contact

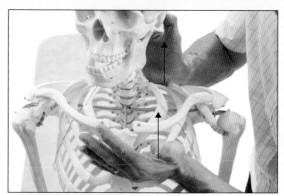

Figure 8.13
Upper rib MWM: model view

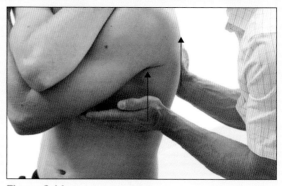

Figure 8.14
Lower rib MWM: hand contact

- The patient sits astride one end of a treatment plinth facing the opposite end of the plinth.
- The ulnar border of each of the therapist's hands contacts the anterior and posterior aspects of the offending rib.
- It is critical that the therapist carefully takes up the skin slack in a superior direction from below the level of the rib prior to applying the upward (lifting) pressure on the rib.
- Pressure is applied and maintained upwardly with both hands, while the patient actively performs the offending movement or breathing, as the case may be.
- The provocative movement should be rendered pain-free with over-pressure being applied with the therapist's hands (see Figs 8.12–8.14).

INDICATION

Pain arising from the rib articulation and experienced in the thorax with physiological thoracic movement or deep breathing.

POSITIONING

Patient:	Sitting on the edge of a treatment plinth.
Treated body part:	Thoracic spine in neutral with arms crossed in front of body or arms up with fingers interlocked behind the neck if applicable.
Therapist:	Standing posterolateral to the patient on the symptomatic side.
Hands/contact points:	Identify the specific area/rib level of the symptoms. The therapist's ulnar border of each hand makes contact with the appropriate rib cage level from a posterior and anterior aspect of the thorax. Use the ulnar border of the hands to first draw up the skin and soft tissue from below in a superior direction. Maintaining the soft tissue lift, direct a superior lifting force to elevate the contacted rib. While the pain-free lifting force is maintained, have the patient perform the offending movement or deep breathing as the case may be. This activity should now be rendered pain-free.

APPLICATION GUIDELINES

- Apply a superiorly directed glide onto the inferior aspect of the offending rib.
- While sustaining the superior gliding force, have the patient repeat the offending movement or deep breathing.
- Apply 6–10 repetitions in a set, with 3–5 sets in a treatment session, but only if there is a substantial increase in pain-free movement or breathing during the application of the technique and no latent pain responses.
- The therapist must maintain the superior glide on the rib during the entire physiological movement as well as the return movement to a neutral thoracic position.

VARIATIONS

- For a patient who complains/presents with more lateral rib cage pain, an alternative is that the ulnar border of both hands contact the left and right lateral rib cage area at the appropriate rib level.
- Maintaining the soft tissue lift, direct a superior lifting force to elevate the contacted ribs together. The patient then carries out the relevant painful or restricted movement (Fig. 8.15).

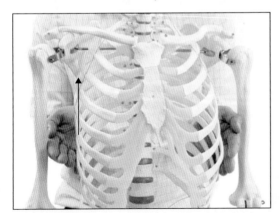

Figure 8.15A
Rib MWM – bilateral contact: model view

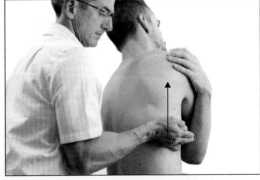

Figure 8.15B
Rib MWM – bilateral contact: lateral flexion end range

(continued next page...)

- For a patient whose shoulder movement is limited by pain or immobility of the rib cage, a unilateral rib MWM can be performed concomitant with shoulder elevation or abduction (Fig. 8.16).

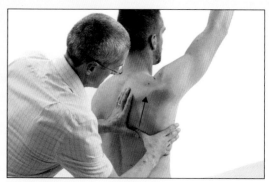

Figure 8.16
Rib MWM using thumbs combined with shoulder elevation

COMMENTS

- Ensure that the skin and soft tissue slack is taken up in a superior direction prior to the application of the superior force on the rib. This will permit good rib contact and a more efficient technique.
- If the rib contact causes some contact discomfort, a thin piece of foam may be used to ensure maximum comfort for the patient.
- If pain-free movement is not achieved on the first attempt, the therapist should assess the effect of the technique on adjacent ribs until the offending movement is rendered pain-free.

ANNOTATIONS

sit L 2nd rib MWM Inspiration×6
sit L 6th rib MWM Inspiration×6
sit L 6th rib MWM LF R×6
sit R 7th rib MWM E×6
sit R 5th rib MWM Rot R×10(3)
sit Bilat 7th CV MWM LF L×6(3)
sit R 6th rib MWM R Sh El×10(3)

8

Costovertebral MWM for first or second rib

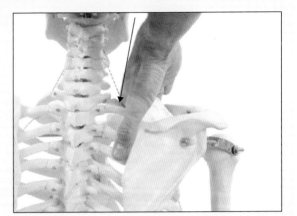

Figure 8.18
First and second rib MWM: model view

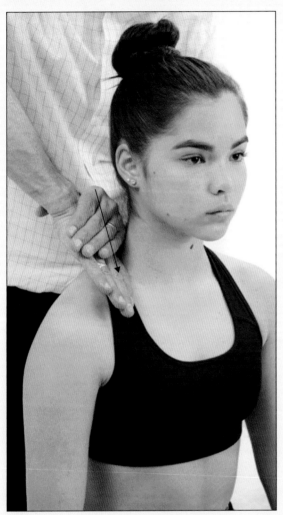

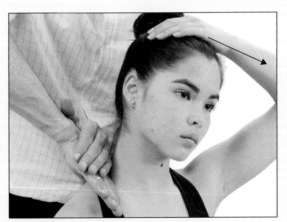

Figure 8.17
First and second rib MWM: start position

Figure 8.19
First and second rib MWM: end point

- The patient sits with head/neck in neutral.
- The therapist stabilises the first or second rib anterolaterally.
- It is critical that the therapist takes up the skin slack towards the base of the neck from below the level of the rib, prior to applying the caudad pressure on the rib.
- Pressure is maintained caudally, while the patient actively side flexes the head to the contralateral side.
- The above movement should be performed without pain with the patient applying over-pressure at the end of active side flexion.
- See Figs 8.17–8.19.

INDICATION

Pain in the root of the neck or in the region of the upper trapezius with contralateral cervical side flexion.

POSITIONING

Patient:	Sitting preferably in a chair supported by the back of a chair.
Treated body part:	Cervical spine neutral.
Therapist:	Standing behind the patient.
Hands/contact points:	Stabilising/gliding hand: use the radial border of the second metacarpophalangeal joint to first draw up the skin and soft tissue from the level of the clavicle in a proximal direction. Maintaining the soft tissue lift, redirect the force in a caudal orientation onto the superior aspect of the first or second rib.
	Use the hand on the same side – e.g. the left hand of the therapist to the left ribs of patient to ensure effective contact.

APPLICATION GUIDELINES

- Apply a caudally directed glide onto the superior aspect of the first or second rib.
- While sustaining the caudal glide force, have the patient repeat the contralateral side flexion.
- Apply 6–10 repetitions in a set, with 3–5 sets in a treatment session, but only if there is a substantial increase in pain-free contralateral side flexion during the application of the technique and no latent pain responses.
- The therapist must maintain the caudal glide on the rib during the entire contralateral side flexion movement as well as the return movement to neutral cervical position.
- The patient may apply over-pressure to the contralateral cervical flexion with the contralateral arm.

COMMENTS

- Ensure that the skin and soft tissue slack is taken up in a proximal direction prior to the application of the caudal force on the rib. This will allow full possible range of cervical contralateral flexion.
- The therapist can use their other hand to assist in applying the glide.
- If the caudal contact on the rib causes some contact discomfort, a thin piece of foam may be used to ensure maximum comfort for the patient.
- This technique is useful as a differential diagnosis for the patient's pain disorder. If this technique does not eliminate the patient's pain then the patient's pain may be generated from an alternative structure where a different Mulligan Concept technique may be effective in eliminating the pain (e.g. cervical or upper thoracic spine SNAG).

ANNOTATIONS

sit L 1st CV MWM×6
sit R 2nd CV MWM +OP×6(3)

References

Andrews, D.P., Odland-Wolf, K.B., May, J., Baker, R., Nasypany, A., 2018. The utilization of Mulligan Concept thoracic sustained natural apophyseal glides on patients classified with secondary impingement syndrome: a multi-site case series. Int. J. Sports Phys. Ther. 13 (1), 121–130.

Briggs, A.M., Smith, A.J., Straker, L.M., Bragge, P., 2009. Thoracic spine pain in the general population: prevalence, incidence and associated factors in children, adolescents and adults. A systematic review. BMC Musculoskelet. Disord. 10, 77.

Crosbie, J., Kilbreath, S.L., Hollmann, L., York, S., 2008. Scapulohumeral rhythm and associated spinal motion. Clin. Biomech. (Bristol, Avon) 23 (2), 184–192.

8

Cross, K.M., Kuenze, C., Grindstaff, T.L., Hertel, J., 2011. Thoracic spine thrust manipulation improves pain, range of motion, and self-reported function in patients with mechanical neck pain: a systematic review. J. Orthop. Sports Phys. Ther. 41 (9), 633–642.

Edmondston, S.J., Singer, K.P., 1997. Thoracic spine: anatomical and biomechanical considerations for manual therapy. Man. Ther. 2 (3), 132–143.

Edmondston, S.J., Aggerholm, M., Elfving, S., Flores, N., Ng, C., Smith, R., et al., 2007. Influence of posture on the range of axial rotation and coupled lateral flexion of the thoracic spine. J. Manipulative Physiol. Ther. 30 (3), 193–199.

Geelhoed, M.A., McGaugh, J., Brewer, P.A., Murphy, D., 2006. A new model to facilitate palpation of the level of the transverse processes of the thoracic spine. J. Orthop. Sports Phys. Ther. 36 (11), 876–881.

Hinkley, H., Drysdale, I., 1995. Audit of 1000 patients attending the clinic of the British College of Naturopathy and Osteopathy. Br. Osteopath. J. XVI, 17–27.

Horton, S.J., 2002. Acute locked thoracic spine: treatment with a modified SNAG. Man. Ther. 7 (2), 103–107.

McClatchie, L., Laprade, J., Martin, S., Jaglal, S.B., Richardson, D., Agur, A., 2009. Mobilizations of the asymptomatic cervical spine can reduce signs of shoulder dysfunction in adults. Man. Ther. 14 (4), 369–374.

Mintken, P.E., Cleland, J.A., Carpenter, K.J., Bieniek, M.L., Keirns, M., Whitman, J.M., 2010. Some factors predict successful short-term outcomes in individuals with shoulder pain receiving cervicothoracic manipulation: a single-arm trial. Phys. Ther. 90 (1), 26–42.

Norlander, S., Nordgren, B., 1998. Clinical symptoms related to musculoskeletal neck-shoulder pain and mobility in the cervico-thoracic spine. Scand. J. Rehabil. Med. 30 (4), 243–251.

Occhipinti, E., Colombini, D., Grieco, A., 1993. Study of distribution and characteristics of spinal disorders using a validated questionnaire in a group of male subjects not exposed to occupational spinal risk factors. Spine 18 (9), 1150.

Sobel, J.S., Kremer, I., Winters, J.C., Arendzen, J.H., de Jong, B.M., 1996. The influence of the mobility in the cervicothoracic spine and the upper ribs (shoulder girdle) on the mobility of the scapulohumeral joint. J. Manipulative Physiol. Ther. 19 (7), 469–474.

Strunce, J.B., Walker, M.J., Boyles, R.E., Young, B.A., 2009. The immediate effects of thoracic spine and rib manipulation on subjects with primary complaints of shoulder pain. J. Man. Manip. Ther. 17 (4), 230–236.

Takasaki, H., Hall, T., Kaneko, S., Iizawa, T., Ikemoto, Y., 2009. Cervical segmental motion induced by shoulder abduction assessed by magnetic resonance imaging. Spine 34 (3), E122–E126.

Williams, P.I., Warwick, R., Dyson, M., Bannister, L.H., 1989. Gray's Anatomy, 37th ed. Churchill Livingstone, Edinburgh.

8

Sacroiliac joint

TECHNIQUES FOR THE SACROILIAC JOINT

Posterior glide MWM innominate in relation to sacrum with trunk extension in prone lying
  Addition of rotation component to the posterior glide for prone-lying SIJ MWM
Lateral glide MWM innominate in relation to sacrum with trunk extension in prone lying
  Addition of rotation component to SIJ lateral glide innominate
Posterior glide and / or posterior rotation MWM innominate in relation to sacrum during walking
Taping: posterior glide and / or posterior rotation innominate in relation to sacrum
Taping: anterior glide and / or anterior rotation innominate in relation to sacrum
Home exercise: posterior rotation innominate MWM in step standing
Posterior rotation innominate / anterior rotation sacrum with appropriate glides for trunk extension
  Four-point kneeling SIJ MWM with posterior rotation / posterior glide innominate and anterior rotation sacrum for hip flexion in four-point kneeling
  Standing SIJ MWM with posterior rotation innominate and anterior rotation / anterior glide sacrum for trunk flexion
Anterior rotation innominate for trunk movement in standing
Posterior rotation innominate / anterior rotation sacrum with appropriate glides for hip flexion in step standing
Posterior rotation innominate / anterior rotation sacrum with appropriate glides for hip extension in step standing

INTRODUCTION

The sacroiliac joints (SIJs) are essential for effective transfer of load between the spine and the lower limbs (Vleeming et al., 2012). Although there is limited movement at the SIJs, the movement present is sufficient and required to complement hip joint motion and influence motion at the lumbosacral junction (Smidt et al., 1997). The innervation of the joint is integrally linked to the surrounding musculature and insufficient or excessive SIJ force closure can adversely affect the function of the pelvis (Vleeming et al., 2012). There is suggestion that mobilisation or manipulation itself may not alter the positional relationship between the sacrum and the ilium, measured through roentgen stereophotogrammetric analysis (Tullberg et al., 1998). Authors seem to agree that the positive effects of both techniques may stem from their influence on the soft tissue structures (i.e. joint capsules, muscles, ligaments, tendons and postural neuromuscular reflex patterns).

SIJ MWM techniques can be used to identify and treat elements of failed SIJ force closure. If performance of a painful restricted movement or functional activity involving the SIJ can be rendered pain-free when an SIJ MWM is applied, and if repetition of the MWM 'immediately' addresses aspects of maladaptive compensatory movement patterns including 'bracing' and 'fear avoidance', then it could be argued that the SIJ had been a contributing factor to the clinical presentation.

The anatomy, biomechanics and neuromuscular control mechanisms of the pelvis related to form and force closure are described and discussed in detail elsewhere (Vleeming et al., 2012). However, the magnitude and directions of MWM force required to restore pain-free function may provide an insight into the force closure insufficiencies or excesses that were part of a presenting trunk and femoropelvic functional problem. The periarticular tissues of the SIJ, like those of other synovial joints, contain mechanoreceptors and nociceptors (Fortin et al., 1999; Grob et al., 1995; Sakamoto et al., 2001; Szadek et al., 2008, 2010; Vilensky et al., 2002; Yin et al., 2003). Vleeming and colleagues (Vleeming et al., 2012) concluded that the findings of these studies indicate that the outer border of the SIJ receives innervation from the posterior primary rami of the lower lumbar and upper sacral segments.

Stimulation of SIJ mechanoreceptors can alter motor responses in the pelvis and lumbar spine (Indahl & Holm, 2007; Indahl et al., 1999, 2001). In these studies, SIJ involvement in activation of porcine spinal and gluteal musculature using EMG was examined. On stimulation within the ventral area of the SIJ, predominant responses occurred in the gluteus maximus and quadratus lumborum muscles. When stimulating the joint capsule, the greatest muscular responses were detected in the multifidus muscles. These studies suggest that mechanical or chemical stimulation or irritation of SIJ nociceptors and mechanoreceptors may potentially alter muscle function in the low back and pelvic region.

Although movement of the SIJ is limited, the magnitude and direction of sacroiliac motion is sufficient and required to complement hip joint motion and influence motion at the lumbosacral junction (Smidt et al., 1997).

According to Vleeming and colleagues (Vleeming et al., 2012), degenerative damage to the SIJ may result from trauma or microtrauma secondary to having either excessive laxity or compressional stiffness in the joint, either of which can be the result of structural aetiology or neuromuscular control aetiology. Excessive laxity or stiffness of the SIJs, pubic symphysis and related ligamentous and neuromuscular structures would influence the 'relative flexibility' between the pelvis, hips and lumbar spine.

Although the reasons for pregnancy-related pelvic girdle pain (PPGP) remain unclear, non-optimal stability resulting from impaired motor control and/or maladaptive behaviour is proposed as a likely cause (Aldabe et al., 2012; O'Sullivan & Beales, 2007; Vermani et al., 2010; Vleeming et al., 2008). MWMs can be used for women with PPGP if there are mechanical SIJ factors. Gentle, pain-free MWM techniques performed in four-point kneeling and performed short of end range may immediately restore pain-free function.

Sahrmann (2002) suggests that abnormal 'relative flexibility' of adjacent spinal motion segments or body segments may result in accumulation of stress at the most flexible segment during movement or in sustained end-of-range positions. If there is restricted movement due to involvement of the SIJs, pubic symphysis or related ligamentous and neuromuscular structures, the alteration in relative flexibility may be sufficient to cause excessive loading on other regions, particularly the hip and lumbar spine. The excessive loading may elicit pain from innervated structures in the low back or hip regions, particularly at end-of-range positions. MWM techniques applied to the SIJ may restore sufficient pelvic movement to 'unload' the hip and/or lumbar spine, rendering the movement symptom-free (Oliver, 2011).

Altered SIJ movement patterns have been demonstrated between individuals with pelvic girdle pain (PGP) and matched controls (Hungerford et al., 2004). In the standing flexion test, healthy controls demonstrated

9

posterior rotation of the innominate in relation to the sacrum on the weight-bearing side. Conversely, in subjects with PGP, the innominate rotated anteriorly in relation to the sacrum. MWM techniques applied to the SIJ aim to reverse abnormal SIJ movement patterns and restore normal recruitment of neuromuscular patterns and arthrokinematics.

A cross-sectional study of electromyographic onsets in the same study group demonstrated delayed onset of internal obliques, multifidus and gluteus maximus activity in the supporting leg during hip flexion with earlier onset of biceps femoris (Hungerford et al., 2003). The authors concluded that the results suggest an alteration in the strategy for lumbopelvic stabilisation that may disrupt load transference through the pelvis. Thus, when applying MWM techniques to the SIJ, posterior rotation of the innominate in relation to the sacrum is usually a major component of a successful technique to facilitate the return of successful load transference.

The SIJ plane is variable between individuals, between sides and in the transverse and coronal planes (Solonen, 1957). Therefore, it is vital to establish the angle of the joint plane relative to the sagittal plane when considering performing an SIJ MWM (refer to Fig. 16.2 in Solonen, 1957) because it is usually applied with mobilisation forces parallel or perpendicular to the joint plane (Mulligan, 2010; Vicenzino et al., 2011). The SIJ joint plane is parallel to the applied line of anteroposterior force where the greatest amount of movement with the least amount of resistance is elicited. Further, as extreme hip positions are necessary to achieve full ROM at the SIJ (Bussey et al., 2009; Smidt et al., 1997), MWM of the SIJ most often utilises end-of-range hip movement or end-of-range lumbar movement to restore SIJ range.

Levels of evidence

Level 2: three RCTs, one case series and two case studies

The three RCTs available support the use of MWM in the treatment of SIJ dysfunctions. Alkady and colleagues (Alkady et al., 2017) compared the use of MWM and muscle energy technique (MET), both coupled with conventional physiotherapy (including strengthening exercises, stretches, ultrasound treatment and infrared therapy) in the treatment of chronic SIJ dysfunction. While both interventions were more successful in reducing pain intensity levels and anterior pelvic tilting angle than conventional physiotherapy alone, the MWM group showed greater increases in SIJ mobility (measured through Doppler imaging) than MET and conventional physiotherapy. Interestingly, Shinde and Jagtap (2018) highlighted the importance of MWM technique in increasing ROM. This group demonstrated that the combined treatment of MET, Mulligan taping and MWM is more effective than MET and Mulligan taping alone in the treatment of SIJ dysfunction. Further, the use of the posterior and anterior innominate MWM technique throughout an 8-week treatment programme has been shown to reduce pelvic obliquity and improve balance and static stability control in female university students with SIJ dysfunction (Son et al., 2014).

A case series ($n=3$) demonstrated the efficacy of MWM intervention in reducing SIJ impairment (Disablement in the Physically Active scale and pain (numerical pain rating scale, NPRS) in female dancers (Krzyzanowicz et al., 2015)). There are two case studies that report on the efficacy or effects of the SIJ MWM in promoting trunk mobility (Oliver, 2011) and in the treatment of asymmetrical hip rotation (Bindra, 2014).

POSTERIOR GLIDE MWM INNOMINATE IN RELATION TO SACRUM WITH TRUNK EXTENSION IN PRONE LYING

TECHNIQUE AT A GLANCE

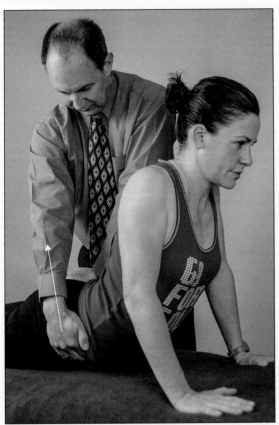

Figure 9.1
SIJ posterior glide of innominate with trunk extension in prone lying

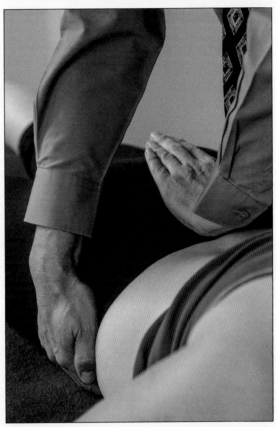

Figure 9.2
SIJ posterior glide of innominate with trunk extension in prone lying: close view

- The patient lies prone with hands under their shoulders (Fig. 9.1).
- The therapist stands facing the patient on the opposite side of the pelvis to the SIJ to be mobilised.
- The ulnar border of one hand is used to fixate the sacrum (Fig. 9.2).
- The fingers of the other hand are wrapped around the anterior border of the anterior superior iliac spine (ASIS) and are used to produce a posterior translation and/or rotation of the innominate in relation to the sacrum.
- The patient then performs extension in the lying movement by extending the elbows.

INDICATION

Pain during and/or movement limitation of trunk extension attributed to SIJ involvement.

POSITIONING

Patient:	Prone lying on treatment table. Hands positioned in preparation to perform passive extension in lying.
Therapist:	Standing on the opposite side to the involved SIJ directly facing the patient's pelvis.
Hands/contact points:	Stabilising hand: palm down on the sacrum so that the ulnar border of the hand lies immediately adjacent to the SIJ on the side to be mobilised with the fingers pointing caudad. Mobilising hand: the fingers are curled around the anterior aspect of the ASIS on the side of the involved SIJ. The anterior aspect of the ASIS is the application point for the mobilising force.

APPLICATION GUIDELINES

- The stabilising hand is used to apply an anteriorly directed force to fixate the sacrum.
- The mobilising hand is used to apply a posterior glide and/or rotation to the innominate.
- These forces are maintained and the patient is asked to perform an extension in lying movement.
- As long as no pain is produced during the manoeuvre, up to 3 sets of 10 repetitions can be performed.

VARIATIONS

- The amount of force and the direction of the therapist's force are determined by the patient's response during the extension movement.
- A rotation component can also be applied to the innominate with the mobilising hand. This can be used in combination with the glide to 'fine-tune' the technique (see Fig. 9.3).
- The technique can also be performed in standing using similar directions of force.
- If necessary, advanced techniques using combinations of rotations and glides applied to the sacrum and innominate simultaneously can be used (Oliver, 2011).

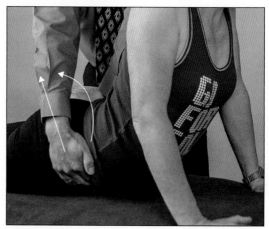

Figure 9.3
Addition of rotation component to the posterior glide for prone-lying SIJ MWM

COMMENTS

- The extension in lying component of the mobilisation can be performed passively or can be performed with an active contribution from the trunk and pelvic muscles.
- Care is taken to avoid 'digging in' with the fingertips, as the region directly medial to the ASIS is very pain-sensitive.
- The direction of the posterior glide of the innominate can be varied to produce the best possible result.

ANNOTATION

 pr ly R SIJ Post gl Inn MWM EIL×10(3)

LATERAL GLIDE MWM INNOMINATE IN RELATION TO SACRUM WITH TRUNK EXTENSION IN PRONE LYING

TECHNIQUE AT A GLANCE

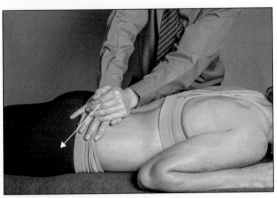

Figure 9.4
Prone-lying SIJ MWM with lateral glide of innominate for trunk extension (in start position)

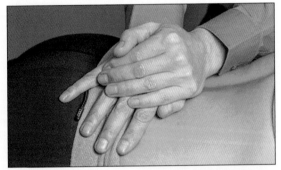

Figure 9.5
SIJ MWM lateral glide of innominate for trunk extension in prone lying: close view

- The thenar eminence of the lowermost hand is placed just medial to the prominent part of the posterior innominate crest.
- The heel of this hand is used to place a lateral glide and/or rotation of the innominate in relation to the sacrum.
- The palm of the other hand assists in application of the lateral glide or can be used to stabilise the rest of the pelvis (Figs 9.4 and 9.5).
- The patient then performs extension in lying movement by extending the elbows.

INDICATION

Pain during and/or movement limitation of trunk extension attributed to SIJ involvement.

POSITIONING

Patient:	Prone lying on treatment table.
	Hands positioned in preparation to perform passive extension in lying movement.
Therapist:	Standing on the opposite side to the involved SIJ directly facing the patient's pelvis.
Hands/contact points:	Mobilising hand: the thenar eminence of the lowermost hand is placed just medial to the prominent part of the posterior innominate crest so that the fingers are pointing laterally. The heel of this hand is used to perform a lateral glide and/or rotation to the innominate in relation to the sacrum. The palm of the other hand may be used to reinforce the mobilising hand and assist in application of the lateral glide or may be used to stabilise the rest of the pelvis.

(continued next page...)

APPLICATION GUIDELINES

- These forces are maintained and the patient asked to perform an extension in lying exercise.
- Apply 6–10 repetitions in a set, with 3–5 sets in a treatment session.

VARIATIONS

- The amount of force and the direction of the therapist's force are determined by the patient's response during the extension movement.
- A medial rotation component is often useful in combination with the lateral glide and can be applied to the innominate with the mobilising hand (Fig. 9.6).

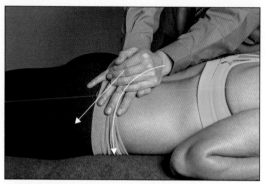

Figure 9.6A
Addition of rotation component to SIJ lateral glide innominate

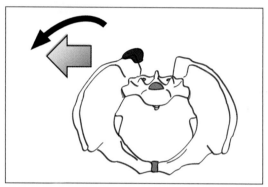

Figure 9.6B
Schematic of rotation component added to lateral glide innominate

- Glide or rotation or forces in other directions can also be used to 'fine-tune' the technique.
- The technique can be performed in standing using combinations of rotations and glides applied to the sacrum and innominate simultaneously (Oliver, 2011).

COMMENTS

- The extension in lying component of the mobilisation can be performed passively or can be performed with an active contribution from the trunk and pelvic muscles.
- The direction of the lateral glide force can be varied to produce the best possible result.
- Altering the point of force application may also be useful.
- This technique can easily be taught to another person so that it can be performed at home.

ANNOTATION

pr ly R SIJ Lat gl Inn MWM EIL×10(3)

POSTERIOR GLIDE AND / OR POSTERIOR ROTATION MWM INNOMINATE IN RELATION TO SACRUM DURING WALKING

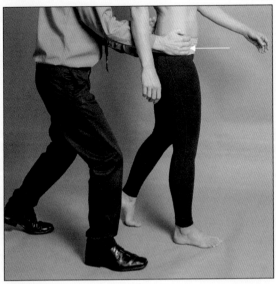

Figure 9.7A
Walking SIJ MWM with posterior glide innominate in relation to the sacrum

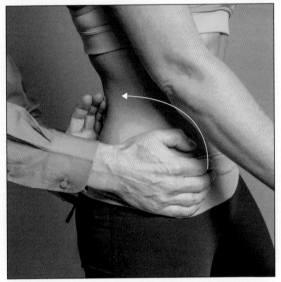

Figure 9.7B
Hand position for walking SIJ MWM with posterior rotation innominate in relation to the sacrum

- The therapist has the ulnar border of one hand over the sacrum immediately adjacent the SIJ to be mobilised (see Fig. 9.7A and B).
- The fingers of the other hand are wrapped around the anterior and pull the innominate to produce a posterior glide and / or rotation of the innominate in relation to the sacrum (Fig 9.7B).
- While maintaining this mobilisation, the patient and the therapist walk.

INDICATION

Pain or limitation of trunk, pelvis or hip movement or pain during gait attributed to SIJ involvement.

POSITIONING

Patient:	Standing.
Therapist:	Standing behind the patient.
Position of hands:	Stabilising hand: the ulnar border of one hand is placed over the sacrum immediately adjacent to the involved SIJ.
	Mobilising hand: the fingers of the other hand are wrapped around the anterior aspect of the ASIS and pull the innominate posteriorly to produce a posterior glide and/or rotation of the innominate in relation to the sacrum.
	If the right SIJ is to be mobilised, the therapist's right hand is on the innominate, and the left hand is on the sacrum (Fig. 9.7).

APPLICATION GUIDELINES

- The ulnar border of the stabilising hand is used to apply an anteriorly directed force to fixate the sacrum.
- The force should ideally be applied parallel to the SIJ plane (Oliver, 2011).
- The mobilising hand is used to apply a posterior glide and/or posterior rotation of the innominate.
- These forces are maintained while the patient and therapist walk.
- If walking has been painful, when the appropriate forces are maintained then walking should be pain-free.
- After 30 seconds or more of walking, the symptomatic trunk or hip movement is retested.
- The walking with mobilisation can be repeated until a marked improvement in the symptomatic movement has been achieved.

VARIATIONS

- If a treadmill is available the patient can be asked to walk on the treadmill while the therapist stands to the side of the track and maintains the mobilisation.

COMMENT

- Care is taken to avoid 'digging in' with the fingertips, as the region directly medial to the ASIS is very pain-sensitive.
- The direction of the posterior glide of the innominate can be varied to produce the best possible result.

ANNOTATIONS

st R SIJ Post gl Inn MWM walk 30 sec
st R SIJ Post gl/Post rot Inn MWM walk 30 sec

TAPING: POSTERIOR GLIDE AND/OR POSTERIOR ROTATION INNOMINATE IN RELATION TO SACRUM

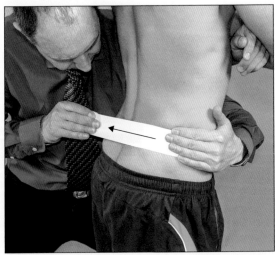

Figure 9.8
Tape innominate posterior glide and/or rotation in relation to the sacrum

- A section of the sports tape is applied without tension across the ASIS (see Fig. 9.8).
- The therapist places one hand over the tape around the ASIS to apply a glide or rotation in the appropriate direction.
- Tape is applied from medial to the ASIS, laterally around the pelvis to the sacrum aligned to follow the direction of force that significantly improves performance of the symptomatic movement.

INDICATION

Pain or limitation of trunk, pelvis or hip movement improved by posterior glide and/or posterior rotation of the innominate in relation to the sacrum.

POSITIONING

Patient:	Standing.
Therapist:	Standing or kneeling on the opposite side of the pelvis to the SIJ being taped.

APPLICATION GUIDELINES

- The tape is aligned to follow the direction of force that significantly improves performance of the symptomatic movement.
- Initially 50-mm-wide sports tape is applied (without tension) extending from medial to the ASIS around the lateral aspect of the pelvis to the sacrum.
- 38-mm-wide rigid sports tape is then applied in two layers. The first section of the sports tape is fixed without tension across the ASIS. The therapist places one hand over the tape around the ASIS to perform a glide or rotation in the appropriate direction.
- The tape is then tensioned using the other hand and wrapped around the pelvis to anchor over the sacrum.
- The patient may need to rest their hands on a wall for support as the tape is applied.
- Wrinkles in the skin are largely unavoidable, and some think they are important, but in any case minimise them at points of increased tape tension on the skin and over areas of potential compression compromise of underlying tissues and bone.
- Check for skin allergies before applying tape.
- Warn the patient about potential skin irritation.
- Remove the tape if allergies arise (skin itch, burning or other sensations).

VARIATIONS

- If it is difficult to apply the tape in the standing position, the patient can be placed in the prone-lying position.
- Tape is initially applied over the anterior ASIS and smoothed down to gain contact. The therapist then uses one hand around the anterior aspect of the ASIS and over the tape to pull the innominate in the appropriate direction while the other hand is used to apply tension to the tape, which is then wrapped around the pelvis and over the sacrum.
- As with SIJ MWM techniques, the direction of the posterior glide and rotation of the innominate in relation to the sacrum can be varied to produce the best possible result.

COMMENT

- The purpose of the tape is not necessarily to forcibly posteriorly translate or rotate the innominate on the sacrum. The restraint may act to control or prevent inappropriate anterior rotation or translation occurring at certain times.

ANNOTATIONS

R SIJ Post gl Inn tape
R SIJ Post rot Inn tape

TAPING: ANTERIOR GLIDE AND/OR ANTERIOR ROTATION INNOMINATE IN RELATION TO SACRUM

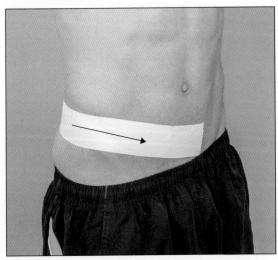

Figure 9.9
Tape innominate anterior glide and/or rotation in relation to the sacrum: anterior view

- The patient is standing and the therapist standing or kneeling on the opposite side of the pelvis to the SIJ being taped.
- A section of the sports tape is fixed without tension across the posterior aspect of the iliac crest (Fig. 9.9).
- The therapist wraps one hand around the patient's waist for stabilisation and the heel of their other hand is placed over the posterior iliac crest to apply anterior glide and/or anterior rotation force in the appropriate direction.
- An assistant applies tension to the tape, which is then pulled anteriorly and wrapped around the lower abdominal wall to finish in the midline below the umbilicus.

INDICATION

Pain or limitation of trunk, pelvis or hip movement improved by anterior glide and/or anterior rotation of the innominate in relation to the sacrum.

POSITIONING

Patient:	Standing.
Therapist:	Standing or kneeling on the opposite side of pelvis to the SIJ being taped.

APPLICATION GUIDELINES

- Application of the tape is more effective if an assistant is available to affix the tape while the therapist maintains the corrected position.
- The tape is aligned to follow the direction of force that significantly improves performance of the symptomatic movement.
- Initially 50-mm-wide hypoallergenic tape is applied (without tension).
- 38-mm-wide rigid sports tape is then applied. The section of the sports tape is applied without tension behind the iliac crest.
- The therapist stands or kneels on opposite side of pelvis to the SIJ being taped. One hand is wrapped around the waist for stabilisation and the heel of the other hand is placed over the posterior iliac crest to apply anterior translation and/or anterior rotation force in the appropriate direction.
- The assistant applies tension to the tape and applies it over the hypoallergenic tape.
- The patient may need to rest their hands on a wall for support as the tape is applied.
- Wrinkles in the skin are largely unavoidable, and some think they are important, but in any case minimise them at points of increased tape tension on the skin and over areas of potential compression compromise of underlying tissues and bone.
- Check for skin allergies before applying tape.
- Warn patient about potential skin irritation.
- Remove the tape if allergies arise (skin itch, burning or other sensations).

COMMENT

- The purpose of the tape is not necessarily to forcibly anteriorly translate or rotate the innominate, but the restraint may act to control or prevent inappropriate posterior rotation or translation occurring at certain times.

ANNOTATIONS

R SIJ Ant gl Inn tape
R SIJ Ant rot Inn tape

HOME EXERCISE: POSTERIOR ROTATION INNOMINATE MWM IN STEP STANDING

TECHNIQUE AT A GLANCE

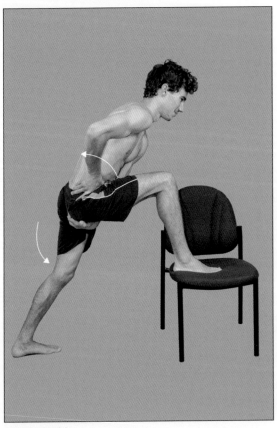

Figure 9.10A
SIJ self-MWM innominate posterior rotation home exercise: side view

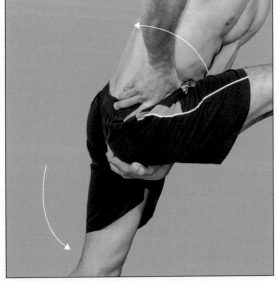

Figure 9.10B
SIJ self-MWM innominate posterior rotation home exercise: close view

9

- The patient reaches across with the opposite arm, medial to inner thigh of the involved side to wrap their hand inferiorly and posteriorly around the ischial tuberosity (see Fig. 9.10).
- The first web-space of the other hand is spread over the involved ASIS so that the fingers are around the lateral aspect of the pelvis with the fingertips pointing posteriorly.
- The patient pulls the ischial tuberosity forwards and pushes the ASIS backwards to posteriorly glide / rotate the innominate.
- The patient then flexes their hip by leaning forwards, and may add additional end-of-range over-pressure by flexing the trunk.

INDICATION

Pain or limitation of trunk, pelvis or hip movement attributed to SIJ involvement and improved by posterior rotation of the innominate.

POSITIONING

Patient:	Step standing with the foot of the involved side on a chair or lowered plinth.
Treated body part:	Pelvis in relaxed upright position.
Patient's hand position:	For a right SIJ, the left arm passes medial to the left inner thigh so that the left hand is wrapped inferiorly and posteriorly around the right ischial tuberosity. The first web-space of the right hand is spread over the right ASIS so that the fingers are around the lateral aspect of the pelvis with the fingertips pointing posteriorly.

APPLICATION GUIDELINES

- The patient pulls the right ischial tuberosity forwards and pushes the right ASIS backwards to produce appropriate posterior glide and/or posterior rotation of the right innominate.
- While maintaining the mobilisation, the patient flexes the right hip by leaning forwards and if indicated applies additional end-of-range over-pressure by flexing the trunk.
- The patient must maintain the mobilisation forces until returning to the start position.
- The effect of the technique is greatly enhanced by maintaining the movement at end range for 3–5 seconds.
- Repeat 6 times in a session, with 2–3 sessions per day.

VARIATIONS

- If focusing on hip and SIJ movement, the patient maintains a neutral spine position.
- If inclusion of spinal flexion is indicated, the patient can be encouraged to flex the spine while flexing the hip.

COMMENTS

- This technique is very useful as a follow up to SIJ MWM techniques performed by the therapist.
- The placement of the hand around the ASIS is to prevent the hip joint from reaching end-of-range flexion. This helps protect the joint and assists in localisation of the mobilisation to the SIJ.

ANNOTATION

step st R Foot on chair R SIJ self Post rot/Post gl Inn MWM Hip F×6

9

POSTERIOR ROTATION INNOMINATE / ANTERIOR ROTATION SACRUM WITH APPROPRIATE GLIDES FOR TRUNK EXTENSION

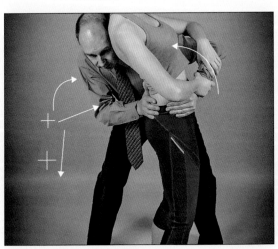

Figure 9.11A
Standing SIJ MWM with posterior rotation innominate and anterior rotation / anterior glide / inferior glide sacrum for trunk extension

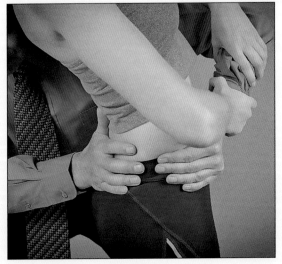

Figure 9.11B
Hand position for SIJ MWM for trunk extension

- The therapist's foremost hand is placed over the anterior aspect of the ASIS on the involved side and the heel of the rearmost hand is placed over the sacrum as close as possible to the involved SIJ (see Fig. 9.11).
- The hands are used to apply appropriate mobilising forces to the involved SIJ.
- The patient holds the therapist's forearm for support and then extends the spine actively.
- The side of the therapist's head, neck and upper shoulder provide light support and guidance for the patient as the spine is extended.

INDICATION

Pain and/or limitation of trunk and/or hip extension or pelvic posterior tilt attributed to SIJ involvement.

POSITIONING

Patient:	Standing.
Therapist:	Standing to the side of the patient, opposite the side to be treated.
Position of hands:	If applying the technique to the right SIJ, the left hand is placed over the anterior aspect of the right ASIS. The heel of the right hand is placed over the sacrum as close as possible to the right SIJ (Fig. 9.11).

(continued next page...)

APPLICATION GUIDELINES

- In this example, the therapist uses the left hand over the right ASIS to apply posterior rotation and posterior glide forces to the right innominate, and the heel of the right hand on the sacrum to apply anterior rotation and anterior glide/inferior glide forces to the sacrum.
- The forces are applied parallel to the SIJ treatment plane.
- If the joint plane is found to be orientated slightly oblique to the sagittal plane, the hand over the sacrum will direct force anterolaterally and the hand over the ASIS will direct force posteromedially, parallel to the plane of the SIJ.
- The patient is instructed to hold the therapist's left forearm for support and then to extend the spine actively.
- The left lateral aspect of the therapist's head, neck and upper shoulder should make contact with the patient's back to provide gentle guidance as the spine is extended.
- The patient is instructed to avoid cervical extension during the manoeuvre.
- To avoid stress on the therapist and to ensure effectiveness of the technique, it is important that the patient posteriorly tilts the pelvis while extending the spine and does not just lean backwards.
- The therapist's hands can help guide the pelvis into posterior pelvic tilt.
- Sometimes asking the patient to 'drop the tail-bone then extend the spine' helps.
- Full-range and pain-free lumbar extension should be possible.
- Apply 6–10 repetitions in a set, with 3–5 sets in a treatment session.

VARIATIONS

- This SIJ MWM can be performed in sitting or four-point kneeling (Fig. 9.12).
- An alternative four-point kneeling hand position can be used for pregnant patients. Four-point kneeling is ideal for treatment during pregnancy, and the therapist stands on the side of the SIJ to be treated (Fig. 9.13).

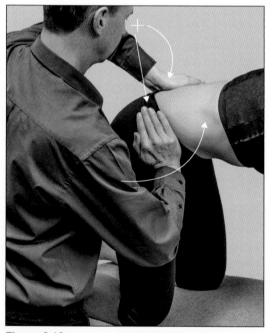

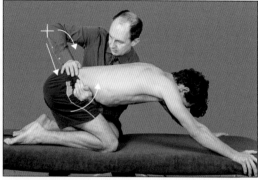

Figure 9.12
Four-point kneeling SIJ MWM with posterior rotation/posterior glide innominate and anterior rotation sacrum for hip flexion

Figure 9.13
Alternative four-point kneeling hand position used for pregnant patients

COMMENTS

- The weight and leverage of the trunk are sufficient to apply end-of-range over-pressure.

- Any combination of rotation and glide forces can be applied simultaneously to the sacrum and innominate. These include glides that add compression or distraction to the involved SIJ.

- As with all MWM techniques, the combination of rotation and glide forces used and the magnitude of force applied will be that which renders the movement or functional activity pain-free.

- If force applied in a medial direction to the ASIS improves the active straight leg raising (ASLR) response, as described by Mens and colleagues (Mens et al., 1999), applying the same force will often improve the effectiveness of the SIJ MWM technique. The patient can apply the medially directed force by placing one hand over each ASIS and 'squeezing' the innominates towards each other. The therapist then places one hand over the patient's hand on the side to be treated and applies additional rotation or glide components. Conversely, if force applied in a medial direction to the lateral aspect of the posterior iliac crests (near the posterior superior iliac spine (PSIS)) improves the ASLR response, this can be incorporated into the SIJ MWM technique.

- The SIJ MWM can be performed for painful limitation of trunk movement in any direction. If the movement is trunk flexion and pelvic anterior tilt (Fig. 9.14), it is important that the patient flexes the knees and uses the back of a chair for support.

- The point of force application to the sacrum can be varied according to patient's response.

- If necessary, the innominate can be taped into posterior or anterior rotation, medial or lateral rotation.

- If the patient is large, the therapist can apply the technique standing on the same side as the involved SIJ.

- If the patient is short in relation to the therapist, the therapist can sit on the arm of a chair or plinth.

- If there is a restriction of trunk flexion as well as extension, it is likely that the same combination of mobilisation forces will improve movement in both directions.

- If it is difficult to improve trunk extension, an SIJ MWM into trunk flexion may assist restoration of extension, even if trunk flexion was not painful or restricted.

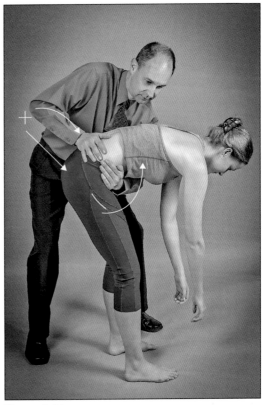

Figure 9.14
Standing SIJ MWM with posterior rotation innominate and anterior rotation/anterior glide sacrum for trunk flexion

ANNOTATIONS

st R SIJ Post rot Inn+Ant rot/Ant gl/Inf gl Sx MWM Trunk E×6(3)
st R SIJ Post rot Inn+Ant rot/Ant gl/Inf gl Sx MWM Trunk F×6(3)
4 point kneel R SIJ Post rot Inn+Ant rot Sx MWM Trunk E×6(3)

ANTERIOR ROTATION INNOMINATE FOR TRUNK MOVEMENT IN STANDING

TECHNIQUE AT A GLANCE

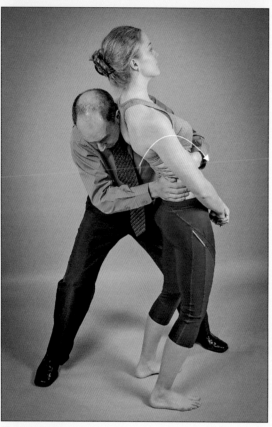

Figure 9.15A
Standing SIJ MWM with anterior rotation innominate for trunk extension

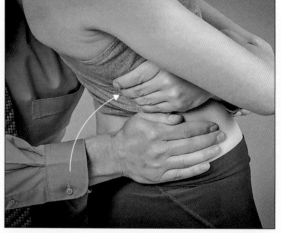

Figure 9.15B
Hand position for standing SIJ MWM with anterior rotation innominate for trunk extension

9

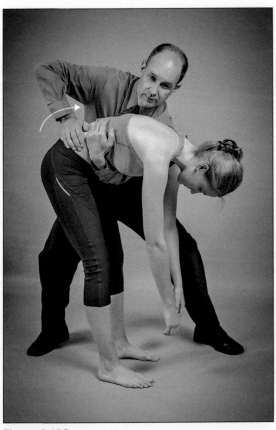

Figure 9.15C
Standing SIJ MWM with anterior rotation innominate
for trunk flexion

9

- The therapist is standing or kneeling on the opposite side to the SIJ to be treated (see Fig. 9.15).
- The therapist places a forearm across the anterior pelvis and lower abdomen so that the hand is wrapped around the waist of the side to be treated.
- The therapist's other hand is wrapped around the posterior aspect of the iliac crest and is used to apply an anterior rotation force to the left innominate.
- If the movement to be performed is trunk extension and posterior tilt of the pelvis, the patient is asked to extend the spine whilst holding the therapist's right arm for support (Fig. 9.15A, B).
- If the movement to be performed is trunk flexion and anterior tilt of the pelvis, the patient is asked to bend the knees then flex the spine using the back of a chair for support (Fig. 9.15C).

INDICATION

Pain or limitation of trunk extension or pelvic posterior tilt attributed to SIJ involvement.

Pain or limitation of trunk flexion, or anterior pelvic tilt attributed to SIJ involvement.

POSITIONING

Patient:	Standing.
Therapist:	Therapist standing or kneeling to the side of the patient opposite the side to be treated and facing slightly backwards in relation to the patient's pelvis.
Position of hands:	If applying the technique to the right SIJ, the left forearm is placed across the anterior pelvis and lower abdomen so the hand is wrapped around the right side of the waist.
	The right hand is wrapped around the posterior aspect of the right iliac crest and used to apply an anterior rotation force to the right innominate.
	The hand position is the same for trunk movement in any direction.

APPLICATION GUIDELINES

- The arm that is placed across the lower abdomen is used to control the trunk during the manoeuvre.
- The right hand that is wrapped around the posterior aspect of the right iliac crest is used to apply an anterior rotation force to the right innominate.
- If the movement to be performed is trunk extension and posterior tilt of the pelvis, the patient is asked to extend the spine whilst holding the therapist's left arm for support.
- If the movement to be performed is trunk flexion and anterior tilt of the pelvis, the patient is asked to bend the knees then flex the spine using the back of a chair for support.
- The end-of-range position is maintained for 1–2 seconds, then the patient returns to the upright position.
- The direction and magnitude of the applied force are maintained throughout the manoeuvre.

COMMENTS

- The weight and leverage of the trunk is sufficient to apply end-of-range over-pressure.
- Usually the desired effect is achieved with 2–3 repetitions.
- For this technique, complete stabilisation of the left and right SIJs is not necessary, but the forearm placed across the lower abdominal wall helps to localise the mobilisation force to the SIJ.
- This technique can be used for limitation of trunk movement (attributed to SIJ involvement) in any direction.

9

ANNOTATION

 st R SIJ Ant rot Inn MWM Trunk F×3

POSTERIOR ROTATION INNOMINATE / ANTERIOR ROTATION SACRUM WITH APPROPRIATE GLIDES FOR HIP FLEXION IN STEP STANDING

TECHNIQUE AT A GLANCE

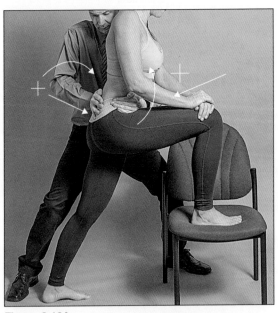

Figure 9.16A
Step-standing SIJ MWM with innominate posterior rotation / posterior glide and sacrum anterior rotation / anterior glide for hip flexion

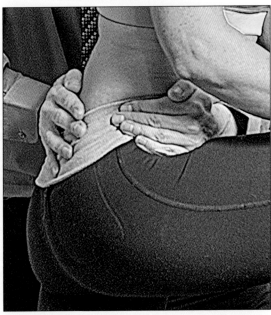

Figure 9.16B
Step-standing SIJ MWM with posterior rotation innominate for hip flexion: close view

- The therapist's foremost hand is placed over the anterior aspect of the ASIS on the involved side and the heel of the rearmost hand is placed over the sacrum as close as possible to the involved SIJ (Fig. 9.16).
- The hands are used to apply appropriate mobilising forces to the involved SIJ.
- The patient is instructed to lunge forwards to flex the hip while the therapist maintains the applied mobilising forces.

INDICATION

Pain and/or limitation of hip and pelvic flexion attributed to right SIJ involvement.

POSITIONING

Patient:	Standing with foot of the involved side on a chair or plinth with both hands placed on the knee of the involved side.
Therapist:	Standing to the side of the patient, opposite the side to be treated.
Position of hands:	If applying the technique to the right SIJ, the left hand is placed over the anterior aspect of the right ASIS. The heel of the right hand is placed over the sacrum as close as possible to the right SIJ.

APPLICATION GUIDELINES

- The therapist applies appropriate rotation and translation forces to the right innominate and to the sacrum.
- In this example, posterior rotation and posterior glide forces are applied to the right innominate using the left hand over the ASIS, and anterior rotation anterior glide forces are applied to the right side of the sacrum through the heel of the right hand.
- The forces are applied parallel to the SIJ treatment plane.
- The patient is instructed to lunge forwards, flexing the right hip.
- The end-of-range position is maintained for 1–2 seconds, and the patient returns to the start position.
- The therapist can guide the patient's pelvis with the hands to ensure the correct movement is performed.
- Full-range and pain-free hip flexion should be possible.
- Apply 6–10 repetitions in a set, with 3–5 sets in a treatment session.

VARIATIONS

- If focusing on hip and SIJ movement, the patient maintains a 'neutral spine' position. If inclusion of spinal flexion is indicated, the patient can be encouraged to flex the spine while flexing the hip.
- If the pelvis is wide or the therapist finds that applying forces to the SIJ on the opposite side of the body is difficult, the therapist can stand on the same side as the SIJ to be treated (Fig. 9.17).

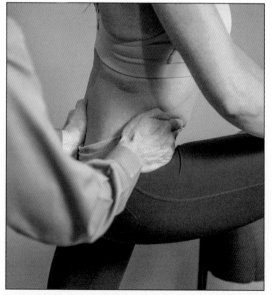

Figure 9.17
Step-standing SIJ MWM for hip flexion with the therapist standing on the same side as the joint to be mobilised

9

COMMENTS

- If the patient requires additional support, their arm closest to the therapist can be rested on the therapist's shoulder.
- The therapist can apply further end-of-range over-pressure using the combined force of the hands around the pelvis.
- Additional end-of-range over-pressure can be applied by flexing the trunk.
- The placement of the hand around the ASIS is used to prevent the hip joint from reaching end-of-range flexion. This helps protect the joint and assists localisation of movement to the SIJ.
- If using an adjustable-height plinth, the height can be altered to fine-tune the start position of the technique.
- The effect of the technique is greatly enhanced by maintaining the movement at end range for 3–5 seconds.

ANNOTATION

 st R foot on chair R SIJ Post rot Inn+Ant rot Sx MWM Hip F×6(3)

POSTERIOR ROTATION INNOMINATE / ANTERIOR ROTATION SACRUM WITH APPROPRIATE GLIDES FOR HIP EXTENSION IN STEP STANDING

TECHNIQUE AT A GLANCE

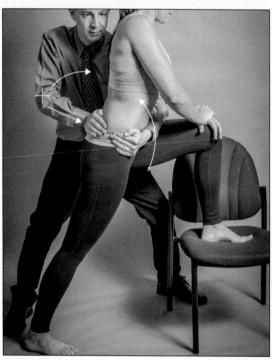

Figure 9.18A
Step-standing SIJ MWM with innominate posterior rotation and sacrum anterior rotation / anterior glide for hip extension

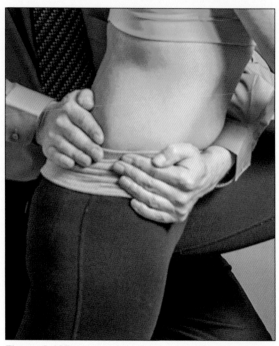

Figure 9.18B
Step-standing SIJ MWM with innominate posterior rotation and sacrum anterior rotation / anterior glide for hip extension: close view

- The therapist's foremost hand is placed over the anterior aspect of the ASIS on the involved side and the heel of the rearmost hand is placed over the sacrum as close as possible to the involved SIJ (see Fig. 9.18).
- The hands are used to apply appropriate mobilising forces to the involved SIJ taking into account the treatment plane of the SIJ.
- The patient is instructed to lunge forwards to extend the hip while the therapist maintains the applied mobilising forces.

INDICATION

Pain and / or limitation of hip and pelvic extension attributed to right SIJ involvement.

POSITIONING

Patient:	Standing with foot of the uninvolved side on a chair or plinth with both hands placed on the knee of the uninvolved side.
Therapist:	Standing to the side of the patient, opposite the side to be treated.
Position of hands:	If applying the technique to the right SIJ, the left hand is placed over the anterior aspect of the right ASIS. The heel of the right hand is placed over the sacrum as close as possible to the right SIJ.

APPLICATION GUIDELINES

- The therapist applies appropriate rotation and translation forces to the right innominate and to the sacrum.
- For this example, posterior rotation and posterior glide forces are applied to the right innominate using the left hand over the ASIS, and anterior rotation anterior glide forces are applied to the right side of the sacrum through the heel of the right hand.
- The forces are applied parallel to the SIJ treatment plane.
- The patient is instructed to lunge forwards, extending the right hip while maintaining a 'neutral spine' position.
- The end-of-range position is maintained for 1–2 seconds, and the patient returns to the start position.
- The therapist can guide the patient's pelvis with the hands to ensure the correct movement is performed.
- Full range and pain-free hip extension should be possible.
- Apply 6–10 repetitions in a set, with 3–5 sets in a treatment session.

VARIATIONS

- If the pelvis is wide or the therapist finds that applying forces to the SIJ on the opposite side of the body is difficult, the therapist can stand on the same side as the SIJ to be treated (Fig. 9.19).

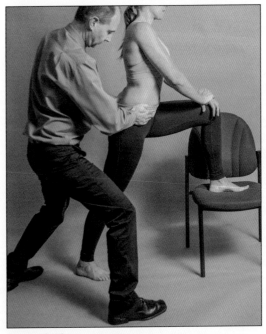

Figure 9.19
Step-standing SIJ MWM for hip extension with the therapist standing on the same side as the joint to be mobilised

9

(continued next page...)

COMMENTS

- If the patient requires additional support, their arm closest to the therapist can be rested on the therapist's shoulder.
- The therapist can apply further end-of-range over-pressure using the combined force of the hands around the pelvis.
- If using an adjustable-height plinth, the height can be altered to fine-tune the start position of the technique.
- The effect of the technique is greatly enhanced by maintaining the movement at end range for 3–5 seconds.

ANNOTATION

 st L foot on chair R SIJ Post rot Inn+Ant rot/Ant gl Sx MWM Hip E×6(3)

References

Aldabe, D., Milosavljevic, S., Bussey, M.D., 2012. Is pregnancy related pelvic girdle pain associated with altered kinematic, kinetic and motor control of the pelvis? A systematic review. Eur. Spine J. 21 (9), 1777–1787.

Alkady, S.M.E., Kamel, R.M., AbuTaleb, E., Lasheen, Y., Alshaarawy, F.A., 2017. Efficacy of Mulligan mobilization versus muscle energy technique in chronic sacroiliac joint dysfunction. Int. J. Physiother. 4 (5), 311–318.

Bindra, S., 2014. Hip rotation MWM for sacroiliac joint dysfunction: a case report. Ind. J. Physiother. Occup. Ther. 8 (3), 8–11.

Bussey, M.D., Bell, M.L., Milosavljevic, S., 2009. The influence of hip abduction and external rotation on sacroiliac motion. Man. Ther. 14 (5), 520–525.

Fortin, J.D., Kissling, R.O., O'Connor, B.L., Vilensky, J.A., 1999. Sacroiliac joint innervation and pain. Am. J. Orthop. 28 (12), 687–690.

Grob, K.R., Neuhuber, W.L., Kissling, R.O., 1995. Innervation of the sacroiliac joint of the human. Zeitschr. Rheumatol. 54 (2), 117–122.

Hungerford, B., Gilleard, W., Hodges, P., 2003. Evidence of altered lumbopelvic muscle recruitment in the presence of sacroiliac joint pain. Spine 28 (14), 1593–1600.

Hungerford, B., Gilleard, W., Lee, D., 2004. Altered patterns of pelvic bone motion determined in subjects with posterior pelvic pain using skin markers. Clin. Biomech. (Bristol, Avon) 19 (5), 456–464.

Indahl, A., Holm, S., 2007. The sacroiliac joint: sensory-motor control and pain. In: Vleeming, A., Mooney, V., Stoekart, R. (Eds.), Movement, Stability and Lumbopelvic Pain. Churchill Livingstone Elsevier, Edinburgh, pp. 101–111.

Indahl, A., Kaigle, A., Reikeras, O., Holm, S., 1999. Sacroiliac joint involvement in activation of the porcine spinal and gluteal musculature. J. Spin. Dis. 12 (4), 325–330.

Indahl, A., Kaigle, A., Reikeras, O., Holm, S., 2001. Pain and muscle responses of the sacroiliac joint. In: 4th Interdisciplinary World Congress on Low Back and Pelvic Pain, Montreal, pp. 134-136.

Krzyzanowicz, R., Baker, R., Nasypany, A., Gargano, F., Seegmiller, J., 2015. Patient outcomes utilizing the selective functional movement assessment and Mulligan mobilizations with movement on recreational dancers with sacroiliac joint pain: a case series. Int. J. Athletic Ther. Training 20 (3), 31–37.

Mens, J.M., Vleeming, A., Snijders, C.J., Stam, H.J., Ginai, A.Z., 1999. The active straight leg raising test and mobility of the pelvic joints. Eur. Spine J. 8 (6), 468–473.

Mulligan, B.R., 2010. Manual Therapy: 'NAGs', 'SNAGs', 'MWMs', etc. 6th ed. Orthopedic Physical Therapy Products, Wellington, NZ.

Oliver, M., 2011. Restoration of trunk extension twenty three years after iatrogenic injury. In: Vicenzino, B., Hing, W., Rivett, D., Hall, T. (Eds.), Mobilisation With Movement: the Art and the Science. Elsevier, Sydney, pp. 179–191.

O'Sullivan, P.B., Beales, D.J., 2007. Diagnosis and classification of pelvic girdle pain disorders – Part 1: a mechanism based approach within a biopsychosocial framework. Man. Ther. 12 (2), 86–97.

Sahrmann, S.A., 2002. Diagnosis and Treatment of Movement Impairment Syndromes. Mosby, St Louis, MO.

9

Sakamoto, N., Yamashita, T., Takebayashi, T., Sekine, M., Ishii, S., 2001. An electrophysiologic study of mechanoreceptors in the sacroiliac joint and adjacent tissues. Spine 26 (20), E468–E471.

Shinde, M., Jagtap, V., 2018. Effect of muscle energy technique and Mulligan mobilization in sacroiliac joint dysfunction. Global J. Res. Analysis 7 (3), 79–81.

Smidt, G.L., Wei, S.H., McQuade, K., Barakatt, E., Sun, T., Stanford, W., 1997. Sacroiliac motion for extreme hip positions. A fresh cadaver study. Spine 22 (18), 2073–2082.

Solonen, K.A., 1957. The sacroiliac joint in the light of anatomical, roentgenological and clinical studies. Acta Orthop. Scand. Suppl. 27, 1–127.

Son, J.H., Park, G.D., Park, H.S., 2014. The effect of sacroiliac joint mobilization on pelvic deformation and the static balance ability of female university students with sacroiliac joint dysfunction. J. Phys. Ther. Sci. 26 (6), 845–848.

Szadek, K.M., Hoogland, P.V., Zuurmond, W.W., de Lange, J.J., Perez, R.S., 2008. Nociceptive nerve fibers in the sacroiliac joint in humans. Reg. Anesth. Pain Med. 33 (1), 36–43.

Szadek, K.M., Hoogland, P.V., Zuurmond, W.W., De Lange, J.J., Perez, R.S., 2010. Possible nociceptive structures in the sacroiliac joint cartilage: an immunohistochemical study. Clin. Anat. 23 (2), 192–198.

Tullberg, T., Blomberg, S., Branth, B., Johnsson, R., 1998. Manipulation does not alter the position of the sacroiliac joint. A roentgen stereophotogrammetric analysis. Spine 23 (10), 1124–1129.

Vermani, E., Mittal, R., Weeks, A., 2010. Pelvic girdle pain and low back pain in pregnancy: a review. Pain Pract. 10 (1), 60–71.

Vicenzino, B., Hing, W., Hall, T., Rivett, D., 2011. Mobilisation with Movement: the art and science of its application. In: Vicenzino, B., Hing, W., Rivett, D., Hall, T. (Eds.), Mobilisation With Movement: The Art and the Science. Churchill Livingstone Australia, Chatswood, NSW, pp. 9–23.

Vilensky, J.A., O'Connor, B.L., Fortin, J.D., Merkel, G.J., Jimenez, A.M., Scofield, B.A., et al., 2002. Histologic analysis of neural elements in the human sacroiliac joint. Spine 27 (11), 1202–1207.

Vleeming, A., Albert, H.B., Ostgaard, H.C., Sturesson, B., Stuge, B., 2008. European guidelines for the diagnosis and treatment of pelvic girdle pain. Eur. Spine J. 17 (6), 794–819.

Vleeming, A., Schuenke, M.D., Masi, A.T., Carreiro, J.E., Danneels, L., Willard, F.H., 2012. The sacroiliac joint: an overview of its anatomy, function and potential clinical implications. J. Anat. 221 (6), 537–567.

Yin, W., Willard, F., Carreiro, J., Dreyfuss, P., 2003. Sensory stimulation-guided sacroiliac joint radiofrequency neurotomy: technique based on neuroanatomy of the dorsal sacral plexus. Spine 28 (20), 2419–2425.

9

Lumbar spine

TECHNIQUES FOR THE LUMBAR SPINE

LUMBAR SNAGS
L1–5 SNAGS for lumbar motion pain and/or restriction for extension (or flexion and lateral flexion) – central or unilateral
  Lumbar extension SNAG in sitting
  Lumbar flexion SNAG in sitting
  Lumbar extension SNAG in standing
  Lumbar flexion SNAG in standing
SNAG in four-point kneeling ('lion position')
  Lumbar flexion SNAG in four-point kneeling
  Lumbar extension SNAG in four-point kneeling
  Lumbar SNAG into extension in prone lying
  Lion position – self-treatment

LUMBAR SPINE PAIN WITH LEG SYMPTOMS
SLR-induced symptoms proximal to the knee
  Gate (two-leg rotation) technique
  Gate (two-leg rotation) – self-management
  Bent leg raise (BLR)
  Traction straight leg raise (TrSLR)

SPINAL MOBILISATION WITH LEG MOVEMENT (SMWLM) FOR SLR
SLR-induced distal leg symptoms
  SLR SMWLM in side lying
  SLR SMWLM in prone position
  SMWLM ('unilateral SNAG') for SLR in prone position
  SMWLM ('unilateral SNAG') for SLR in slump position
Femoral nerve test-induced anterior leg symptoms
  Femoral SMWLM in side lying
  SNAG SMWLM in prone position
  SNAG SMWLM for PKB in standing

INTRODUCTION

Lumbar spine pain disorders may involve any innervated structure, but essentially low back pain (LBP) arises from myofascial, articular (facet joint, disc and supporting ligaments) or neuro-meningeal structures (Bogduk, 2012). In the Mulligan Concept, low-back-related pain disorders are managed through a range of quite diverse, but useful, techniques (SNAGs, SMWLM, etc.) when used in the right context.

However, choosing the right technique can be confusing for the inexperienced practitioner. Clinical experience indicates that lumbar spine MWM techniques can be broadly grouped into three categories according to their responsiveness in different pain presentations: (1) localised back / buttock pain, (2) low back referred pain in the posterior thigh, proximal to the knee, and (3) low back referred pain radiating distal to the knee or to the anterior thigh.

Lumbar SNAG techniques (Figs 10.1–10.5) are better suited for localised low back / buttock pain, but pain does not have to relate to a specific structure for SNAGs to be effective. Mulligan hypothesised that SNAGs may be helpful for pain arising from either the intervertebral disc or the facet joints (Mulligan, 2010) – the explanation being that hypomobility of the facet joints distorts the intervertebral disc. The lumbar motion segment is a triad of joints involving the central intervertebral disc and the two posterolaterally placed facet joints. For normal movement to occur at a specific lumbar segment there must be adequate movement of each joint. For example, during lumbar flexion, if the opposing surfaces of the facet joints don't glide sufficiently on each other this may induce excessive 'wedging' and anterior compression of the intervertebral disc. Such abnormal movement patterns in the presence of a weakened internally disrupted and fissured annulus may further stress the damaged disc and cause or perpetuate pain.

A SNAG is thought to improve gliding and translation of facet articular surfaces, thereby reducing the 'wedging' effect on the disc. Although no studies have specifically investigated the biomechanical effects of lumbar SNAGs, one study reported that a posteroanterior pressure on the L5 spinous process induced translation and flexion of the L5 / S1 motion segment (Lee & Evans, 1997). The biomechanical effects of a SNAG may be enhanced by the cephalad direction of glide force employed in this technique, and there is at least some conceptual evidence to support this (Allison et al., 1998).

One study found that lumbar flexion SNAGs improved ROM, but not pain in a small sample of people with LBP (Konstantinou et al., 2007). In asymptomatic people, lumbar flexion SNAGs did not differ in their biomechanical (Moutzouri et al., 2008) or sympathoexcitation (Moutzouri et al., 2012) effects when compared with a sham treatment. It is, however, not possible to relate this information to people with LBP as the effect may be very different in the presence of pain and limitation of movement.

The second and third category assigned to lumbar MWM techniques are for referred leg pain. In this case it is important to identify a pain-provocative movement. Typically sciatic or femoral nerve neurodynamic tests are symptomatic and can be the basis for the CSIM. The MWM is intended to directly improve the neurodynamic movement and eliminate pain either by directly influencing the affected spinal motion segment (SMWLM) at the source of symptoms or indirectly (gate, bent leg raise (BLR) or traction straight leg raise (TrSLR)). These techniques are also used to improve hamstring and rectus femoris muscle extensibility. The evidence for these techniques is presented at the end of this chapter.

Levels of evidence

Level 2: five RCTs and two pilot RCTs

There are four placebo-controlled clinical trials investigating lumbar SNAG techniques (Hidalgo et al., 2015; Konstantinou et al., 2007; Moutzouri et al., 2008, 2012), but only two of these (Hidalgo et al., 2015; Konstantinou et al., 2007) investigated symptomatic people. In the latter study, MWM had a significant effect on lumbar ROM, but not on pain. Recently, Subarna Das and colleagues (Subarna Das et al., 2018) have provided evidence on the superior effects of the combination of SMWLM with neural mobilisation and conventional physiotherapy in decreasing pain (numerical pain rating scale (NPRS)) and back-specific disability scores (Modified Oswestry Low Back Pain Questionnaire) as well as increasing straight leg raise (SLR) ROM compared with conventional physiotherapy alone or combined only to neural mobilisation. A number of studies have investigated the effects of BLR and TrSLR either for low-back-related leg pain (Hall et al., 2006a, 2006b) or to improve muscle length (Hall, 2001; Nijskens et al., 2013). These studies have reported significant effects on improving ROM, muscle length and pain.

Nijskens and colleagues (Nijskens et al., 2013), in their controlled trial, also found that gains in flexibility following MWM were significantly better than a control and a single 30-second static stretch. These improvements were maintained even after 1-week follow-up and were not helped by the incorporation of home exercise.

Utilising validated kinematic algorithms for ROM and speed (Hidalgo et al., 2012, 2014), Hidalgo and colleagues (Hidalgo et al., 2015) demonstrated quantitatively the efficacy of MWM compared with sham technique in restoring trunk ROM in patients with LBP. Further, this group demonstrated significant differences in favour of the group treated with SNAGs compared with sham in the reduction of self-reported pain at rest and during active trunk flexion, as well as functional disability with large clinical effect sizes.

LUMBAR SNAGS

L1–5 SNAGs for lumbar motion pain and/or restriction for extension (or flexion and lateral flexion) – central or unilateral

TECHNIQUE AT A GLANCE

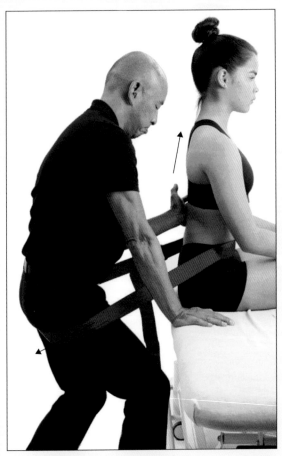

Figure 10.1
Lumbar extension SNAG: side view

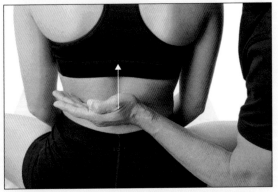

Figure 10.2
Lumbar extension SNAG: start position

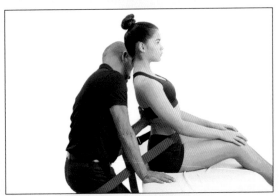

Figure 10.3
Lumbar extension SNAG: end position side view

- The patient is sitting on a treatment table.
- The patient's palms rest on their anterior thighs.
- The therapist is standing behind and slightly to one side of the patient.
- A belt is wrapped around the patient's pelvis and therapist's upper thighs.
- The therapist places one hand on the table for support.
- The ulnar border of the contact hand is placed under the spinous (central) or transverse process (unilateral) L1–4, thumbs on L5.
- See Figs 10.1–10.3.

INDICATION

Localised lumbar spine pain/restriction with lumbar spine movement in sitting.

POSITIONING

Patient:	Sitting on a couch, both hands resting on their thighs.
Treated body part:	Neutral lumbar spine position.
Therapist:	Standing behind the patient, slightly to one side. Knees bent and elbow held beside the body. A belt is wrapped around the patient's pelvis anteriorly and therapist's hips (Fig. 10.1). A towel is used for belt contact comfort.
Hands/contact points:	Stabilising hand: on the table for support. Gliding hand: hypothenar eminence is in contact under the spinous (central) or transverse process (unilateral) of the appropriate vertebral level.

APPLICATION GUIDELINES

- Instruct the patient to arch their back but avoid leaning backwards from the hips.
- Before proceeding, apply a cranially directed glide of sufficient force to be pain-free.
- Maintain the glide while the patient extends the lumbar spine until pain/restriction is felt and maintain the glide until resuming the start position.
- If pain persists during the movement try adjusting the vertebral level, glide direction and/or force.
- Note that when the lumbar spine is extended the pelvis tilts anteriorly, which needs to be accommodated by the therapist's body movement. It is important that the therapist moves slightly forwards during extension and reciprocally on return to maintain stabilising belt tension and avoiding restricting the movement.

COMMENTS

- After completing the SNAG evaluate the opposite movement (flexion in sitting in this case) to ensure that the mobilisation did not aggravate the previously pain-free movement. This occurs occasionally; if that is the case then try to mobilise through the whole range of flexion and extension in sitting or in a different start position such as four-point kneeling (see Fig. 10.4).
- Asking the patient to keep hand contact on their thighs during extension maximises lumbar extension.
- If the extension SNAG does not seem to improve range, try a flexion SNAG immediately followed by extension.
- When pain-free end range cannot be achieved, consider variations in the vertebral level of contact, contact direction, direction of mobilisation, speed of movement and start position.
- Other factors may also strongly influence the choice of mobilising position, for example: body composition of the patient relative to therapist (tall/short, big/small), therapist preference and technical ability, confidence and level of expertise in using SNAGs or specific concurrent injury (pelvis, hip/knee pathology may hinder SNAG in four-point kneeling).

10

- In principle, the therapist should choose the SNAG technique based on the movement and position that replicates the patient's main complaint. See SNAG into flexion (Fig. 10.4). However, a SNAG in sitting may be preferable to in standing when pain and limitation are more severe.

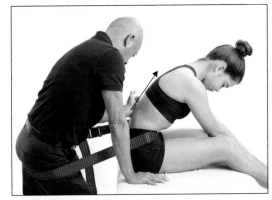

Figure 10.4
Lumbar flexion SNAG in sitting

- The technique may be progressed into standing when full range in sitting is achieved (see Fig. 10.5).
- A SNAG in standing would be the first choice if the patient does not have limitation or pain during sitting.

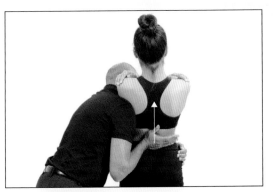

Figure 10.5A
Lumbar extension SNAG in standing

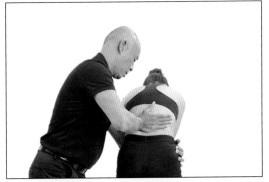

Figure 10.5B
Lumbar flexion SNAG in standing

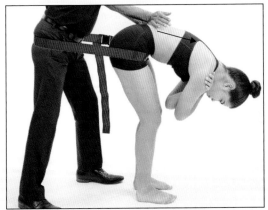

Figure 10.5C
Lumbar flexion SNAG in standing: using a belt

10

(continued next page...)

- For a flexion SNAG in standing, greater movement may be achieved with the patient's knees slightly flexed (Fig. 10.5C). The patient may also prefer to stand beside a table with one hand on the table for support. The patient begins with a neutral lumbar spine position.

- The application guidelines are as described for a SNAG in sitting. A belt can be used to stabilise the pelvis also (Fig. 10.5C). Apply a cranially directed glide, either centrally or unilaterally depending on pain location. Maintain the glide while the patient flexes their lumbar spine until pain/restriction is felt and maintain the glide until resuming the start position.

Unilateral SNAG for L5/S1

- For a unilateral SNAG at the L5/S1 segment a different grip is needed to achieve the required effect (Fig. 10.6A). The medial edge of the thumb is used to contact the transverse process of L5. This thumb is reinforced with the opposite thumb to create the glide force in the direction of the facet plane. This technique is most easily applied in a four-point kneeling position (Fig. 10.6B).

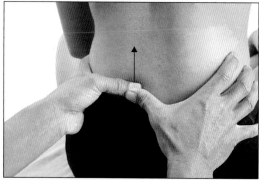

Figure 10.6A
L5/S1 unilateral SNAG with therapist hand contact: thumb position

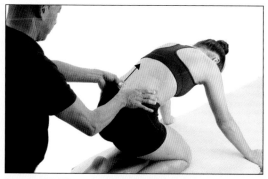

Figure 10.6B
L5/S1 unilateral SNAG with therapist hand contact: four-point kneeling end range

- The above sitting and standing start position is the basic method for applying a SNAG. However, based on other factors in the presentation, therapist confidence and skill, the therapist may choose between several alternative start positions such as four-point kneeling or prone lying (see Figs 10.8 and 10.12).

10

SELF-MANAGEMENT

- Self-treatment may be applied in a standing or sitting position with a self-SNAG strap or other narrow cloth belt.
- The patient hooks the strap around the spinous process of the superior vertebrae and grasps the strap in both hands. Both elbows should be maximally flexed and the belt in a vertically orientated direction to follow the facet plane.
- Maintaining tension on the belt, the patient moves the spine in the appropriate direction (i.e. flexion or extension, Fig. 10.7A and B). No pain should be experienced during the movement. An alternative is for the patient to utilise their fist to apply the glide (Fig. 10.7C).

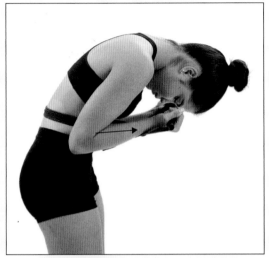

Figure 10.7A
Self-SNAG into flexion

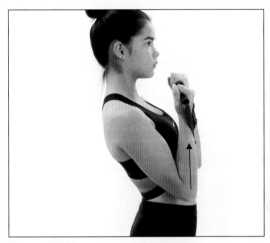

Figure 10.7B
Self-SNAG into extension

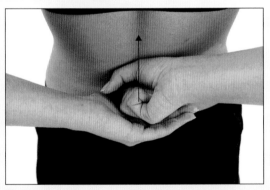

Figure 10.7C
Use of fist for L5/S1 self-SNAG

ANNOTATIONS

sit L3 belt SNAG E×3
sit L3 belt SNAG F×6(3)
st L4 SNAG E×3
st L4 SNAG F×6(3)
st L4 belt SNAG F×10(3)
4 point kneel L L5 SNAG F×10
st L4 self strap SNAG F×10
st L4 self strap SNAG E×10
st L5 self fist SNAG E×10

SNAG in four-point kneeling ('lion position')

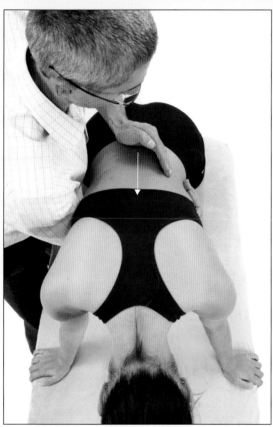

Figure 10.8
Lumbar flexion SNAG in four-point kneeling: start position

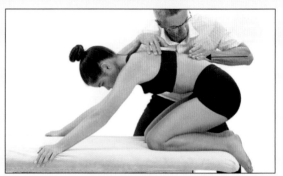

Figure 10.9
Lumbar flexion SNAG in four-point kneeling: end position

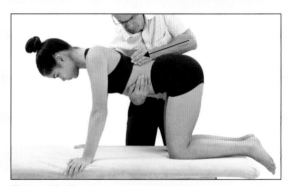

Figure 10.10
Lumbar extension SNAG in four-point kneeling: side view with hand position

10

- The patient is in four-point kneeling, close to the side and end of the table, with feet over the edge and knees apart (see Figs 10.9 and 10.11).
- The therapist is standing facing the patient's head at their side.
- The therapist 's hand is wrapped under the patient's abdomen for counterforce and stabilisation.
- The contact hand's hypothenar eminence glides the spinous or transverse process of the involved segment.
- The contact point is for L5 (spinous process if central SNAG or over transverse process if unilateral).
- See Figs 10.8–10.10.

INDICATION

Localised LBP/limitation with lumbar spine flexion or extension.

POSITIONING

Patient:	Four-point kneeling close to the edge and end of a treatment table, feet over the edge.
Treated body part:	Neutral lumbar spine position.
Therapist:	Standing at the side of the treatment table, facing the patient's head.
Hands/contact points:	Stabilising hand: one arm is wrapped around the patient's abdomen. Gliding hand: hypothenar eminence contacts under the target spinous or transverse process.

APPLICATION GUIDELINES

- Instruct the patient to flex their back slightly to separate the spinous process to allow a good contact with the gliding hand.
- Before proceeding, apply a cranially directed glide that is of sufficient force to be pain-free. For unilateral pain a unilateral SNAG is usually effective, whereas for bilateral or central pain a central SNAG could be more effective.
- Maintain the glide while the patient sits back towards their heels (for flexion) until pain/restriction is felt and maintain the glide until resuming the start position. For extension ask the patient to hollow their back and tilt the pelvis anteriorly.
- If pain persists during the movement try adjusting the vertebral level, glide direction and/or force.
- Encourage the patient to achieve the maximum available range.
- Apply only 3 repetitions on the first occasion; subsequently 3–5 sets of 6–10 repetitions can be used.

COMMENT

- For a unilateral SNAG at L5/S1 only, it is difficult to contact the transverse process of L5 due to the iliac crest being 'in the way'. In this case use the medial (ulnar) side of the thumb to contact the transverse process and reinforce the pressure with the pad of the opposite thumb. For this technique, stand at the foot of the table. The glide direction is along the facet plane (see Fig. 10.6).

VARIATIONS

- An alternative hand position for the stabilising the hand/arm (rather than around the abdomen) is on the shoulder of the patient (see Fig. 10.11).

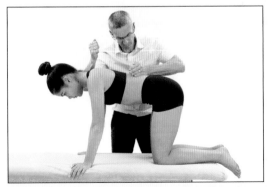

Figure 10.11
Lumbar flexion SNAG in four-point-kneeling variation

10

(continued next page...)

Lumbar SNAG into extension in prone lying

- Another variation is to perform the SNAG in a non-weight-bearing prone position. This can be an alternative for pain or restriction into extension where a sitting, four-point kneeling or standing start position is less preferred or not achievable.
- Based on other factors in the presentation, therapist confidence and skill, the therapist may choose between several alternative start positions (i.e. four-point kneeling or in prone lying – see Figs 10.8–10.12).

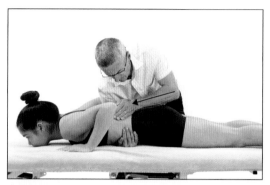

Figure 10.12A
Lumbar extension SNAG in prone lying: start position

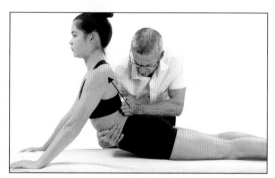

Figure 10.12B
Lumbar extension SNAG in prone lying: end position

SELF-MANAGEMENT

Lion position – self-treatment

- The patient is in four-point kneeling with the lumbar spine flexed and pelvis posteriorly rotated. A self-SNAG strap is placed at the involved level (a small piece of sports tape can be used to indicate the point for the patient at home). Tension is maintained in the strap with both hands fixing the strap to the table.
- They then lower their pelvis towards their feet until strap tension prevents any further movement, inducing a small flexion effect. The patient may also do a simple exercise without the belt.
- See Fig. 10.13.

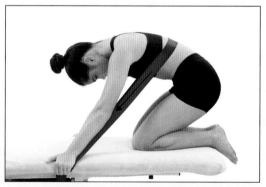

Figure 10.13A
Self-SNAG in four-point kneeling using a strap: start position

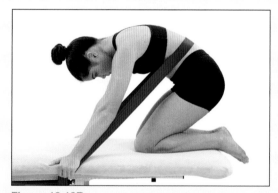

Figure 10.13B
Self-SNAG in four-point kneeling using a strap: end position

10

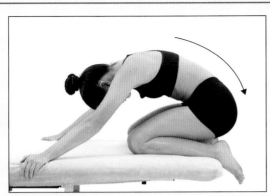

Figure 10.13C
Self-SNAG in four-point kneeling using a strap:
without belt

ANNOTATIONS

4 point kneel L4 SNAG F×3
4 point kneel L4 SNAG E×6(3)
pr ly L4 SNAG E×10
4 point kneel L2 self belt SNAG Lion×10
4 point kneel Lion stretch×10

10

LUMBAR SPINE PAIN WITH LEG SYMPTOMS

SLR-induced symptoms proximal to the knee

Gate (two-leg rotation) technique

TECHNIQUE AT A GLANCE

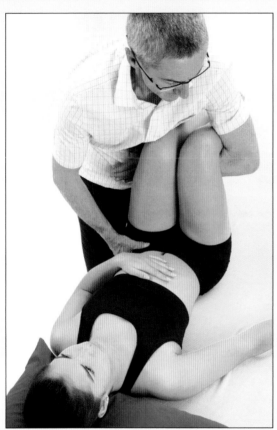

Figure 10.14
Two-leg rotation (gate technique): start position

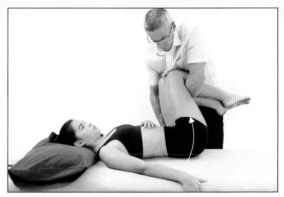

Figure 10.15
Two-leg rotation (gate technique): start position
lateral view

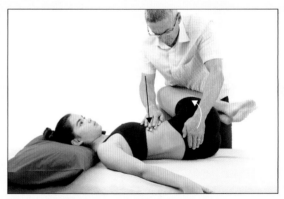

Figure 10.16
Two-leg rotation (gate technique) with left pelvic
rotation: end range

- The patient lies in crook lying. Both hips are flexed to beyond 90° with knees flexed. The pelvis/legs are supported by the therapist.
- The knees are brought to the side of SLR limitation, rotating the pelvis and trunk as far as possible without pain.
- Change the hip/lumbar position (flexion/extension) if pain is provoked. Sustain for 20 seconds and return painlessly to the start position. Reassess SLR in supine.
- See Figs 10.14–10.16.

10

INDICATION

Posterior thigh, buttock or back pain induced by the SLR test.

POSITIONING

Patient:	The patient lies supine with the head supported on a pillow and the contralateral hand holding the side of the table for stability.
Treated body part:	The lower trunk is in flexion (both hips and knees are flexed beyond 90°).
Therapist:	Adjacent to the symptomatic side of the patient, beside the pelvis, facing perpendicular to the patient.
Hands/contact points:	Cranial hand: the cranial hand of the therapist stabilises the patient's trunk. Caudal hand: the caudal hand of the therapist supports the legs keeping the hips and knees in 90° flexion.

APPLICATION GUIDELINES

- Passively rotate the trunk to the involved side, by rolling the knees towards the therapist, while maintaining the angle of the hip and knee flexion. The therapist bends their knees to continue to support the patient's legs to achieve full-range passive trunk rotation.
- If pain is provoked during the trunk rotation, the hip/lumbar spine flexion position is altered to find a 'gate' to go through that allows greater pain-free movement of the trunk.
- Once end range is achieved the position is sustained for up to 20 seconds. Take care when returning to the start position and ensure that the movement is pain-free.
- Apply up to 3 repetitions in the first session, with up to 5 repetitions in subsequent sessions. Reassess the patient's SLR.

COMMENTS

- If pain is provoked during the technique application then subtle changes in hip and lumbar spine flexion position may eliminate pain and allow greater rotation range to be achieved. This may need to be done several times to gain full ROM and to return to the start position.
- The technique should be applied smoothly and slowly to avoid excessive loading of sensitised lumbar spine tissues.
- In some more-sensitised cases of LBP, the patient may be apprehensive and have strong muscle over-activity and guarding. In this case, let the patient actively measure their SLR range and get them to try the technique gently, within a small ROM. Return to the start position and remeasure the active SLR. If the range has visibly improved, the patient's attitude to the next repetition will be free from any apprehension.

VARIATIONS

- In the presence of a more mobile patient, it may be necessary to stabilise the lower ribs to localise the rotation to the lower trunk.
- In addition, over-pressure may be applied by pulling the pelvis into rotation. Furthermore, the trunk may be rotated further as the patient relaxes in the end-range position.

10

(continued next page...)

SELF-MANAGEMENT

- The patient lies supine with hips and knees bent to 90°.
- The patient stabilises the upper trunk with one arm holding the side of the table. The patient actively rotates their trunk with support from their other hand.
- The hip/lower trunk flexion angle is altered if pain is provoked during the movement.
- The end position is maintained for 20 seconds.
- Cautiously return to the start position, to ensure no pain during the exercise.
- Perform 3 repetitions 3 times per day. This frequency can be altered at the therapist's discretion.
- See Fig. 10.17.

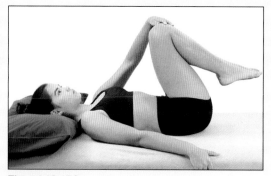

Figure 10.17A
Gate technique: start position

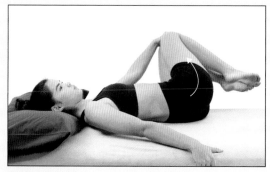

Figure 10.17B
Gate technique: end range

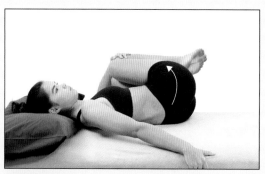

Figure 10.17C
Gate technique: with greater hip flexion

- A wider bed is preferred to give the patient a greater sense of support.
- For more mobile patients, lying on top of one or two pillows will enable the spine to move into a greater range (Fig. 10.18).
- For a stiffer patient, a pillow or two at their side will allow them to rest their legs at their available end range. Advise the patient to move slowly to ensure maximum comfort.

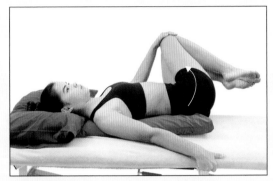

Figure 10.18
Gate technique for more mobile patients

ANNOTATIONS

sup ly L gate×20 sec(3)
sup ly L self gate×20 sec(3)
sup ly L self- gate×20 sec(3)

Bent leg raise (BLR)

TECHNIQUE AT A GLANCE

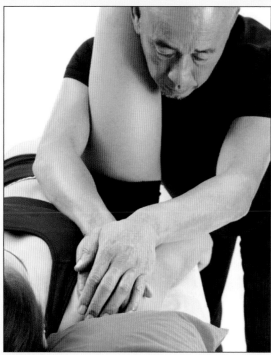

Figure 10.19
Bent leg raise: start position

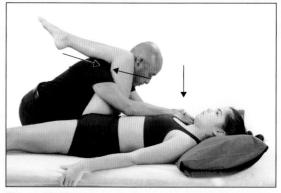

Figure 10.20
Bent leg raise: side view

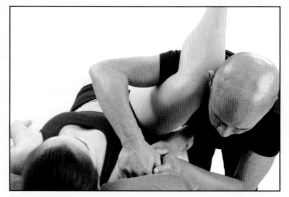

Figure 10.21
Bent leg raise: end position

10

- The patient lies supine close to the edge of a treatment table. The affected hip and knee is flexed and rests over the therapist's shoulder.
- A 5-second submaximal isometric contraction of the hamstrings is performed by the patient pushing down with their hip, which is resisted through the therapist's shoulder, into increasing positions of hip flexion.
- Traction can be applied through the femur (see Fig. 10.20) to help gain range between contractions.
- See Figs 10.19–10.21.

INDICATION

Posterior thigh, buttock or back pain induced by the SLR test.

POSITIONING

Patient:	Supine, close to the edge of the treatment table.
Treated body part:	The involved hip and knee are flexed, supported by the therapist's shoulder.
Therapist:	Stride stance position, knees flexed slightly, adjacent to the affected side facing towards the head of the patient.
Hands/contact points:	The therapist places the patient's flexed knee of the involved side over the therapist's shoulder.

APPLICATION GUIDELINES

- Apply a sustained longitudinal traction to the hip, along the line of the femur.
- A 5-second hamstring isometric contraction is induced by asking the patient to extend their hip into the therapist's shoulder. The patient then relaxes and the hip is moved passively into a new point in range. Repeat the process until maximal hip flexion range is achieved.
- A degree of abduction may also be required as more flexion is gained.
- Sustain the end-range position for several seconds and then return the leg to the start position.
- Repeat the technique 3 times in the first session.
- Reassess the SLR in supine.

COMMENTS

- Every time you ask the patient to contract, use your hand on the patient's shoulder to apply effective resistance.
- If the patient feels pain when the hip is moved into flexion then slight abduction or lateral rotation of the hip or more flexion of the knee may assist in achieving a greater range.
- There is conflicting evidence regarding the length of contraction and relaxation phases for techniques such as this. Based on clinical experience, the optimum time period is 5–10 seconds.

(continued next page...)

SELF-MANAGEMENT

Bent leg raise

- The patient can perform a self-BLR by clasping their hands around the lower thigh and performing an isometric hamstring contraction and then relaxing (see Fig. 10.22).

- The patient moves the leg into increasing hip flexion (with some abduction) range as capable, stopping when they feel discomfort.

- A 5-second hamstring isometric contraction can be incorporated if necessary. In the relaxation phase, the patient pulls the thigh towards their chest. This action may induce traction in the longitudinal axis of the femur. At the point of pain or discomfort, the patient repeats the isometric contraction, repeating the cycle until full-range hip flexion is achieved.

- Repeat the exercise 3 times in a session and 3 times per day. This frequency can be altered at the therapist's discretion.

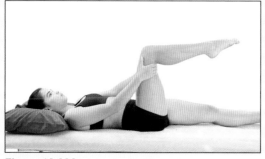

Figure 10.22A
Bent leg raise self-mobilisation: start position

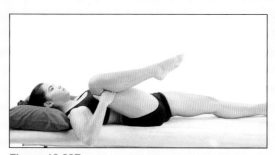

Figure 10.22B
Bent leg raise self-mobilisation: end position with slight hip abduction

Lion exercise

- The lion exercise (see Fig. 10.23) is an addition to the BLR exercise. The patient starts in four-point kneeling with knees well apart and ankles over the edge of the bed for comfort.

- The hip on the affected side is flexed more than on the opposite side to replicate the BLR exercise.

- When the patient lowers their pelvis to their feet and sustains the stretch, the BLR technique is replicated on the affected side.

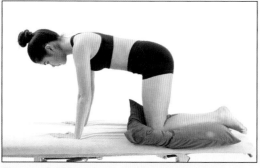

Figure 10.23A
Lion exercise: start position

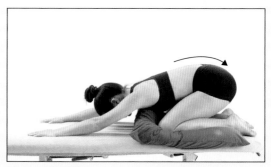

Figure 10.23B
Lion exercise: end position

ANNOTATIONS

sup ly R BLR×3
sup ly R self-BLR×3
4 point kneel L Kn forw Lion×10 sec(3)
4 point kneel L Kn on pillow Lion×10 sec(3)

Traction straight leg raise (TrSLR)

TECHNIQUE AT A GLANCE

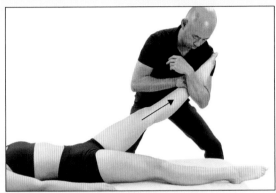

Figure 10.24
Traction straight leg raise: start position

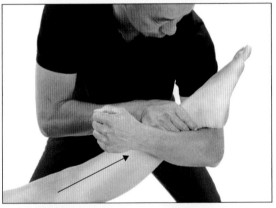

Figure 10.25
Traction straight leg raise: hand position

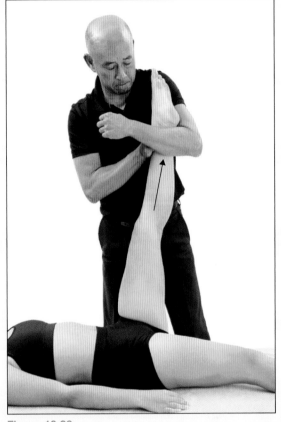

Figure 10.26
Traction straight leg raise: end-range position

- The patient lies supine.
- The therapist grasps around the ankle and lower leg of the patient comfortably.
- The therapist applies a longitudinal glide along the line of the femur, by extending the knees and leaning backwards.
- While maintaining the glide, a longitudinal stretch is applied whilst moving the patient's leg passively into the pain-free range of SLR.
- See Figs 10.24–10.26.

INDICATION

Pain in the posterior thigh reproduced by SLR not extending below the knee.

Tight hamstrings or 'chronic hamstring strain'.

POSITIONING

Patient:	The patient lies supine on a very low plinth or the floor.
Treated body part:	Leg close to the limitation of SLR.
Therapist:	The therapist stands on the affected side in lunge stance, knees flexed, facing the patient's head.
Hands/contact points:	The patient's leg is grasped proximal to the ankle, in the crook of the therapist's elbow with the other hand grasping the anterior shin. Use a towel or pad for contact comfort.

APPLICATION GUIDELINES

- Apply a longitudinal glide along the line of the femur, by extending the knees and leaning backwards.
- While maintaining the glide, move the patient's leg passively into the pain-free range of SLR.
- If pain is provoked, try to eliminate it by moving the hip into abduction and/or external or internal rotation while repeating the movement into SLR.
- Apply 3 repetitions on the first treatment occasion, with 6–10 repetitions subsequently.
- Hold the stretch at the ROM for up to 10 seconds.
- Return to neutral position before reducing the longitudinal glide force.

10

COMMENTS

- The pain should be in the posterior thigh and not below the knee for the technique to be successful.
- If the patient is tall, have the patient lie on a mat on the floor rather than on a plinth (Fig. 10.27).
- Maintain the glide force throughout the technique until resuming the neutral position.
- If symptoms are made worse by this manoeuvre, compression along the line of the femur may be used instead of traction.
- This technique may also be used as a treatment for chronic low back, buttock and posterior thigh pain in patients presenting with limitation of SLR.
- This technique can be used prior to training and exercising in patients where hamstring muscle length appears to be affecting training ability. Clinical experience suggests it is very useful in patients with 'hamstring'-related pain around the ischial tuberosity, often (mis)diagnosed as tendinosis and sometimes irritated by stretching. In those patients, the combination of the traction SLR technique and eccentric loading can be effective.

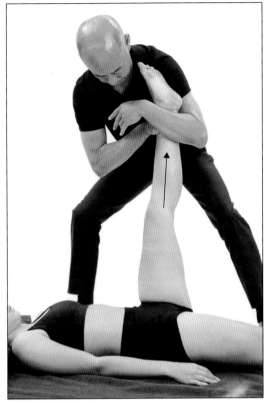

Figure 10.27
Traction straight leg raise on a mat

ANNOTATION

 sup ly L Tr SLR×10 sec(3)

SPINAL MOBILISATION WITH LEG MOVEMENT (SMWLM) FOR SLR

SLR-induced distal leg symptoms

SLR SMWLM in side lying

TECHNIQUE AT A GLANCE

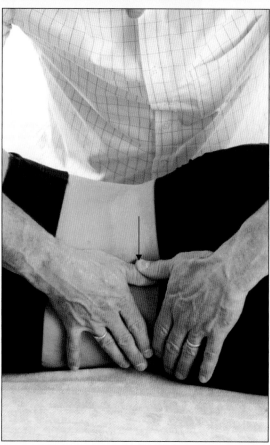

Figure 10.28
Spinal mobilisation with leg movement: hand position

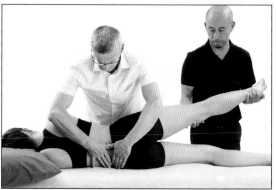

Figure 10.29
Spinal mobilisation with leg movement: start position

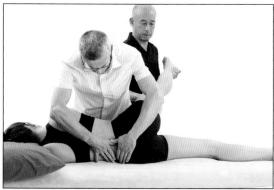

Figure 10.30
Spinal mobilisation with leg movement: end position

- This technique requires two therapists, A and B. Therapist A is considered the lead.
- The patient is in side-lying position, with their affected leg uppermost, close to edge of the treatment table. The affected leg is extended with slight abduction at the hip and held by therapist B. Therapist A applies and sustains a transverse glide of the spinous process towards the floor of the cranial vertebra at the involved segment.
- The patient actively moves the leg into SLR, with the assistance of therapist B. Reassess the SLR in supine position.
- See Figs 10.28–10.30.

10

INDICATION

Leg pain and other symptoms extending below the knee induced by the SLR test.

POSITIONING

Patient:	Side lying with symptomatic side uppermost. Close to the edge of the treatment table.
Treated body part:	Contralateral hip and knee flexed to 45°. The affected leg is extended with approximately 10° of abduction.
Therapists:	This technique requires two therapists, A and B. Therapist A faces the patient's pelvis and leans over their lower trunk. Therapist B remains caudally, towards the patient's feet.
Hands contact points:	Therapist A places their thumbs, reinforced one on top of the other, on the lateral aspect of the spinous process of L4 or L5 (Fig. 10.28). Therapist B supports the involved leg and thigh.

APPLICATION GUIDELINES

- Therapist A applies a strong transverse glide of the involved level, by pressure against the side of the spinous process (typically L4 or L5).
- Sustain the glide and have the patient actively SLR, with the assistance of therapist B, ensuring that no symptoms are provoked during the movement.
- Repeat 3 times and retest the SLR in supine.
- On subsequent visits, as the patient improves, therapist B can apply over-pressure into the SLR range, again provided that there are no symptoms.
- The spinous process of the L5 vertebra is chosen if the patient has an L5/S1 lesion.

COMMENTS

- Use sponge rubber to minimise vertebral contact discomfort.
- Mobilise the L4 or L3 vertebra if the first attempt at L5 does not improve the SLR range.
- This technique can be applied without an assistant. In this case, the patient moves their involved leg actively through the range of SLR.
- A further alternative is to have the patient support their thigh on a pillow, with the hip flexed to 90° and the hip 10° abducted. The patient actively extends their knee, while the therapist applies the transverse glide.

10

(continued next page...)

SMWLM ('unilateral SNAG') for SLR in prone position

- The patient lies prone and slightly oblique with their pelvis close to the edge of the treatment table. The affected leg (extended at the hip and knee) is held by the other therapist, who remains caudally of the ipsilateral side (therapist B) (Fig. 10.31).
- Therapist A stands on the involved side and applies a superior/cranial glide (SNAG) of the transverse process of the cranial vertebra of the involved segment.
- Note the SNAG mobilisation should be sustained during the whole process.
- Therapist B simultaneously lowers the patient's involved leg into SLR (towards the floor), provided there are no symptoms.
- Use sponge rubber to minimise vertebral contact discomfort.
- This technique is particularly helpful for L4/L5 and L5/S1 lesions.
- Repeat 3 times and reassess SLR in supine.
- Do not apply more than 6 repetitions in the subsequent sessions.

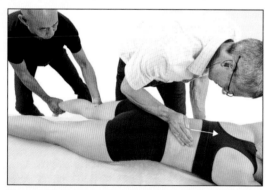

Figure 10.31
Spinal mobilisation with leg movement ('unilateral SNAG') for SLR in prone position

SMWLM ('unilateral SNAG') for SLR in slump position

- Another option is to perform the above technique with the patient in a sitting position. The patient sits on the side of the treatment table with their involved leg flexed at the knee and foot resting on a chair in front of them.
- The therapist stands beside the patient, on the involved side, contacting the transverse process of the involved vertebra, applying a SNAG.
- The pelvis is stabilised by the use of a mobilisation belt (Fig. 10.32B).
- The patient flexes the trunk with the leg fixed, provided there are no symptoms.
- An adjustable height treatment table helps in the correct positioning prior to the SNAG. This technique is particularly helpful for L4/L5 and L5/S1 lesions.
- If the involved segment is L5/S1 then the SNAG can be applied with contact using the ulnar side of the therapist's thumb reinforced by the other (see Fig. 10.6A). The remaining fingers of both hands spread around the posterior aspect of the patient's pelvis and trunk.
- Use sponge rubber to minimise contact discomfort on the vertebra.
- This technique can be undertaken in a sitting slump position, where the neuromeningeal tract would be under greater tension, increasing the provocative nature of the movement.
- See Fig. 10.32.

10

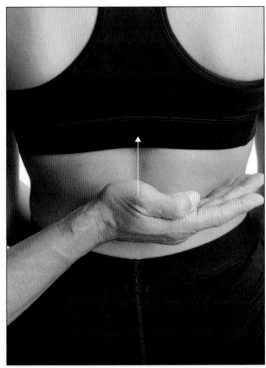

Figure 10.32A
Slump spinal mobilisation with leg movement: hand position

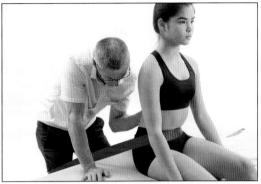

Figure 10.32B
Slump spinal mobilisation with leg movement: start position

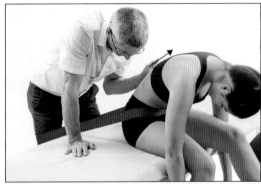

Figure 10.32C
Slump spinal mobilisation with leg movement: end position

ANNOTATIONS

L s ly R L5 SMWLM SLR +A×3
pr ly L L4 SNAG SMWLM SLR +A×3
sit L L4 SNAG SMWLM Slump×3

10

Femoral nerve test-induced anterior leg symptoms

Femoral SMWLM in side lying

TECHNIQUE AT A GLANCE

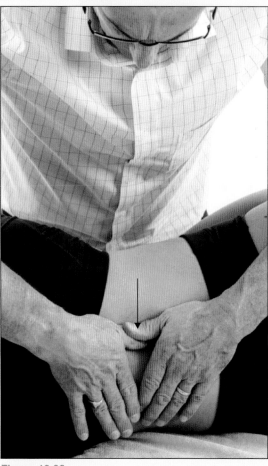

Figure 10.33
Femoral spinal mobilisation with leg movement: hand position

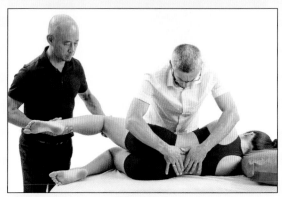

Figure 10.34
Femoral spinal mobilisation with leg movement: start position

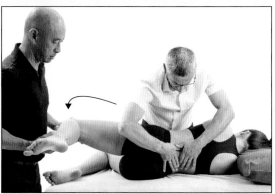

Figure 10.35
Femoral spinal mobilisation with leg movement: end position

- This technique requires two therapists, A and B.
- The patient is in side-lying position, close to the edge of the treatment table with the affected leg uppermost. Therapist A applies and sustains a transverse glide of the spinous process towards the floor of the cranial vertebra at the involved segment.
- Therapist B supports the affected leg in 90° knee flexion and moves the hip into extension concurrently with the glide from therapist A.
- See Figs 10.33–10.35.

10

INDICATION

Groin and anterior thigh symptoms induced by a femoral neurodynamic test.

POSITIONING

Patient:	Side lying with symptomatic side uppermost, close to the edge of the treatment table.
Treated body part:	The patient's contralateral hip and knee are flexed to 45°. The affected leg is in slight flexion and abduction with the knee in 90° flexion.
Therapist:	This technique requires two therapists, A and B.
	Therapist A faces the patient's pelvis and leans over their lower trunk.
	Therapist B stays caudally, towards the patient's feet.
Hands contact points:	Therapist A places their thumbs, reinforced one on top of the other, on the lateral aspect of the spinous process of the involved vertebra.
	Therapist B supports the affected leg and thigh.

APPLICATION GUIDELINES

- Therapist A applies a strong transverse glide of the involved level, by pressure against the side of the transverse process (typically L2 or L3).
- Therapist A sustains the glide while therapist B assists the patient into hip extension with knee flexion, ensuring no symptoms are provoked during the movement.
- Repeat 3 times and retest the femoral neurodynamic test in prone.
- On subsequent visits, as the patient improves, therapist B can apply over-pressure into hip extension with knee flexion, again with the understanding that there are no symptoms.
- The spinous process of the L2 vertebra is chosen if the patient has an L2/3 lesion.

COMMENTS

- Use sponge rubber to minimise contact discomfort on the spinous process.
- Mobilise the L3 or L4 vertebra if the first attempt at L2 does not improve the range. If muscle contraction from patient's active hip extension prevents the therapist from making good contact with the spinous process then a passive movement should be introduced.
- SMWLM is useful for pain or other symptoms provoked during femoral nerve neurodynamic tests, such as prone knee bend (PKB) or femoral slump in side lying. This might include LBP as well as symptoms that follow the course of the femoral nerve such as in the inguinal and hip regions as well as symptoms in the anterior thigh and knee.

10

(continued next page...)

VARIATIONS

This technique can also be performed in both a prone position and a standing position.

SNAG SMWLM in prone position

- The patient lies prone close to the edge of the treatment table.
- The affected leg is flexed to 90° at the knee and held by therapist B, who stays caudally.
- Therapist A stands at the patient's involved side, mobilising the cranial vertebra by applying a SNAG on the transverse or spinous process of the involved vertebra.
- Therapist B assists the patient to flex their knee eventually to the end range with over-pressure (heel to the buttock) provided that there is no pain.
- Putting a pillow under the patient's thigh to increase hip extension can be used as a progression or for the more mobile person.
- Make sure that the patient has no knee joint problems.
- Use sponge rubber to minimise contact discomfort on the vertebra.
- Sometimes the patient requires more than one pillow under their abdomen for comfort or to allow access to the spinous process.
- This technique is typically used at L2/3, L3/4 or L4/5 vertebral levels.
- See Fig. 10.36.

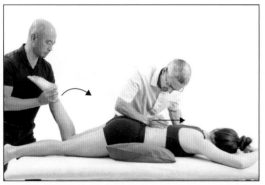

Figure 10.36A
Femoral nerve spinal mobilisation with leg movement in prone: start position

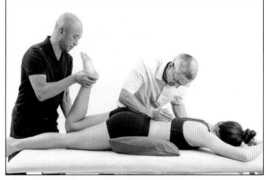

Figure 10.36B
Femoral nerve spinal mobilisation with leg movement in prone: end position

10

SNAG SMWLM for PKB in standing

- This technique requires two therapists, A and B, with the patient in standing position.
- Therapist A stands to the side of the patient and applies a central or unilateral SNAG to the involved segment.
- Concurrently, therapist B assists the patient to flex their knee and extend their hip.
- Make sure that the patient has no knee joint problems.
- Use sponge rubber to minimise contact discomfort on the vertebra.
- Performing the SMWLM in standing replicates a more functional position. This technique is successful with L2/3, L3/4 or L4/5 lumbar levels.
- See Fig. 10.37.

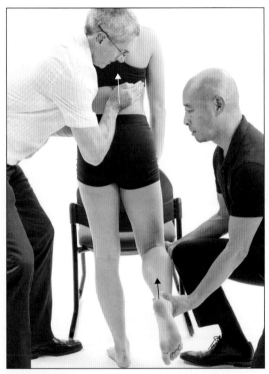

Figure 10.37A
Femoral nerve spinal mobilisation with leg movement in standing: start position

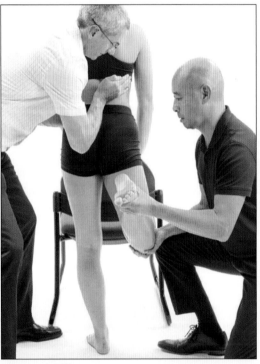

Figure 10.37B
Femoral nerve spinal mobilisation with leg movement in standing: end position

10

ANNOTATIONS

R s ly L L2 SMWLM PKB +A×3
pr ly L L3 SNAG SMWLM L PKB +A×3
st R L2 SNAG SMWLM R PKB +A×3

References

Allison, G.T., Edmondston, S.J., Roe, C.P., Reid, S.E., Toy, D.A., Lundgren, H.E., 1998. Influence of load orientation on the posteroanterior stiffness of the lumbar spine. J. Manipulative Physiol. Ther. 21 (8), 534–538.

Bogduk, N., 2012. Clinical and Radiological Anatomy of the Lumbar Spine, 5th ed. Churchill Livingstone, Edinburgh.

Hall, T., Cacho, A., McNee, C., Riches, J., Walsh, J., 2001. Effects of the Mulligan traction straight leg raise technique on range of movement. J. Man. Manipulative Ther. 9 (3), 128–133.

Hall, T., Beyerlein, C., Hansson, U., Lim, H.T., Odermark, M., Sainsbury, D., 2006a. Mulligan traction straight leg raise: a pilot study to investigate effects on range of motion in patients with low back pain. J. Man. Manipulative Ther. 14 (2), 95–100.

Hall, T., Hardt, S., Schafer, A., Wallin, L., 2006b. Mulligan bent leg raise technique – a preliminary randomized trial of immediate effects after a single intervention. Man. Ther. 11 (2), 130–135.

Hidalgo, B., Gilliaux, M., Poncin, W., Detrembleur, C., 2012. Reliability and validity of a kinematic spine model during active trunk movement in healthy subjects and patients with chronic non-specific low back pain. J. Rehabil. Med. 44 (9), 756–763.

Hidalgo, B., Hall, T., Nielens, H., Detrembleur, C., 2014. Intertester agreement and validity of identifying lumbar pain provocative movement patterns using active and passive accessory movement tests. J. Manipulative Physiol. Ther. 37 (2), 105–115.

Hidalgo, B., Pitance, L., Hall, T., Detrembleur, C., Nielens, H., 2015. Short-term effects of Mulligan mobilization with movement on pain, disability, and kinematic spinal movements in patients with nonspecific low back pain: a randomized placebo-controlled trial. J. Manipulative Physiol. Ther. 38 (6), 365–374.

Konstantinou, K., Foster, N., Rushton, A., Baxter, D., Wright, C., Breen, A., 2007. Flexion mobilizations with movement techniques: the immediate effects on range of movement and pain in subjects with low back pain. J. Manipulative Physiol. Ther. 30 (3), 178–185.

Lee, R., Evans, J., 1997. An in vivo study of the intervertebral movements produced by posteroanterior mobilization. Clin. Biomech. (Bristol, Avon) 12 (6), 400–408.

Moutzouri, M., Billis, E., Strimpakos, N., Kottika, P., Oldham, J.A., 2008. The effects of the Mulligan Sustained Natural Apophyseal Glide (SNAG) mobilisation in the lumbar flexion range of asymptomatic subjects as measured by the Zebris CMS20 3-D motion analysis system. BMC Musculoskelet. Disord. 9, 131.

Moutzouri, M., Perry, J., Billis, E., 2012. Investigation of the effects of a centrally applied lumbar sustained natural apophyseal glide mobilization on lower limb sympathetic nervous system activity in asymptomatic subjects. J. Manipulative Physiol. Ther. 35 (4), 286–294.

Mulligan, B.R., 2010. Manual Therapy: 'NAGs', 'SNAGs', 'MWMs', etc., 6th ed. Orthopedic Physical Therapy Products, Wellington, NZ.

Nijskens, S., Hing, W., Steele, M., 2013. The effect of Mulligan's bent leg raise. In: Australian Physiotherapy Association Conference, Melbourne.

Subarna Das, M.S., Dowle, P., Iyengar, R., 2018. Effect of spinal mobilization with leg movement as an adjunct to neural mobilization and conventional therapy in patients with lumbar radiculopathy: randomized controlled trial. J. Med. Sci. Clin. Res. 6 (4), 356–364.

10

11

Hip region

TECHNIQUES FOR THE HIP REGION

Lateral glide MWM for hip flexion and internal/external rotation in supine lying
   Lateral glide MWM for hip flexion in supine lying
   Lateral glide MWM for internal rotation
   Lateral glide MWM for external rotation
   Hip quadrant
   Hip FABER (flexed, abducted and externally rotated)
   Hip flexion MWM self-treatment
Lateral glide MWM for hip extension in weight-bearing
   Lateral glide for hip extension: alternative technique leaning back from upper body – combined with resistance band to activate contralateral abductors
Lateral glide MWM for hip flexion in weight-bearing
   Hip flexion MWM in four-point kneeling
   Hip flexion self-treatment MWM in four-point kneeling
Lateral glide MWM for hip internal and external rotation in weight-bearing
Hip MWM in supine lying for abduction and adduction
   Posterior glide MWM for hip abduction in weight-bearing
   Bilateral hip abduction MWM in supine lying
   Bilateral hip abduction MWM in sitting
Hip extension and rectus femoris/hip flexor MWM in prone, supine and side lying (one and two therapists)
   Hip extension and rectus femoris MWM in prone lying
   Hip MWM with longitudinal belt traction into hip extension – rectus femoris stretch in supine lying
   Hip extension and rectus femoris/hip flexor stretch MWM in side lying

INTRODUCTION

The hip joint is one of the largest synovial joints of the human body and is perfectly designed to allow for a wide range of motion while at the same time supporting the weight of the body. The articular surfaces are highly reciprocally shaped, being a ball-and-socket joint comprising the ball-like end of the femur, which articulates with the socket-like acetabulum of the pelvic girdle. The ball-and-socket articulation is sealed by a synovial capsule and anchored firmly with strong ligaments and muscles. Unlike the majority of the other joints in the body, the very tight, reciprocal-shaped nature of the hip joint articular surfaces minimises the potential for translation (Loubert et al., 2013), hence impacting on the choice of gliding techniques with hip MWM.

Osteoarthritis is a common and typically localised degenerative joint disease that causes substantial musculoskeletal pain and disability (Bennell, 2013). In 2007, 8% of Australians had osteoarthritis and this is projected to increase to 11% by 2050 owing to an ageing population, sedentary lifestyle and rising obesity rates and, as such, osteoarthritis is a rising public health issue (Bennell & Hinman, 2011). The prevalence of hip osteoarthritis varies according to differences in definition, with estimates as high as 45% according to one review (Pereira et al., 2011).

The characteristic changes associated with hip osteoarthritis include loss of articular cartilage, joint space narrowing, sclerosis of subchondral bone, ostephyte formation and capsule contracture and fibrosis (Sokolove & Lepus, 2013). These changes will often result in pain, impaired mobility, reduced muscle strength, limitation in activities of daily living (Steultjens et al., 2000) and reduced quality of life (Salaffi et al., 2005). Individuals suffering from hip osteoarthritis often report extreme functional limitation. The predominant feature is pain becoming more persistent and more limiting as the disease progresses. Typically, patients report difficulty with activities of daily living such as walking, climbing stairs, driving a car and performing general housework (Guccione et al., 1994). As well as these functional limitations, people also present with higher levels of anxiety and depression (Murphy et al., 2012).

Manual therapy is a commonly used form of treatment for hip osteoarthritis, with a survey of Irish physiotherapists reporting that 96% used this form of treatment in their management for this condition (French, 2007). A recent narrative review identified a number of randomised controlled trials (RCTs), the results of which support the use of manual therapy for hip osteoarthritis (Bennell, 2013). Interestingly, in that review, manual therapy was found to be more effective than exercise, and the addition of exercise to manual therapy reduced the effectiveness of the latter form of treatment, thus suggesting that one form of therapy should be used. The benefits of manual therapy were still maintained in one clinical trial at 29-week follow-up (Hoeksma et al., 2004). This evidence provides some justification for clinicians considering techniques of the Mulligan Concept in the management of hip osteoarthritis. Other pathologies affecting the hip include femoroacetabular impingement syndrome, labral tears, bursal lesions, tendinopathy of the hip abductor and adductor muscles, and muscle tears among others. Restrictions of hip rotation and of flexion movement have been suggested as clinical indicators of hip disorders (Ellenbecker et al., 2007). Hence, bilateral measurement of hip joint ROM should be performed to identify impairments for injury prevention, manual therapy management and performance enhancement. A recent case series reported substantial improvement in pain and disability following multimodal management (manual therapy and exercise) of patients with acetabular labral tears (Yazbek et al., 2011).

The Mulligan Concept is ideally suited to the management of a range of hip disorders as the techniques can be carefully graduated from non-weight-bearing positions to full weight-bearing as the condition improves and allows. In this chapter, techniques are described to improve ROM at the hip joint in various directions and positions as well as to improve length of muscles surrounding and controlling the hip. These techniques may therefore be useful in hip conditions with muscle imbalances, as well as those involving movement impairment and pain. Although there are no studies that have specifically investigated the effects of Mulligan techniques in isolation for hip disorders, clinical anecdotal evidence suggests substantial benefits from such techniques. The proposed mechanisms underlying improvements with MWM include mechanical alteration of tissues and neurophysiological effects, as well as a psychological influence (Vicenzino et al., 2011).

Levels of evidence

Level 2: four RCTs and one case report

In an RCT with two interventions and one control group, Walsh and Kinsella (2016) demonstrated that both caudal MWM and self-MWM improved hip internal rotation (IR) of healthy males with reduced hip IR, with

11

no significant difference in the results of a seated internal rotation test between the two treatment groups. Interestingly, therapist-induced MWM was more effective than self-MWM in restoring functional internal rotation (Walsh & Kinsella, 2016). Such effects of MWM were also observed in patients with hip osteoarthritis (OA).

Beselga and colleagues (Beselga et al., 2016) reported immediate pain relief (assessed via NRS) and an 11.0° (95% CI 8.2–13.7) and 4.4° (95% CI 2.4–6.4) between-group difference in hip flexion and internal rotation, respectively, favouring the group treated with two MWM techniques (hip flexion and IR) compared with the sham MWM group.

Utilising the same lateral glide hip MWM as Beselga and colleagues (Beselga et al., 2016), Smith and colleagues (Smith et al., 2018) examined the effect of MWM on vibration threshold (VT) in asymptomatic individuals compared with placebo and control. VT has been postulated to allow quantification of changes to sensory processing in patients presenting with musculoskeletal pain (Laursen et al., 2006). Although no statistically significant change in VT was found between the groups, Smith and colleagues (Smith et al., 2018) suggested that future studies recruiting symptomatic patients may have different outcomes.

The use of TrSLR technique was shown to be superior to both static stretching and no intervention in a study of 40 students with bilateral hamstring tightness (Yıldırım et al., 2016). In this study, a 4-week intervention increased hip flexion ROM by more than 15° in the groups treated with either MWM or proprioceptive neuromuscular facilitation (PNF) stretching, with no statistically significant difference between the two interventions (Yıldırım et al., 2016).

A single case report (Carpenter, 2008) describes the favourable response of a 53-year-old woman with a 3-month history of lateral hip pain to a 4-week programme of passive mobilisation, hip MWM and therapeutic exercise, which is level 4 evidence.

11

LATERAL GLIDE MWM FOR HIP FLEXION AND INTERNAL / EXTERNAL ROTATION IN SUPINE LYING

Lateral glide MWM for hip flexion in supine lying

TECHNIQUE AT A GLANCE

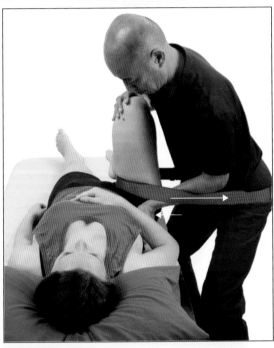

Figure 11.1
Hip flexion MWM in supine lying: start position

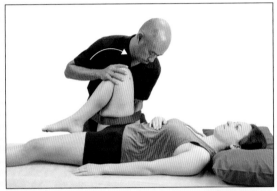

Figure 11.2
Hip flexion MWM in supine lying: start position side view

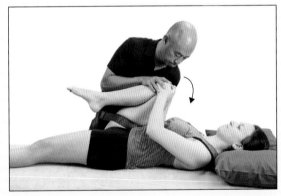

Figure 11.3
Hip flexion MWM in supine lying: end position

- The patient lies supine at the edge of the treatment table nearest to the therapist with their hip in 90° flexion, knee flexion and neutral hip rotation.
- The patient's pelvis is stabilised by the therapist's hand on the ilium, and the distal femur by the therapist's other hand or their sternum.
- A belt is looped around the proximal end of the patient's thigh (with a folded towel or rubber pad to soften the belt contact) and around the therapist's pelvis.
- With the lateral glide force sustained, the patient actively flexes the hip with therapist's assistance if necessary. Over-pressure is applied and the patient is then returned to the start position.
- See Figs 11.1–11.3.

INDICATION

Limitation of hip flexion in supine lying due to pain or stiffness.

POSITIONING

Patient:	Supine and as close as possible to the edge of the treatment table on the therapist's side.
Treated body part:	90° hip flexion, neutral hip rotation with knee flexed.
Therapist:	Adjacent and perpendicular to the affected hip, knees slightly flexed.
Hands/belt contact points:	Belt looped around the therapist's pelvis and as high as possible on the patient's inner proximal thigh. The belt lies flat on the skin.
	Proximal stabilising hand: palm of the hand making broad contact with the patient's ilium, immediately proximal to the greater trochanter.
	Distal stabilising hand: the therapist's hand grasps the distal femur and the elbow contacts the medial aspect of the distal leg. The patient's lateral aspect of the knee can be held against the therapist's sternum.

APPLICATION GUIDELINES

- Apply a lateral glide force using the manual therapy belt at the hip joint with the pelvis stabilised by the proximal hand on the ilium and the therapist's sternum preventing hip abduction.
- While sustaining the lateral glide force with the belt, have the patient actively flex the hip.
- Apply 6–10 repetitions in a set, with 3–5 sets in a treatment session, but only if there is a substantial increase in range of hip pain-free flexion.
- Apply over-pressure using the distal arm on the distal leg only if full-range flexion can be achieved. The patient can also pull their knee into further flexion and apply over-pressure themself.

COMMENTS

- Do not compress the hip joint by leaning on the femur during the technique, as this can provoke more pain.
- Likewise do not adduct the hip joint, as this might compress the anterior joint.
- Alter the angle of glide with the belt and the degree of force if pain-free movement cannot be achieved.
- Use a folded towel or sponge rubber pad to soften the contact of the belt on the patient's thigh.

11

This belt lateral glide technique can be modified to improve internal and external rotation. As movement increases and pain reduces, the MWM can also be applied during a combination of movements such as the hip quadrant or flexion/abduction/external rotation.

Lateral glide MWM for internal rotation

- The patient's position is as for the flexion technique.
- The therapist's distal stabilising hand grasps the patient's distal femur and the elbow contacts the medial aspect of the patient's distal leg. The patient's lateral aspect of the knee is held against the therapist's sternum.
- Upon application of the sustained lateral glide force, either the patient can actively rotate their hip (with therapist assistance if necessary) or the therapist can apply a passive internal rotation to the femur (Fig. 11.4A).
- Over-pressure is applied; then return to the start position.
- If the patient has knee pathology an alternative hand hold of the femur can be used (Fig. 11.4B).
- Apply 6–10 repetitions in a set, with 3–5 sets in a treatment session, but only if there is a substantial increase in range of hip pain-free internal rotation.
- Apply over-pressure using the elbow on the distal leg only if full-range hip rotation can be achieved.

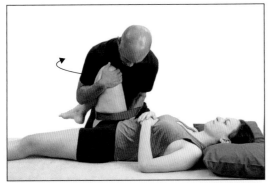

Figure 11.4A
Hip internal rotation MWM in supine lying: end position

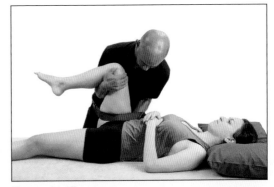

Figure 11.4B
Hip flexion MWM in supine lying: alternative hand hold

Lateral glide MWM for external rotation

- The patient lies supine at the edge of the treatment table nearest the therapist with the hip in 90° flexion, knee 90° flexion and neutral hip rotation, as for the flexion and internal rotation techniques previously described.
- The patient's pelvis is stabilised by the therapist's hand on the ilium inside the belt, and the distal femur by the therapist's sternum, while the patient's leg is supported by the therapist's distal hand around the thigh.
- A belt is looped around the proximal end of the patient's thigh and the therapist's pelvis.
- With the lateral glide force sustained, either the patient actively rotates the hip or the therapist can apply passive external rotation through the distal leg acting as a lever.
- Over-pressure is applied; then return to the start position.
- See Fig. 11.5.

11

(continued next page...)

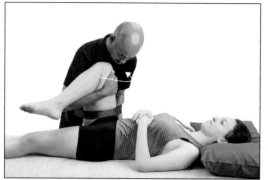

Figure 11.5A
Hip external rotation MWM in supine lying: end position

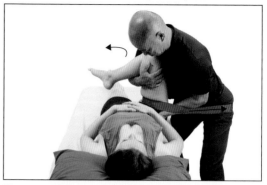

Figure 11.5B
Hip external rotation MWM in supine lying: alternative view

Hip quadrant

- The patient lies supine at the edge of the treatment table nearest the therapist with their hip in 90° flexion and the knee flexed.
- A low table height such that the therapist's knees are flexed is preferable.
- The patient's pelvis is stabilised by the therapist's hand on the ilium inside the belt, and the patient's distal femur by the therapist's other hand.
- A belt is looped around the proximal end of the patient's thigh and the therapist's upper body.
- With the lateral glide force sustained, the therapist passively moves the hip into flexion and adduction with assistance from the patient (Fig. 11.6).
- Over-pressure is applied; then return to the start position.

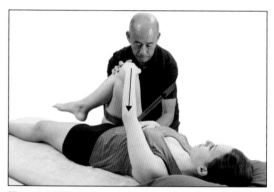

Figure 11.6
Hip quadrant MWM

Hip FABER (flexed, abducted and externally rotated)

- The patient lies supine at the edge of the treatment table nearest the therapist with their hip in flexion/abduction and with the foot resting on the opposite knee.
- The patient's pelvis is stabilised by the therapist's hand on the ilium inside the belt and the patient's distal femur by the therapist's other hand.
- A belt is looped around the proximal end of the patient's thigh and the therapist's pelvis.
- With the lateral glide force sustained, the therapist passively moves the hip into abduction and external rotation.
- Over-pressure is applied; then return to the start position (Fig. 11.7).

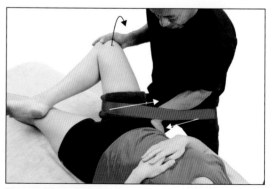

Figure 11.7
Hip FABER MWM

11

SELF-MANAGEMENT

- In supine lying, the patient can perform self-treatment into flexion, flexion/adduction or flexion/rotation (Fig. 11.8) by using a loop of strong resistance band to replicate the belt glide.

- The patient should ensure that the resistance band is placed high into the groin at the proximal end of the femur as close as possible to the hip joint and the other end is firmly attached to a secure anchor.

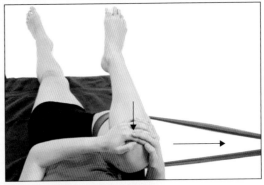

Figure 11.8
Hip flexion MWM self-treatment in supine lying

ANNOTATIONS

sup ly R Hip belt Lat gl MWM F×6(3)
sup ly R Hip belt Lat gl MWM F +OP×10(5)
sup ly R Hip belt Lat gl MWM IR×6(3)
sup ly R Hip belt Lat gl MWM ER×6(3)
sup ly R Hip belt Lat gl MWM quadrant +OP×10(5)
sup ly R hip belt Lat gl MWM FABER×10(5)
sup ly R hip self resistance band Lat gl MWM F +OP×6(3)

LATERAL GLIDE MWM FOR HIP EXTENSION IN WEIGHT-BEARING

TECHNIQUE AT A GLANCE

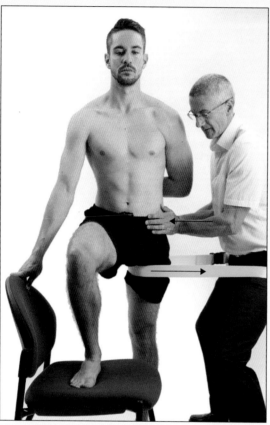

Figure 11.9
Lateral glide for hip extension in weight-bearing

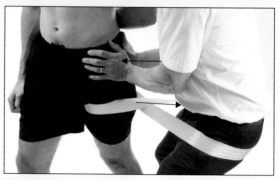

Figure 11.10
Hip extension: early restriction stride stance with alternative figure-of-eight belt technique

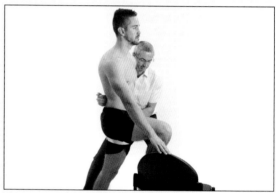

Figure 11.11
Lateral glide for hip extension in weight-bearing: side view

- The patient stands with the unaffected leg positioned farthest from the therapist on a chair in hip flexion and forwards while the affected leg is in a hip-neutral position.
- The therapist performs a hip lateral glide using a belt while stabilising the patient's pelvis with both hands on the lateral side.
- While the glide is sustained, the patient moves forwards with their pelvis, bringing the involved hip into extension.
- See Figs 11.9–11.11.

INDICATION

Pain or limitation of movement into hip extension in standing.

POSITIONING

Patient:	Standing facing a chair, with the unaffected leg forwards, foot on the chair.
Treated body part:	The affected leg bears most of the weight, starting in a neutral position. The patient should hold the chair back for stability (see Fig. 11.9).
Therapist:	The therapist stands perpendicular to the patient and adjacent to the hip to be treated, with knees slightly bent to allow the therapist's sideways body movement, and hands stabilising the patient's pelvis laterally.
Hands/belt contact points:	A treatment belt is looped around the therapist's hips/thighs and the patient's proximal thigh. The belt is applied as proximally as comfortably possible in the groin.

APPLICATION GUIDELINES

- The therapist applies lateral glide force by shifting their weight backwards, pulling through the treatment belt. Sponge rubber/padding between the belt and inner thigh can be used to maximise comfort.
- The patient extends their hip by lunging forwards, hence shifting their weight forwards.
- Return to the start position before removing the lateral glide force.
- The therapist moves their pelvis so as to maintain alignment of the glide force, thereby moving in coordination with the patient's movements forwards and backwards.
- If the belt slips on the patient's thigh, a figure-of-eight technique is recommended (see Fig. 11.10).
- Apply 6–10 repetitions in a set, with 3–5 sets in a treatment session, but only if the extension ROM is pain-free when applying MWM and no latent pain responses occur.

COMMENTS

- Ensure that the belt is parallel to the floor, and flat on the patient's thigh, before applying the lateral glide force.
- If pain is not eliminated fully or considerably reduced, adjustment can be made by altering the glide force or by altering the angle of the belt a few degrees ventrally or dorsally, or by rotating the effected hip externally or internally.
- Consider patient's normal hip resting position before applying the technique (i.e. if the normal resting position is somewhat flexed or rotated, then commence from that position).

(continued next page...)

VARIATIONS

- An alternative start position is in lunge standing with the affected leg more posterior (i.e. greater hip extension). Progression is achieved by going further into hip extension, increasing the load by moving the shoulders backwards and rotating the hip into internal or external rotation depending on patient's pain-provocative movement (see Fig. 11.12).

- Adding muscle contraction / control during the MWM by bringing in contralateral active / resisted stabilisation using pulleys and weights or resistance bands may also be clinically effective (see Fig. 11.13).

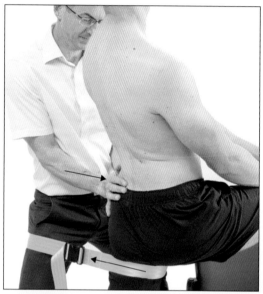

Figure 11.12

Lateral glide for hip extension: alternative technique leaning back from upper body

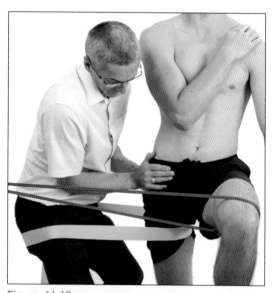

Figure 11.13

Lateral glide with belt for hip extension combined with a resistance band to activate contralateral hip abductors

ANNOTATIONS

st R Foot on chair L Hip belt Lat gl MWM E×6

st R Foot on chair L Hip belt Lat gl MWM E×10(3)

st R Foot on chair L Hip belt lat gl MWM E+Trunk E×6

st R foot on chair R hip res Ab (resistance band) L Hip belt Lat gl MWM E×6

11

LATERAL GLIDE MWM FOR HIP FLEXION IN WEIGHT-BEARING

TECHNIQUE AT A GLANCE

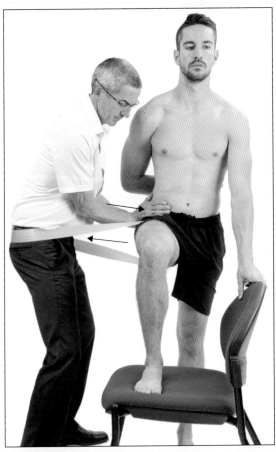

Figure 11.14
Lateral glide MWM for hip flexion in weight-bearing

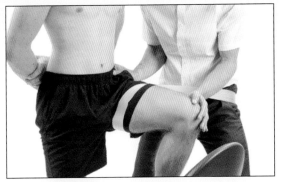

Figure 11.15
Lateral glide MWM for hip flexion in weight-bearing:
alternative hand position

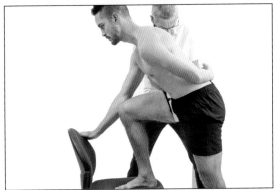

Figure 11.16
Lateral glide MWM for hip flexion in weight-bearing:
end range

- The patient stands facing a chair with the affected leg positioned forwards and the foot on a chair in hip flexion.
- The unaffected leg is in hip-neutral position with the foot on the floor.
- The therapist performs a hip lateral glide using a belt while stabilising the patient's pelvis with both hands on the lateral side.
- While the glide is sustained, the patient moves forwards with their pelvis, bringing the involved hip into flexion.
- See Figs 11.14–11.16.

INDICATION

Pain or limitation of movement into hip flexion in standing.

POSITION

Patient:	Standing facing a chair, with the affected leg forwards, foot on the chair.
Treated body part:	The affected leg bears the majority of the weight, starting in a neutral position. The patient should hold the chair back for stability.
Therapist:	The therapist stands perpendicular to the patient, with knees slightly bent to allow movement, and hands stabilising patient's pelvis laterally.
Hands/belt contact points:	A treatment belt is looped around the therapist's hips/thighs and around the patient's proximal thigh. The belt is applied as proximally as comfortably possible in the groin.

APPLICATION GUIDELINES

- Ask the patient to increase the load on their affected limb, which is on the chair.
- The therapist applies lateral glide force by shifting their weight backwards pulling through the treatment belt. Sponge rubber can be used to maximise comfort.
- Maintain glide force throughout the mobilisation.
- The patient moves their hip into flexion by shifting their weight forwards onto the chair.
- The therapist moves their pelvis in coordination with the patient's pelvis to maintain constant direction of glide force.
- Apply 6–10 repetitions in a set, with 3–5 sets in a treatment session, but only if flexion ROM is pain-free when applying MWM and no latent pain responses occur.

COMMENTS

- Ensure that the belt is parallel to the floor, and flat on the patient's thigh, before applying the lateral glide force.
- If pain is not eliminated fully, adjustment can be made by altering the glide force, or by altering the angle of the belt a few degrees ventrally or dorsally, or by taking the affected leg into slight horizontal abduction or adduction depending on the response.
- Do not release the lateral glide before the patient returns to neutral.
- If the belt slips on the patient's thigh a figure-of-eight technique is recommended.

11

- Progression is achieved by going further into hip flexion, increasing the load by moving the shoulders forwards (flexing the pelvis on the femur) and moving the hip into horizontal adduction or abduction depending on the patient's pain-provocative movement.

- The therapist can also guide the hip flexion movement via the patient's flexed knee while maintaining stabilisation of the pelvis with their other hand (Fig. 11.15).

- A variation of the technique can be done in four-point kneeling (Fig. 11.17). This position allows for easier variation into various degrees of hip rotation and flexion, but requires the patient to have good knee flexion ROM. This position is relevant for patients who report pain or impaired function in this combined hip movement direction, such as cyclists or field hockey players.

- Also, as previously mentioned for extension in weight-bearing, an elastic band can be used to promote/facilitate muscle stabilisation such as when hip rotator imbalance is evident, or to enhance the treatment effect or progress treatment.

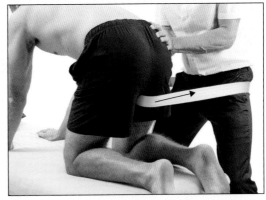

Figure 11.17
Hip flexion MWM in four-point kneeling: start position

SELF-MANAGEMENT

- In four-point kneeling, the patient can perform self-treatment into flexion, flexion/adduction or flexion/rotation (Fig. 11.18) by using a loop of a strong resistance band to replicate the belt glide.

- Ensure that the resistance band is placed high into the groin at the proximal end of the femur as close as possible to the hip joint and the other end is firmly attached to a secure anchor.

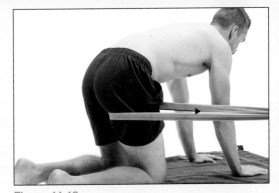

Figure 11.18
Hip flexion self-treatment MWM in four-point kneeling

ANNOTATIONS

st R Foot on chair R Hip belt Lat gl MWM F×6
4 point kneel R Hip belt Lat gl MWM F×6(3)
4 point kneel R Hip self resistance band Lat gl MWM F×6(3)

LATERAL GLIDE FOR HIP INTERNAL AND EXTERNAL ROTATION IN WEIGHT-BEARING

TECHNIQUE AT A GLANCE

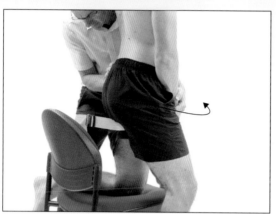

Figure 11.19
Lateral glide MWM for internal rotation of hip: start position

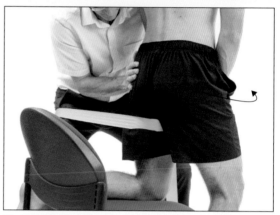

Figure 11.20
Lateral glide MWM for internal rotation of hip: end position

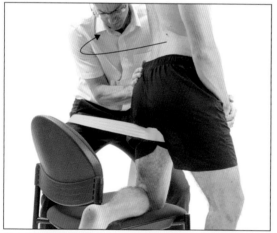

Figure 11.21
Lateral glide MWM for external rotation of hip

- The patient kneels with the affected leg on a chair, positioned in either internal or external rotation. The chair back stabilises against the medial or lateral aspect of the ankle.
- A belt is looped horizontally around the proximal end of the patient's thigh and the therapist's pelvis.
- The therapist stabilises the lateral aspect of the patient's pelvis with two hands.
- With the lateral glide force sustained, the patient actively rotates their hip either internally or externally with assistance if necessary.
- Over-pressure is applied; then return to the start position.
- See Figs 11.19–11.21.

11

INDICATION

Limitation of hip internal or external rotation in standing due to pain or stiffness.

POSITIONING

Patient:	Standing with the support of a high-backed chair or plinth for stability.
Treated body part:	Hip in extension, hip rotated to the point of limitation or pain.
Therapist:	Adjacent and perpendicular to the affected hip, knees slightly flexed.
Hands/belt contact points:	Belt looped around the therapist's pelvis/proximal thighs and as high as comfortably possible on the patient's inner proximal thigh. The belt lies flat, immediately distal to the patient's groin. Stabilising hands: palm of both hands making broad contact with the ilium/lateral pelvis proximal to the greater trochanter.

APPLICATION GUIDELINES

- Apply a laterally directed glide force using the manual therapy belt at the hip joint with the pelvis stabilised by the therapist's hands on the ilium/lateral aspect of the pelvis.
- While sustaining the lateral glide force with the belt, have the patient actively internally or externally rotate the hip by turning the body towards or away from the weight-bearing leg.
- Apply 6–10 repetitions in a set, with 3–5 sets in a treatment session, but only if there is a substantial increase in range of hip pain-free rotation.
- Apply over-pressure using the patient's pelvis as the lever.

COMMENTS

- Alter the angle of glide with the belt and the degree of force if pain-free movement cannot be achieved.
- Use a folded towel or large piece of sponge rubber to soften the contact of the belt on the patient's thigh and the back of the chair against the malleolus.

11

(continued next page...)

Lateral glide MWM for internal or external rotation in standing

- Weight-bearing hip rotation may also be achieved in standing, without kneeling on a chair (Fig. 11.22).
- While standing on the affected leg, and sustaining the lateral glide force with the belt, the patient actively rotates the hip internally or externally by turning the body towards or away from the weight-bearing leg.

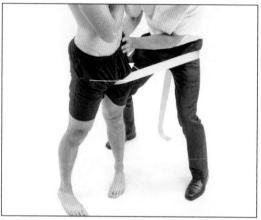

Figure 11.22A
Lateral glide MWM for internal rotation of hip using a belt

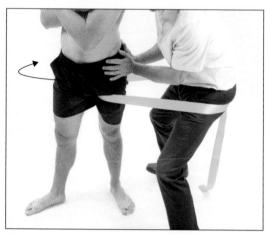

Figure 11.22B
Lateral glide MWM for external rotation of hip using a belt

ANNOTATIONS

st L knee on chair L hip belt Lat gl MWM IR×6
st L knee on chair L hip belt Lat gl MWM ER×10(3)
st L Hip belt Lat gl MWM IR×6
st L hip belt Lat gl MWM ER×10(3)

11

HIP MWM IN SUPINE LYING FOR ABDUCTION AND ADDUCTION

TECHNIQUE AT A GLANCE

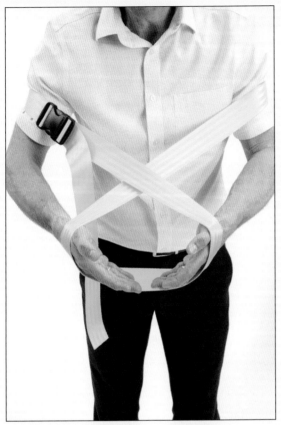

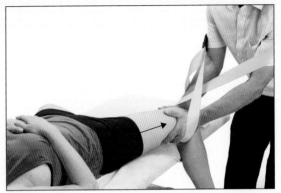

Figure 11.24
Hip abduction MWM with longitudinal traction

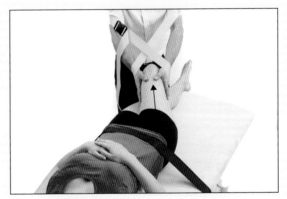

Figure 11.25
Hip adduction MWM with longitudinal traction

Figure 11.23
Hip abduction MWM: belt set-up for longitudinal traction

11

- The patient lies supine.
- The contralateral leg is abducted with the knee flexed and the leg hanging off side of the table.
- The treated hip is slightly flexed with the joint in the loose-packed position.
- Longitudinal traction is applied along the line of the femur to create the stretch using a treatment belt.
- While maintaining the stretch, the hip is taken into abduction or adduction.
- See Figs 11.23–11.25.

INDICATION

Limitation of hip abduction or adduction due to pain or muscle tightness.

POSITIONING

Patient:	The patient lies supine with their contralateral leg hanging over the side of the treatment table to act as a stabiliser of the pelvis.
Treated body part:	The treated hip is in a loose-packed position with the knee flexed (see Fig. 11.24).
Therapist:	The therapist stands on the affected side, close to the patient's knee.
Hands/belt contact points:	A treatment belt in a figure of eight is looped around the therapist's shoulders, with their hands inside the distal loop. The patient's femur is inserted into the distal loop of the belt. The therapist's hands hold the patient's thigh proximal to the knee, with the belt around the hands.

APPLICATION GUIDELINES

- Grasp the distal femur above the knee, with the distal loop of the treatment belt around the therapist's hands.
- Apply a longitudinal traction along the line of the femur by leaning backwards, tensioning the belt (Fig. 11.24).
- While maintaining the traction, move the hip into abduction (Fig. 11.24) or adduction (Fig. 11.25).
- Apply 6–10 repetitions. Hold each stretch at maximal ROM for up to 10 seconds. If applied correctly, the stretching sensation should be felt in the opposite limb (non-stretched limb).
- Return to neutral position before reducing the longitudinal glide force.

COMMENTS

- If pain is not eliminated fully, adjustment can be made by altering the position of hip flexion and/or external rotation.
- Abduction/adduction can be combined with flexion/extension and with rotation to mimic the patient's functional requirements.
- Progression is achieved by moving further into hip abduction or adduction, or by adjusting the degree of hip flexion and rotation to allow for maximal ROM.
- If a therapist finds it difficult to stabilise a patient's pelvis, an extra belt can be used looped around the patient's pelvis and the treatment table.

11

VARIATIONS

VARIATIONS

- This technique can also be performed in weight-bearing for hip abduction (Fig. 11.26).
- This technique for abduction can be performed bilaterally by two therapists with the patient either lying flat in supine (Fig. 11.27) or sitting forwards (Fig. 11.28).

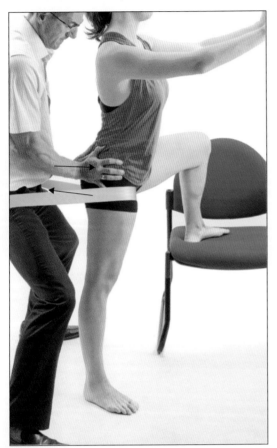

Figure 11.26
Posterior glide MWM for hip abduction in weight-bearing

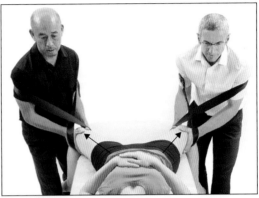

Figure 11.27
Bilateral hip abduction MWM in supine lying

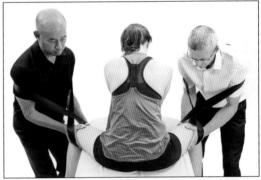

Figure 11.28
Bilateral hip abduction MWM in sitting

ANNOTATIONS

sup ly R hip belt Tr MWM Ab×10 sec(10)
sup ly R hip belt Tr MWM Ab×10 sec(6)
st L foot on chair R hip belt post gl MWM Ab×10
sup ly bilat hip belt Tr MWM Ab +A×10 sec(10)
sit bilat hip belt Tr MWM Ab +A×10 sec(10)

HIP EXTENSION AND RECTUS FEMORIS/HIP FLEXOR MWM IN PRONE, SUPINE AND SIDE LYING

Hip extension and rectus femoris MWM in prone lying

TECHNIQUE AT A GLANCE: SINGLE THERAPIST

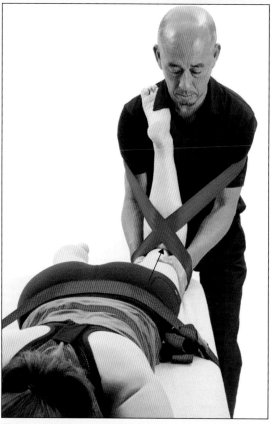

Figure 11.29
Hip MWM with longitudinal traction and rectus femoris stretch into hip extension

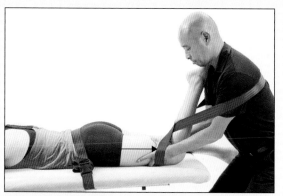

Figure 11.30
Hip MWM with longitudinal traction into hip extension: rectus femoris stretch start position

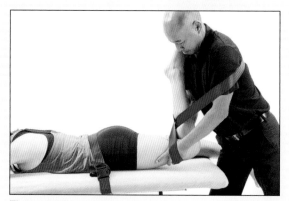

Figure 11.31
Hip MWM with longitudinal traction into hip extension: rectus femoris stretch end range

11

- The patient lies prone with knee flexed.
- Longitudinal traction is applied along the line of the femur to create the stretch using a treatment belt applied at the distal femur.
- The patient's hip with knee flexed is moved into extension.
- See Figs 11.29–11.31.

INDICATION

Pain during hip extension, or tightness of rectus femoris.

POSITIONING

Patient:	The patient lies prone with knees at the end of the treatment table.
Treated body part:	Knee flexed and hip extended (Figs 11.29 and 11.30).
Therapist:	The therapist is standing on the affected side.
Hands/belt contact points:	The treatment belt is in a figure-of-eight loop, with one part around the therapist's shoulders and the other with the hands around the distal femur.

APPLICATION GUIDELINES

- The therapist grasps the distal femur above the patient's knee, with the distal loop of the treatment belt around the therapist's hands.
- Apply a longitudinal traction along the line of the femur by leaning backwards, tensioning the belt.
- While maintaining the force, move the hip into extension, keeping the knee flexed.
- Apply 6–10 repetitions, holding each stretch at maximal ROM for up to 10 seconds.
- Return to neutral position before reducing the longitudinal traction force.

COMMENTS

- If the pain is not eliminated fully, adjustments can be made by adding degrees of slight rotation of the hip or by altering the degree of force.
- An additional belt can be used to stabilise the patient's pelvis to the treatment table.
- A pillow may be placed under the patient's abdomen to reduce excessive lordosis if required.

VARIATIONS

- To apply over-pressure in flexible patients an additional belt may be attached to the patient's ankle and over-pressure into knee flexion applied by the patient.
- An alternative start position is where the patient is lying supine with their pelvis at the end of a treatment table and the unaffected leg flexed (see Fig. 11.32). The treated leg hangs over the treatment table (as in the Thomas test). The pelvis can be stabilised with a treatment belt. In this position the stretch can easily be adjusted to adduction/abduction and rotation.

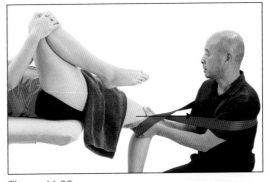

Figure 11.32
Hip MWM with longitudinal belt traction into hip extension: rectus femoris stretch in supine lying – Thomas test position

ANNOTATIONS

pr ly L hip belt Tr MWM hip E/Kn F×10 sec(6)
sup ly L hip belt Tr MWM hip E/Kn F×10 sec(6)

Hip extension and rectus femoris / hip flexor stretch MWM in side lying

TECHNIQUE AT A GLANCE

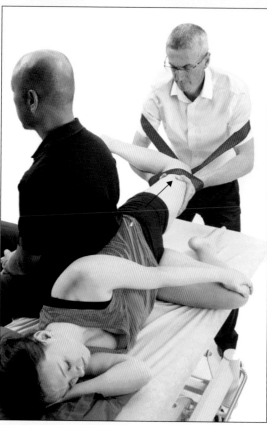

Figure 11.33
Hip longitudinal traction MWM for hip extension and rectus femoris / hip flexor stretch in side lying: therapist stabilisation

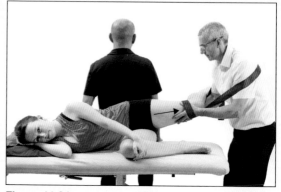

Figure 11.34
Hip longitudinal traction MWM for hip extension and rectus femoris / hip flexor stretch in side lying: therapist stabilisation side view

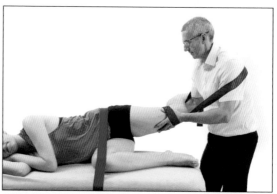

Figure 11.35
Hip longitudinal traction MWM for hip extension and rectus femoris / hip flexor stretch in side lying: belt stabilisation

- This technique requires a therapist and an assistant.
- The patient is in side-lying position, with their affected leg uppermost.
- The affected leg is extended at the hip and flexed at the knee and held by the therapist, who uses a belt to apply a longitudinal traction to the involved leg while at the same time moving the hip into extension.
- The assistant stabilises the patient's pelvis (alternatively a second belt can be used to stabilise the pelvis).
- See Figs 11.33–11.35.

INDICATION

Muscle tightness or symptom provocation during hip extension associated with rectus femoris or hip flexor muscle stretch.

POSITIONING

Patient:	Side lying with symptomatic side uppermost.
Treated body part:	The patient grasps underneath their thigh (of the unaffected side) for stability. The involved hip is slightly flexed, while the knee is flexed to approximately 60°.
Therapist:	The therapist is in step-standing position behind the patient.
Hands contact points:	The therapist, using a figure-of-eight treatment belt, grasps around the patient's thigh. The patient's distal leg is tucked under the therapist's arm to control knee flexion. The assistant is in step-standing position behind and next to the patient's pelvis. Using both hands or their body, the assistant stabilises the patient's pelvis (see Fig. 11.33). Alternatively a second belt can be used to stabilise the pelvis (Fig. 11.35).

APPLICATION GUIDELINES

- The therapist applies a longitudinal traction with the belt along the line of the femur, by leaning backwards.
- The assistant maintains stabilisation of the patient's pelvis, or a second belt is employed for pelvis stabilisation.
- The therapist sustains the force, and moves the patient's hip passively into extension, provided there are no symptoms.
- Apply up to 3 repetitions in the first session.
- On subsequent visits apply 6–10 repetitions depending on the response of the patient.

COMMENT

- Extension can be combined with knee flexion or with hip abduction/adduction and with rotation to mimic the patient's functional requirements.

ANNOTATIONS

R s ly Pelvis stabilised (A) L Hip belt Tr MWM Hip E/Kn F×3
R s ly Pelvis stabilised (belt) L Hip belt Tr MWM Hip E/Kn F×3

References

Bennell, K., 2013. Physiotherapy management of hip osteoarthritis. J. Physiother. 59 (3), 145–157.

Bennell, K.L., Hinman, R.S., 2011. A review of the clinical evidence for exercise in osteoarthritis of the hip and knee. J. Sci. Med. Sport 14 (1), 4–9.

Beselga, C., Neto, F., Alburquerque-Sendín, F., Hall, T., Oliveira-Campelo, N., 2016. Immediate effects of hip mobilization with movement in patients with hip osteoarthritis: a randomised controlled trial. Man. Ther. 22, 80–85.

Carpenter, G., 2008. The effects of hip mobilisation and mobilisation with movement in the physical therapy management of a person with lateral hip pain: a case report. J. Man. Manipulative Ther. 16 (3), 170.

Ellenbecker, T.S., Ellenbecker, G.A., Roetert, E.P., Silva, R.T., Keuter, G., Sperling, F., 2007. Descriptive profile of hip rotation range of motion in elite tennis players and professional baseball pitchers. Am. J. Sports Med. 35 (8), 1371–1376.

French, H.P., 2007. Physiotherapy management of osteoarthritis of the hip: a survey of current practice in acute hospitals and private practice in the Republic of Ireland. Physiotherapy 93 (4), 253–260.

Guccione, A.A., Felson, D.T., Anderson, J.J., Anthony, J.M., Zhang, Y., Wilson, P.W., et al., 1994. The effects of specific medical conditions on the functional limitations of elders in the Framingham Study. Am. J. Public Health 84 (3), 351–358.

11

Hoeksma, H.L., Dekker, J., Ronday, H.K., Heering, A., van der Lubbe, N., Vel, C., et al., 2004. Comparison of manual therapy and exercise therapy in osteoarthritis of the hip: a randomized clinical trial. Arthritis Rheum. 51 (5), 722–729.

Laursen, L.H., Jepsen, J.R., Sjøgaard, G., 2006. Vibrotactile sense in patients with different upper limb disorders compared with a control group. Int. Arch. Occup. Environ. Health 79 (7), 593–601.

Loubert, P.V., Zipple, J.T., Klobucher, M.J., Marquardt, E.D., Opolka, M.J., 2013. In vivo ultrasound measurement of posterior femoral glide during hip joint mobilization in healthy college students. J. Orthop. Sports Phys. Ther. 43 (8), 534–541.

Murphy, L.B., Sacks, J.J., Brady, T.J., Hootman, J.M., Chapman, D.P., 2012. Anxiety and depression among US adults with arthritis: prevalence and correlates. Arthritis Care Res. 64 (7), 968–976.

Pereira, D., Peleteiro, B., Araujo, J., Branco, J., Santos, R.A., Ramos, E., 2011. The effect of osteoarthritis definition on prevalence and incidence estimates: a systematic review. Osteoarthritis Cartilage 19 (11), 1270–1285.

Salaffi, F., Carotti, M., Stancati, A., Grassi, W., 2005. Health-related quality of life in older adults with symptomatic hip and knee osteoarthritis: a comparison with matched healthy controls. Aging Clin. Exp. Res. 17 (4), 255–263.

Smith, D.A., Saranga, J., Pritchard, A., Kommatas, N.A., Punnoose, S.K., Kale, S.T., 2018. Effect of a lateral glide mobilisation with movement of the hip on vibration threshold in healthy volunteers. J. Bodyw. Mov. Ther. 22 (1), 13–17.

Sokolove, J., Lepus, C.M., 2013. Role of inflammation in the pathogenesis of osteoarthritis: latest findings and interpretations. Ther. Adv. Musculoskelet. Dis. 5 (2), 77–94.

Steultjens, M.P., Dekker, J., van Baar, M.E., Oostendorp, R.A., Bijlsma, J.W., 2000. Range of joint motion and disability in patients with osteoarthritis of the knee or hip. Rheumatology 39 (9), 955–961.

Vicenzino, B., Hing, W., Hall, T., Rivett, D., 2011. Mobilisation with movement: the art and science of its application. In: Vicenzino, B., Hing, W., Rivett, D., Hall, T. (Eds.), Mobilisation With Movement: The Art and the Science. Churchill Livingstone Australia, Chatswood, NSW, pp. 9–23.

Walsh, R., Kinsella, S., 2016. The effects of caudal mobilisation with movement (MWM) and caudal self-mobilisation with movement (SMWM) in relation to restricted internal rotation in the hip: a randomised control pilot study. Man. Ther. 22, 9–15.

Yazbek, P.M., Ovanessian, V., Martin, R.L., Fukuda, T.Y., 2011. Nonsurgical treatment of acetabular labrum tears: a case series. J. Orthop. Sports Phys. Ther. 41 (5), 346–353.

Yıldırım, M.S., Ozyurek, S., Tosun, O., Uzer, S., Gelecek, N., 2016. Comparison of effects of static, proprioceptive neuromuscular facilitation and Mulligan stretching on hip flexion range of motion: a randomized controlled trial. Biol. Sport 33 (1), 89–94.

11

Knee

INTRODUCTION

The knee complex comprises the tibiofemoral, patellofemoral and superior tibiofibular joints, each of which may be symptomatic. In younger patients, patellofemoral pain syndrome, fat-pad irritation, meniscal injuries, medial and lateral collateral and cruciate ligament damage as well as joint sprains are more likely to be the predominant reason for consultation. In contrast in older people, knee osteoarthritis is the most common presentation owing to its frequent cause of pain and higher prevalence (Felson et al., 1987). For example, knee osteoarthritis affects 28% of adults over the age of 45 years and more than a third of adults older than 65 years in the United States (Dillon et al., 2006; Jordan et al., 2007). Consequently, due to its high prevalence, knee osteoarthritis is a leading cause of disability among adults (Dillon et al., 2006) and its impact is expected to increase as a greater proportion of the population ages and lives longer. Fortunately, knee osteoarthritis can be successfully managed by physiotherapy (Page et al., 2011). Indeed, a recent RCT showed that physiotherapy was as effective as arthroscopic surgery for meniscal tear and knee osteoarthritis (Katz et al., 2013). Systematic reviews have demonstrated the benefits of manual therapy and exercise for the management of knee osteoarthritis (French et al., 2011).

In addition to other forms of manual therapy, MWM can be an effective treatment modality for knee osteoarthritis. MWM can reduce movement impairment and associated pain and thereby increase the patient's ability to exercise effectively. An illustration of the impact of MWM in knee osteoarthritis is demonstrated by a recent case series in Japan (Takasaki et al., 2013). In that study, participants suffering from chronic knee osteoarthritis pain were given three sessions of MWM in non-weight-bearing and weight-bearing positions prior to their routine treatment in an orthopaedic outpatient clinic. After MWM there was a significant reduction in disability, improved knee range of motion and less pain. Exercise is difficult to perform in the presence of pain. If pain can be eliminated, patients are more likely to exercise and thereby gain long-term benefits.

Similar to MWM at other joints, and in the absence of knee derangement (meniscal disorder), when treating the tibiofemoral joint a lateral or medial glide should be trialled first, followed by rotational glides and finally glides in the sagittal plane if the previous glides have been unsuccessful. For a meniscal disorder, the squeeze technique should be trialled first.

Patellofemoral pain is particularly prevalent in younger persons who are physically active; it affects females more than males and causes substantial pain and disability (Boling et al., 2010). The problem of patellofemoral pain is highlighted by the fact that up to 90% of individuals with this condition have recurrent or chronic pain (Stathopulu & Baildam, 2003). Strengthening exercise does not appear to be a long-term answer to improving pain (Blond & Hansen, 1998), perhaps because pain is associated with poor motor control around the pelvis, hip and knee (Nakagawa et al., 2012). Sufferers of patellofemoral pain typically present with increased medial femoral rotation and external tibial rotation. In the Mulligan Concept, taping is used to correct this alignment and improve motor control, and there is evidence that even a short period of motor control retraining can have sustained long-term benefits on pain (Willy et al., 2012), supporting the MWM concept.

Levels of evidence

Level 3: six RCTs, two case series, two case reports

Six clinical trials report on the efficacy of the application of MWM in treating knee pathologies such as osteoarthritis (OA) (Dabholkar et al., 2014; Kaya Mutlu et al., 2018; Kiran et al., 2018; Nam et al. 2013; Rao et al., 2018) and patellofemoral pain (Demirci et al., 2017).

Four clinical trials comparing MWM with Maitland's mobilisation (Dabholkar et al., 2014; Kaya Mutlu et al., 2018; Kiran et al., 2018; Rao et al., 2018) demonstrate that both techniques are efficient in treating knee OA. Kiran and colleagues (Kiran et al., 2018) and Dabholkar and colleagues (Dabholkar et al., 2014) both identified MWM as more effective than Maitland mobilisation in reducing pain (VAS), perceived change (Global Rating of Change Scale (GRCS)) and knee ROM, albeit lacking data on statistical significance. Similarly, Rao and colleagues (Rao et al., 2018) demonstrated significant increase in pain-free squat angle and timed up-and-go and reduction in pain (NPRS) from pre- to post-session with no statistical difference between the two groups. In agreement with the previously presented studies, Kaya Mutlu and colleagues (Kaya Mutlu et al., 2018) demonstrated the superior efficacy of both manual therapy techniques (plus exercise) compared with the combination of electrotherapy (transcutaneous electrical nerve stimulation (TENS) and therapeutic ultrasound) and exercise in the treatment of knee OA. Interestingly, although knee ROM was improved immediately post treatment in the three

12

intervention groups, the manual therapy groups had significantly better active ROM (flexion and extension) and greater increase in functional score as well as quadriceps muscle strength than the electrotherapy group at the 1-year follow-up.

Similarly, Nam and colleagues (Nam et al. 2013) compared a programme of knee MWM, 10 minutes hot pack, 20 minutes interferential current, 5 minutes ultrasound and trunk stabilisation exercises with a programme of general physiotherapy (not defined by the authors) and trunk stabilisation exercises. Patients received thrice-weekly treatment for 6 weeks. The knee MWM (chair stand med rot gl MWM K F) repetitions, sets or volume were not reported. There was significantly greater improvement in pain (approximately 17 mm / 100 mm on VAS), WOMAC disability score and physical function in the MWM group compared with the usual care group (Nam et al., 2013).

LATERAL AND MEDIAL GLIDE (NON-WEIGHT-BEARING / WEIGHT-BEARING) – FLEXION AND EXTENSION (SUPINE)

Lateral glide MWM for flexion/extension

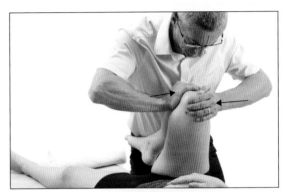

Figure 12.2
Tibiofemoral manual lateral glide MWM: flexion

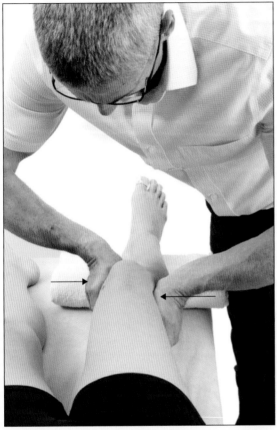

Figure 12.1
Tibiofemoral manual lateral glide MWM: hand position

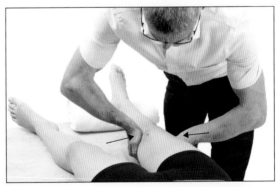

Figure 12.3
Tibiofemoral manual lateral glide MWM: extension

- The patient lies supine with the knee in semi-flexed position.
- The distal femur is stabilised laterally with the therapist's outside hand.
- The therapist glides the proximal tibia laterally with the other (distal) hand.
- While the manual glide is sustained, the patient actively moves the knee into flexion and/or extension and then returns to the start position.
- Full pain-free flexion or extension is complemented with over-pressure from the patient via a strap/belt or from the therapist.
- See Figs 12.1–12.3.

12

INDICATION

Painful and/or restricted knee flexion or extension movement.

POSITIONING

Patient:	Supine, close to edge of treatment table with foot supported on treatment table. The patient can hold a strap/belt placed around their ankle in stirrup position, with both ends of the strap being held medial and lateral to the involved leg.
Treated body part:	Relaxed mid-range position of the knee, prior to any onset of pain.
Therapist:	Adjacent to the affected knee facing the patient.
Hands/contact points:	Stabilising hand: entire palm of the lateral hand placed gently on the lateral surface of the distal femur, fingers directed up, wrist extended and forearm pronated. Gliding hand: entire palm of the medial hand and web-space placed on the medial surface of the patient's tibia just distal to the joint line. The hand is kept in slight supination, with the forearm perpendicular and fingers directed posteriorly.

APPLICATION GUIDELINES

- The therapist applies a laterally directed glide across the knee joint. The therapist's forearms are maintained parallel to each other.
- The therapist maintains the glide while the patient actively moves into flexion or extension.
- Pain-free over-pressure is applied to flexion or extension by the patient or therapist.
- Apply 6–10 repetitions in a set, with 3–5 sets in a treatment session.

COMMENTS

- Ensure that the stabilising and gliding hands have a broad contact so they do not cause pressure pain or that which reproduces the patient's symptoms.
- A foam sponge rubber or a towel may be used under the belt for added comfort.
- A common error made is that the glide is not lateral owing to the therapist referencing the perpendicular force relative to the edge of the table instead of the femur.
- Do not release the glide until the patient returns to the start position.

VARIATIONS

Use of a belt
- A treatment belt may also be used for easier application of the gliding force (see Fig. 12.4A). In this case the patient is positioned in prone lying.
- The patient's distal femur is stabilised laterally with one hand while the therapist pushes their hips backwards, inducing a lateral tibial glide. The position of the lower leg is controlled with the therapist's distal stabilising hand close to the malleolus.
- While the glide is sustained, the therapist passively or actively moves the knee into flexion (Fig. 12.4B) or extension from the start position.
- Full, active pain-free flexion or extension is complemented with over-pressure from the therapist.
- It is essential that the therapist is positioned such that a perpendicular glide is achieved at all times with reference to the femur, and the glide is parallel to the tibial plateau.

12

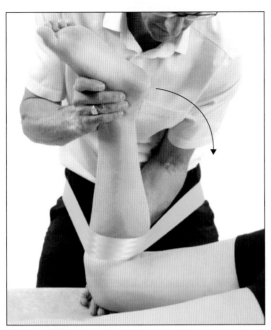

Figure 12.4A
Tibiofemoral lateral glide MWM into knee flexion:
therapist and belt positioning

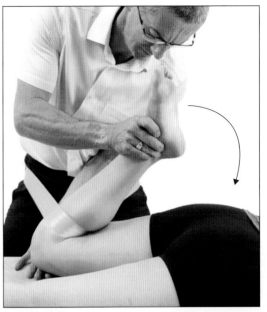

Figure 12.4B
Tibiofemoral lateral glide MWM into knee flexion:
end position

Weight-bearing

- Progression from non-weight-bearing to weight-bearing can occur when there is a substantial improvement with non-weight-bearing movement techniques or if the patient has pain predominantly in weight-bearing activities and movements.

- A lateral or medial glide can be achieved with the therapist's hands directly (Fig. 12.5).

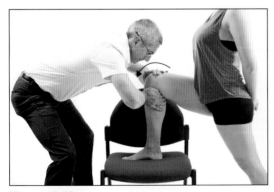

Figure 12.5A
Tibiofemoral lateral glide MWM into knee flexion

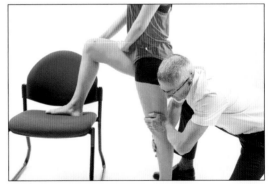

Figure 12.5B
Tibiofemoral lateral glide MWM into knee extension

(continued next page...)

SELF-MANAGEMENT

Self-lateral glide MWM for flexion/extension: home exercise

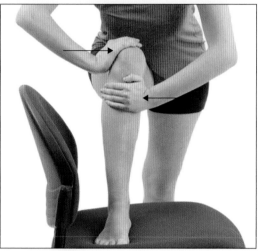

Figure 12.6A
Knee flexion tibiofemoral lateral glide MWM: home exercise with chair

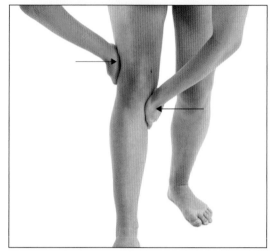

Figure 12.6B
Knee extension tibiofemoral lateral glide MWM: home exercise

- The patient stands with the affected knee flexed, and foot resting on a chair (for flexion) (Fig. 12.6A) or on the ground (for extension) (Fig. 12.6B).
- The distal femur is stabilised laterally with the patient's hand.
- The proximal tibia is mobilised in a lateral direction with the patient's other hand.
- While the glide is sustained, the patient actively moves the knee by 'lunging' into flexion from the start position (for flexion) or extension (for extension) and then returns.
- Full, active pain-free movement is complemented by self-generated over-pressure.

ANNOTATION

sup ly R Kn Lat gl MWM F×6(3)
sup ly R Kn Lat gl MWM E +OP(therapist)×6(3)
pr ly L Kn belt Lat gl MWM F +OP(therapist)×6(3)
st R Foot on chair R Kn Lat gl MWM F×10
st R foot on chair L Kn Lat gl MWM E×10
st R Foot on chair R Kn self Lat gl MWM F×10
st R Kn self Lat gl MWM E×10

12

Medial glide MWM for flexion / extension

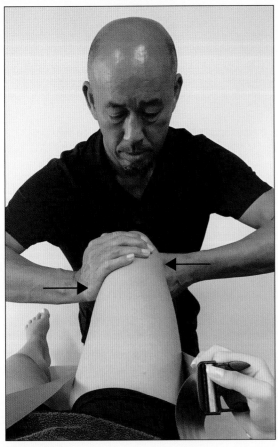

Figure 12.7
Tibiofemoral manual medial glide MWM with a belt

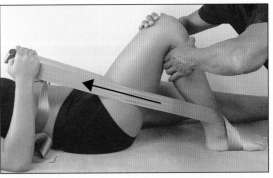

Figure 12.8
Tibiofemoral manual medial glide MWM with a belt: into knee flexion

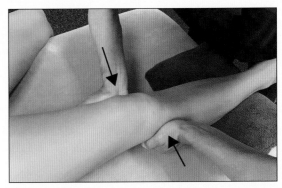

Figure 12.9
Tibiofemoral manual medial glide MWM: into knee extension

- The patient lies supine with the knee semi-flexed, holding a strap placed around the foot.
- The therapist stabilises the distal femur medially with one hand on the patient's inner thigh.
- The therapist glides the tibia medially with the other hand.
- While the glide is sustained, the patient actively moves the knee into flexion (Fig. 12.8) or extension (Fig. 12.9) and then returns to the start position.
- Full pain-free flexion is complemented with over-pressure from the patient via the treatment belt or can be applied by the therapist for extension.
- See Figs 12.7–12.9.

INDICATION

Painful and/or restricted knee flexion or extension movement.

POSITIONING

Patient:	Supine lying, close to the edge of a treatment table with foot fully supported on treatment table.
	For flexion the patient holds a strap placed around their ankle in stirrup position, with both ends of the strap being held medial and lateral to the involved leg.
Treated body part:	Relaxed mid-range position of the knee, prior to any onset of pain.
Therapist:	Adjacent to the affected knee facing the patient.
Hands/contact points:	Stabilising hand: the entire palm of the therapist's medial hand is placed on the medial surface of the patient's distal femur, fingers directed up, wrist extended and forearm pronated.
	Gliding hand: the entire palm of the therapist's hand and web-space are placed on the lateral surface of the patient's tibia just distal to the joint line. The hand is kept in slight supination with fingers directed posteriorly.

APPLICATION GUIDELINES

- The therapist applies a medially directed glide across the knee joint. If the therapist's forearms are parallel, the glide force can be achieved with less effort.
- Pain-free over-pressure is applied to flexion by the patient via the strap, or by the therapist for extension.
- Apply 6–10 repetitions in a set, with 3–5 sets in a treatment session.

COMMENTS

- Ensure that the stabilising and gliding hands have a broad contact so they do not cause pressure pain or that which reproduces the patient's symptoms, particularly with respect to the fibula head and common peroneal nerve.
- Do not release the glide until the patient returns to the start position.

12

● As previously mentioned, altering the glide mechanics, exploring the direction of the glide, utilisation of a treatment belt (Fig. 12.10) and assessing progression into weight-bearing positions can/should be considered.

Use of a belt

● The therapist pushes their hips backwards, inducing a medial tibial glide, while controlling the position of the patient's lower leg with the distal stabilising hand.

● It is essential that the therapist is positioned such that a perpendicular glide is achieved at all times with reference to the femur, and the glide is parallel to the tibial plateau.

● Pain-free over-pressure is applied to flexion or extension by the therapist.

● Note that passive movement is preferred, as excessive hamstring contraction often leads to cramping.

● Maintain belt tension until the patient resumes the start position.

● Apply 6–10 repetitions in a set, with 3–5 sets in a treatment session, but only if there is a substantial increase in knee flexion or extension.

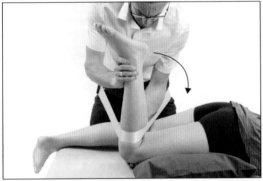

Figure 12.10A
Tibiofemoral medial glide MWM with belt: start position

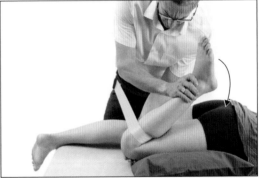

Figure 12.10B
Tibiofemoral medial glide MWM with belt: into knee flexion

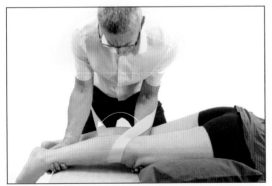

Figure 12.10C
Tibiofemoral medial glide MWM with belt: into knee extension

(continued next page...)

SELF-MANAGEMENT

Self-medial glide MWM for knee flexion/extension: home exercise

- The patient stands with affected knee flexed, foot resting on a chair for flexion or standing for extension (Fig. 12.11A).
- The distal femur is stabilised medially with the patient's hand.
- The proximal tibia is mobilised in a medial direction with the patient's other hand.
- While the glide is sustained, the patient actively moves the knee by 'lunging' into flexion (Fig. 12.11B) or pushing back into extension (Fig. 12.11C) from the start position and then returns.
- Full, active pain-free movement is complemented by self-generated over-pressure.

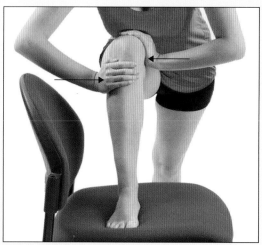

Figure 12.11A
Knee extension tibiofemoral medial glide MWM: start position

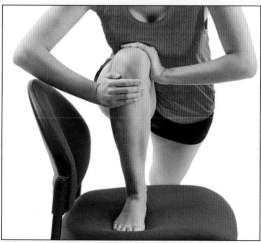

Figure 12.11B
Knee flexion tibiofemoral medial glide MWM: into knee flexion

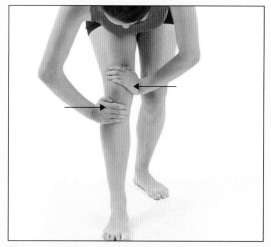

Figure 12.11C
Knee extension tibiofemoral medial glide MWM: into knee extension

12

ANNOTATIONS

sup ly R Kn Med gl MWM F +OP(belt)×6(3)

sup ly R Kn Med gl MWM E +OP(therapist)×6(3)

pr ly R Kn belt Med gl MWM F +OP(therapist)×6(3)

pr ly R Kn belt Med gl MWM F +OP(therapist)×6(3)

st R Foot on chair R Kn self Med gl MWM F×10

st R Kn self Med gl MWM E×10

KNEE ANTEROPOSTERIOR MWM FOR FLEXION AND POSTEROANTERIOR MWM FOR EXTENSION

Knee anteroposterior MWM for flexion

TECHNIQUE AT A GLANCE

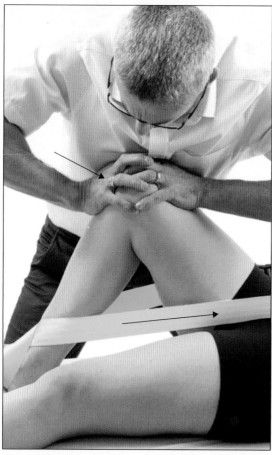

Figure 12.12
Knee flexion tibiofemoral anteroposterior glide MWM: close view

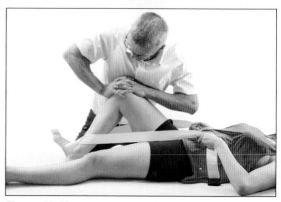

Figure 12.13
Knee flexion tibiofemoral anteroposterior glide MWM: assistance with a belt

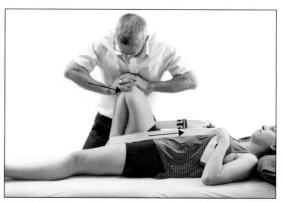

Figure 12.14
Knee flexion tibiofemoral anteroposterior glide MWM: end range

- The patient lies supine at the edge of the treatment table with the hip in flexion, and knee close to the limitation of flexion.
- The therapist stabilises the patient's femur with one hand while the other (contacting the tibia) applies an anteroposterior glide on the tibia.
- A treatment belt is looped around the ankle and foot, to allow the patient to pull the knee into flexion (Figs 12.13 and 12.14).
- While the therapist maintains the anteroposterior glide, the patient pulls their knee into flexion.
- Over-pressure is applied if necessary before returning to the start position.
- See Figs 12.12–12.14.

12

INDICATION

Pain and gross limitation/stiffness of knee flexion.

POSITIONING

Patient:	Supine lying, as close as possible to the edge of the treatment table on the therapist's side.
Treated body part:	Hip flexed, knee close to the limitation of flexion.
Therapist:	Stride standing next to the patient's affected knee.
Hands contact points:	One hand stabilises the patient's distal femur, while the other contacts the proximal end of their tibia, close to the tibial tubercle. The fingers of both hands are interlaced.

APPLICATION GUIDELINES

- The therapist stabilises the patient's femur with one hand to prevent hip rotation and flexion.
- The other hand applies the tibial anteroposterior glide through the heel of the hand over the tibial tubercle.
- Hold the patient's leg close to the therapist's body for control.
- Maintain the anteroposterior tibial glide while the patient pulls their knee into flexion through a treatment belt looped around the ankle and foot.
- Maintain the glide while they return to the start position.
- Apply 6–10 repetitions in a set, with 3–5 sets in a treatment session, but only if there is a substantial increase in the range of knee pain-free flexion.
- Apply over-pressure at the end range if pain-free full range can be achieved.

COMMENTS

- The angle of glide should follow the tibial plateau, which is maintained as the patient flexes their knee.
- Avoid compressing the patella and the patella tendon.

ANNOTATION

sup ly R Kn Tib Post gl MWM F +OP(belt)×6(3)

Knee posteroanterior MWM for extension

TECHNIQUE AT A GLANCE

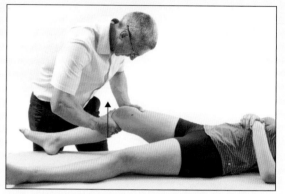

Figure 12.16
Knee extension tibiofemoral posteroanterior manual glide MWM: start position

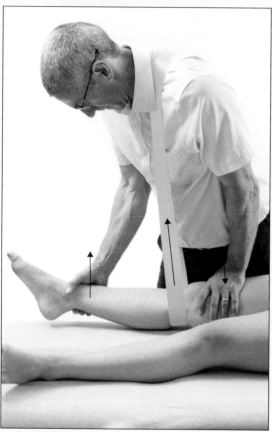

Figure 12.15
Knee extension tibiofemoral posteroanterior glide MWM: with belt

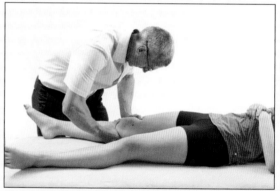

Figure 12.17
Knee extension tibiofemoral posteroanterior manual glide MWM: end position

- The patient lies supine at the edge of the treatment table, knee close to the limitation of extension.
- The therapist stabilises the patient's femur with one hand while the other (contacting the tibia) applies a posteroanterior glide to their tibia.
- A treatment belt can also be utilised where it is looped under the tibia and over the shoulder of the therapist and a posteroanterior glide is applied and sustained.
- While maintaining the posteroanterior glide, the patient actively straightens their knee into extension.
- Over-pressure is applied if necessary before returning to the start position.
- See Figs 12.15–12.17.

12

INDICATION

Pain and gross limitation/stiffness of knee extension.

POSITIONING

Patient:	Supine lying, as close as possible to the edge of the treatment table on the therapist's side.
Treated body part:	Hip neutral, knee close to the limitation of extension.
Therapist:	Stride standing next to the patient's affected knee.
Hands contact points:	One hand stabilises the patient's distal femur, while the other contacts the posterior proximal end of the tibia, around the calf muscle close to the joint line.
	Or use the belt, which is positioned under the proximal tibia and over the therapist's shoulder.

APPLICATION GUIDELINES

- The therapist stabilises the patient's femur with one hand to prevent hip rotation and flexion.
- The other hand applies the tibial posteroanterior glide through the posterior aspect of the knee, or in the case of the belt an upward posteroanterior glide is applied.
- Hold the patient's leg close to the therapist's body for control.
- Maintain the posteroanterior tibial glide while the patient pushes their knee into extension and back to the start position.
- Apply 6–10 repetitions in a set, with 3–5 sets in a treatment session, but only if there is a substantial increase in range of knee pain-free flexion.
- Apply over-pressure at the end range if pain-free full range can be achieved.

COMMENT

- Angle of glide should follow the tibial plateau, which is maintained as the patient extends their knee.

ANNOTATION

sup ly R Kn Tib belt Ant gl MWM E×6(3)
sup ly R Kn Tib Ant gl MWM E +OP(therapist)×6(3)

TIBIAL ROTATION – NON-WEIGHT-BEARING/WEIGHT-BEARING

Internal rotation MWM for flexion

TECHNIQUE AT A GLANCE

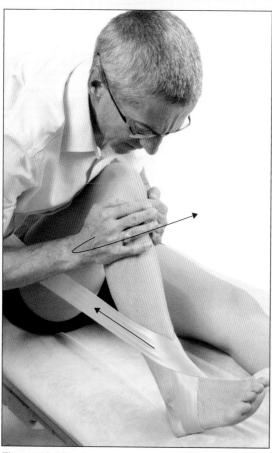

Figure 12.18
Knee flexion tibiofemoral internal rotation MWM: start position

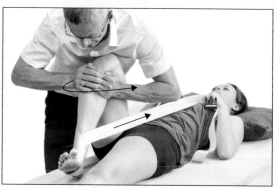

Figure 12.19
Knee flexion tibiofemoral internal rotation MWM: into flexion with belt assistance

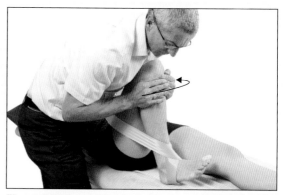

Figure 12.20
Knee flexion tibiofemoral internal rotation MWM: end position

- The patient lies supine with the knee flexed close to the limitation, holding a treatment belt placed around their foot.
- The proximal lower leg is mobilised into internal rotation with both the therapist's hands.
- While the rotational glide is sustained, the patient actively moves the knee into flexion and returns to the start position.
- Full pain-free flexion is complemented with over-pressure by the belt.
- See Figs 12.18–12.20.

12

INDICATION

Painful and/or restricted knee flexion movement.

POSITIONING

Patient:	Supine lying, with the affected knee closest to the side of a treatment table and with the foot supported. The patient holds a strap placed around their ankle in stirrup position, with both ends of the strap being held medially and laterally to the involved leg with both hands.
Treated body part:	Relaxed mid-range position of the knee, prior to any onset of pain.
Therapist:	In step standing adjacent to the affected knee, facing in a caudal direction. Medial and lateral hand placement is 'around' the affected knee.
Hands/contact points:	Medial hand: the therapist's palm is placed on the medial surface of the proximal tibia and their fingers placed over the medial aspect of the tibial spine. Lateral hand: the therapist's palm is placed on the lateral aspect of the fibula and proximal tibia and their fingers anteriorly. The therapist's fingers may be intertwined or overlapped.

APPLICATION GUIDELINES

- Apply an internal rotation mobilisation of the tibia by pulling the tibial spine medially with the medial hand while pushing the posterior–lateral calf in an anterior direction with the lateral hand.
- Pain-free over-pressure is applied to flexion by the patient via the strap.
- Apply 6–10 repetitions in a set, with 3–5 sets in a treatment session, but only if there is a substantial increase in pain-free knee flexion ROM.

COMMENTS

- Ensure that the mobilising hands have a broad contact so they do not cause pressure pain or that which reproduces the patient's symptoms.
- Do not release the rotation until the patient returns to the start position.

(continued next page...)

- The tibial rotation technique can also be carried out into external rotation if internal rotation is not effective or increases symptoms (Fig. 12.21).

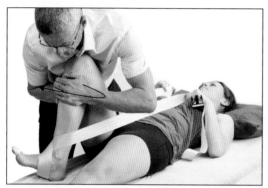

Figure 12.21A
Knee flexion tibiofemoral external rotation MWM: medial view

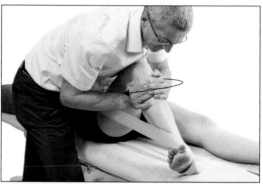

Figure 12.21B
Knee flexion tibiofemoral external rotation MWM: lateral view

- **Tibiofemoral internal or external rotation** can be carried out in a weight-bearing position if required (Fig. 12.22). This may be a functional requirement for some people, such as those who undertake daily prayer in a kneeling position.

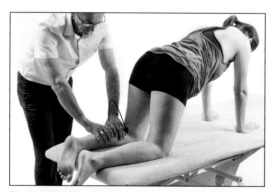

Figure 12.22A
Knee flexion tibiofemoral internal or external rotation MWM: start position

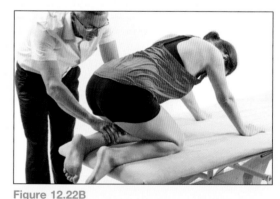

Figure 12.22B
Knee flexion tibiofemoral internal or external rotation MWM: end position

12

SELF-MANAGEMENT

Tibial internal rotation in weight-bearing: home exercise

- The patient stands with their affected knee flexed, and the foot on the floor or resting on a chair or step.
- The patient grasps their fibula and tibia with interlocked fingers and rotates the lower leg into internal rotation. While the internal rotation is sustained, the patient actively moves the knee into extension or by 'squatting' into flexion from the start position of partial flexion and then returns.
- Full, active pain-free flexion is complemented by self-generated over-pressure.
- See Fig. 12.23.

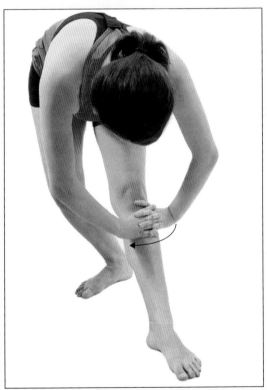

Figure 12.23A
Knee extension tibiofemoral internal rotation in weight-bearing

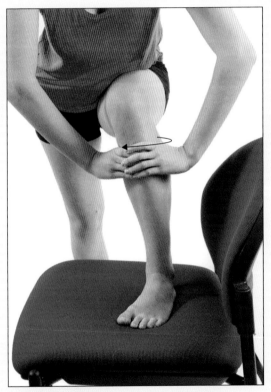

Figure 12.23B
Knee flexion tibiofemoral internal rotation self-MWM on a chair

(continued next page...)

TAPING

Tibial internal rotation weight-bearing

- This taping technique may be useful for tibiofemoral pain responding to tibial rotation MWM or for patellofemoral pain.

- In general the tape is spiralled upwards from the lateral aspect of the fibula immediately below the medial knee joint line, crossing the posterior aspect of the knee and ending on the posterolateral femur. Use 50-mm non-stretch sports tape or flexible tape with near-maximum tension.

- Have the patient stand with their involved foot slightly internally rotated, knee slightly flexed and femur externally rotated relative to the tibia (Fig. 12.24). This position will increase tape tension when they stand in a normal position.

- Start the tape laterally around the lateral aspect of the fibula. Spiral the tape in a proximal direction across the tibial tubercle, around the medial side of the tibia, while assisting the tibia into internal rotation. End the tape on the lateral aspect of the distal femur.

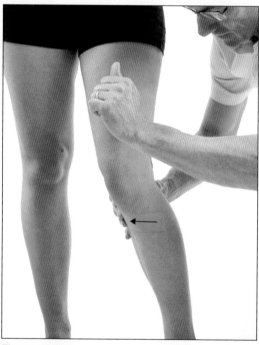

Figure 12.24A
Tibiofemoral internal rotation taping for tibiofemoral and patellofemoral pain: application

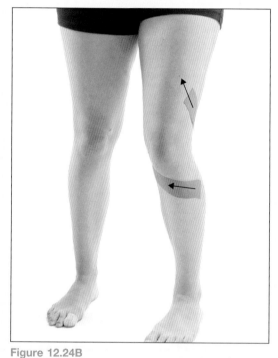

Figure 12.24B
Tibiofemoral internal rotation taping for tibiofemoral and patellofemoral pain: leg position during application

12

- The tension needs to be maximal when the tape crosses the knee joint line.
- Apply two layers of tape in the same location, with equal tension on both layers for maximum effect.
- Patients can be taught to self-apply this taping as part of a home programme.
- A trial of tibiofemoral external rotation taping for tibiofemoral external rotation MWM was found to be effective for knee pain and impairment (Fig. 12.25).

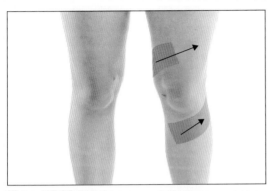

Figure 12.25
Tibiofemoral external rotation taping for tibiofemoral and patellofemoral pain

ANNOTATIONS

sup ly R Kn IR MWM F +OP(belt)×6(3)
sup ly L Kn ER MWM F +OP(belt)×6(3)
st L Foot on chair L Kn self IR MWM F×10
st L Kn self IR MWM E×10
L Kn IR tape
L Kn ER tape

Internal / external rotation MWM for extension

Internal rotation MWM for extension

TECHNIQUE AT A GLANCE

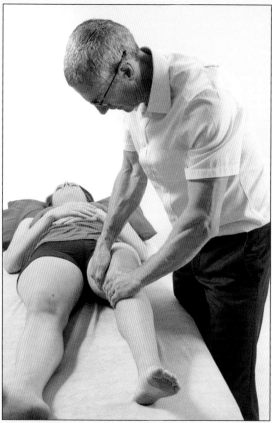

Figure 12.26
Knee extension tibiofemoral internal rotation MWM: start position

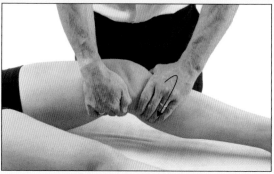

Figure 12.27
Knee extension tibiofemoral internal rotation MWM: start position medial view

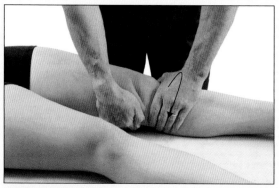

Figure 12.28
Knee extension tibiofemoral internal rotation MWM: end position with over-pressure

- The patient lies supine with the knee extended close to the limitation and elevated sufficiently at the foot such that the posterior knee cannot touch the table upon full extension.
- The therapist stabilises the distal femur medially with their proximal hand.
- The proximal tibia is mobilised internally with the distal hand.
- Return to the start position.
- Full, active pain-free extension is complemented with over-pressure from the therapist.
- See Figs 12.26–12.28.

INDICATION

Painful and / or restricted knee extension movement.

POSITIONING

Patient:	Supine lying, with the affected knee closest to the side of a treatment table and with the ankle resting on a foam roll.
Treated body part:	Relaxed knee extension position, prior to any onset of pain.
Therapist:	Adjacent to the affected knee and facing towards the knee.
Hands / contact points:	Stabilising hand: the entire palm of the therapist's proximal hand placed on the posterior–medial surface of the distal femur, fingers directed posteriorly.
	Mobilising hand: the therapist's palm crossing the spine of the tibia, thumb in contact with the lateral tibial spine and fingers directed posteriorly over the medial calf.

APPLICATION GUIDELINES

- Apply an internal rotation mobilisation of the tibia at the knee joint.
- Pain-free over-pressure is applied to extension by the therapist.
- Apply 6–10 repetitions in a set, with 3–5 sets in a treatment session, but only if there is a substantial increase in pain-free knee extension ROM.

COMMENTS

- Ensure that the stabilising and mobilising hands have a broad contact so they do not cause pressure pain or that which reproduces the patient's symptoms.
- Do not release the rotation until the patient returns to the start position.
- Taping may be a useful adjunct if this technique is found effective (see Fig. 12.24).

(continued next page...)

12

External rotation MWM for extension

- This technique can also be performed by applying an external rotation.
- The patient is positioned as described in the previous technique for internal rotation.
- The patient's proximal tibia is mobilised externally with the therapist's distal hand.
- While the tibial rotation is sustained, the patient actively moves the knee into extension and then returns to the start position (Fig. 12.29).

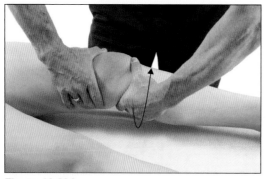

Figure 12.29A
Knee extension tibiofemoral external rotation
MWM: start position

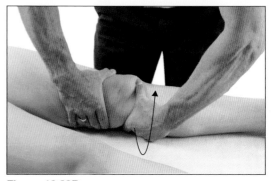

Figure 12.29B
Knee extension tibiofemoral external rotation
MWM: end position

ANNOTATIONS

sup ly L Kn IR MWM E×6(3)
sup ly L Kn ER MWM E×6(3)

KNEE SQUEEZE TECHNIQUE FOR MENISCAL PAIN

TECHNIQUE AT A GLANCE

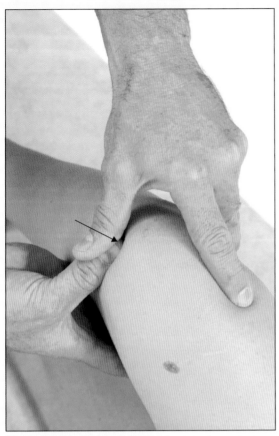

Figure 12.30
Knee meniscal 'squeeze' technique – finger contact: hand position close view

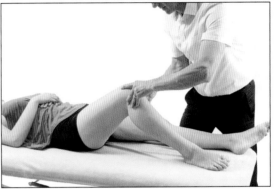

Figure 12.31
Knee meniscal 'squeeze' technique: start position

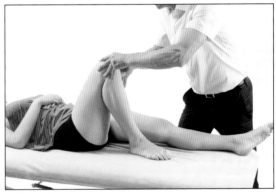

Figure 12.32
Knee meniscal 'squeeze' technique: flexion

- The patient lies supine at the edge of the treatment table with the hip in flexion, knee in flexion and neutral hip rotation.
- The therapist places the medial edge of their thumb on the joint line at the site of maximal tenderness.
- The other thumb reinforces and applies centrally directed force.
- The patient first flexes then extends their knee to the onset of pain, gradually increasing the range in each direction.
- Aim for full-range knee extension or flexion in the first session.
- See Figs 12.30–12.32.

12

INDICATION

Meniscal injury or degenerative change causing joint line pain and limitation of knee flexion and extension; localised point of pain over the anterior or posterior horn of meniscus within the medial or lateral joint line.

POSITIONING

Patient:	Supine lying, as close as possible to the edge of the treatment table on the therapist's side.
Treated body part:	Hip and knee flexed in a pain-free position.
Therapist:	Stride standing next to the patient's affected knee.
Hands contact points:	Medial edge of thumb on the knee joint line, with reinforcement from the opposite thumb (see Fig. 12.30).

APPLICATION GUIDELINES

- Identify the most pain-sensitive point on the knee joint line.
- Place the medial edge of one thumb on the tender point on the side of pain (either the medial or the lateral joint line for the medial or lateral meniscus respectively). The opposite thumb reinforces over the other thumb.
- While sustaining the thumb centrally directed joint line force, ask the patient to flex and then extend their knee to the onset of pain (see Fig. 12.32).
- Repeat the knee movement backwards and forwards while maintaining the thumb pressure.
- The pain-free knee ROM should gradually increase until full range can be achieved into extension.

COMMENTS

- Only the medial border of the thumb should be used, not the pulp of the thumb, as the latter is too large to contact the joint line.
- The thumb should be placed along the joint line and not across it.
- Meniscal pressure should be maintained throughout the movement.
- The patient flexes the knee as the first movement and does not extend it, as flexion will increase the joint space and allow pressure to be maintained on the meniscus.
- The therapist follows the movement of the leg as it moves into flexion/extension to maintain the pressure within the joint line (indirectly on the meniscus).
- The therapist may provide passive over-pressure at the end of the available range.

12

VARIATIONS

- The technique can progress to a weight-bearing position if required. The patient puts their affected foot on the chair and holds onto the chair back for support as they flex the knee with the therapist applying direct pressure to the joint line as described above (Fig. 12.33).

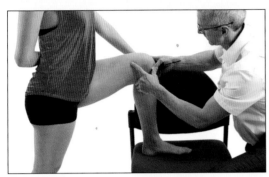

Figure 12.33A
Squeeze technique in weight-bearing: start position

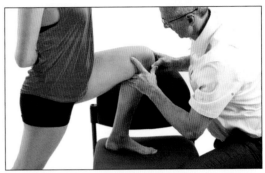

Figure 12.33B
Squeeze technique in weight-bearing: end position

SELF-MANAGEMENT

- The patient can perform self-treatment by placing the medial border of one thumb or index finger over the tender point (similar to the thumb position in Fig. 12.34), which is reinforced by the other thumb, and then carrying out knee movement into flexion and extension.

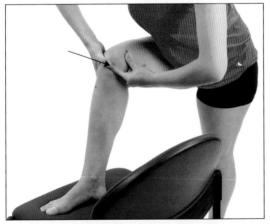

Figure 12.34A
Self-squeeze technique: start position

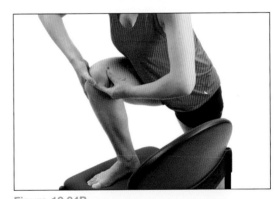

Figure 12.34B
Self-squeeze technique: flexion end position

ANNOTATIONS

sup ly L Kn Med Squeeze F/E×3
sup ly L Kn Lat Squeeze F/E×6
st L foot on chair L Kn Med Squeeze F×6
st R foot on chair R Kn self Lat Squeeze F/E×6

PROXIMAL FIBULAR MWM – VENTRAL OR POSTERIOR GLIDE DURING KNEE FLEXION AND EXTENSION

TECHNIQUE AT A GLANCE

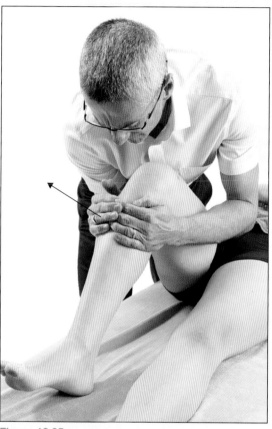

Figure 12.35
Ventral fibular glide during knee flexion: start position medial view

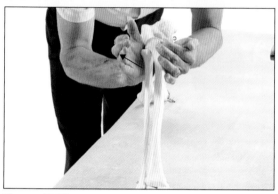

Figure 12.36
Ventral fibular glide during knee flexion: start position model view

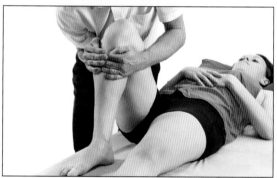

Figure 12.37
Ventral fibular glide during knee flexion: end position

- The patient lies supine at the edge of the treatment table with the hip in flexion, the knee in flexion and neutral hip rotation.
- The therapist places their thenar eminence on the posterior aspect of the proximal aspect of the fibula.
- The other hand provides counterforce to stabilise the tibia.
- The patient flexes or extends their knee to the onset of pain or limitation.
- See Figs 12.35–12.37.

12

INDICATION

Lateral knee pain in proximity to the head of fibula during knee flexion or extension.

POSITIONING

Patient:	Supine lying, as close as possible to the edge of the treatment table on the therapist's side.
Treated body part:	Hip and knee flexed in a pain-free position.
Therapist:	Stride standing next to the patient's affected knee, facing towards the feet.
Hands contact points:	Mobilising hand: the thenar eminence on the posterior aspect of the proximal aspect of the fibula. Stabilising hand: grasp the upper medial aspect of the tibia (see Fig. 12.36).

APPLICATION GUIDELINES

- Contact the posterior aspect of the proximal fibula with the thenar eminence of one hand and glide the fibula anteriorly.
- The opposite hand provides counterforce to stabilise the tibia on the medial side.
- While sustaining the ventral glide force, ask the patient to flex or extend their knee to the onset of pain (see Fig. 12.37).
- Repeat the knee movement backwards and forwards while maintaining the fibular glide.

COMMENTS

- Avoid compression over the common peroneal nerve as it winds around the posterior aspect of the neck of the fibula.
- Be careful not to block the movement into flexion.
- The patient may provide passive over-pressure at the end of the available range with a manual therapy belt looped around the foot.

(continued next page...)

12

Posterior fibula glide

- In the event that a ventral glide is not successful, trial a dorsal fibular glide MWM.
- Face towards the patient's head, and with one hand contact the ventral aspect of the proximal fibula. The other hand stabilises the tibia medially.
- Glide the fibula and ask the patient to flex or extend their knee to the onset of pain.

Posterior and ventral fibula MWM for knee flexion in weight-bearing

- The technique can be progressed to a weight-bearing position if required. The patient puts their affected foot on the chair and holds onto the chair back for support as they flex the knee.
- The therapist stands in front of the patient stabilising the tibia medially with one hand while mobilising the fibula ventrally with their fingers or posteriorly with the thenar eminence (Fig. 12.38).

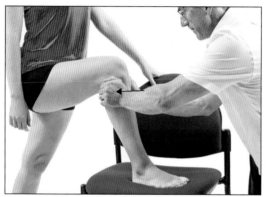

Figure 12.38A
Posterior fibular glide during knee flexion in weight-bearing: start position

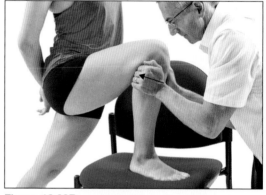

Figure 12.38B
Posterior fibular glide during knee flexion in weight-bearing: end position

SELF-MANAGEMENT

- The patient can perform self-treatment in weight-bearing by placing the thenar eminence of one hand on the posterior aspect of the proximal fibula, stabilising the tibia with the other hand (Fig. 12.39).

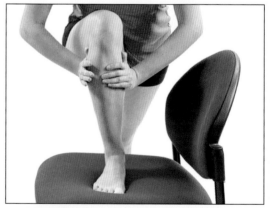

Figure 12.39
Ventral fibula glide self-mobilisation during weight-bearing knee flexion

12

TAPING

- Taping can be used to maintain improvement gained after MWM (Fig. 12.40).
- For a ventral glide, start the tape on the posterior aspect of the fibula, pulling the tape anteriorly to wind around first the fibula and then the tibia just below the tibial tubercle (Fig. 12.40A).
- For a dorsal fibula glide, start the tape anteriorly and wind around the lateral aspect of the fibula and then the posterior aspect of the tibia (Fig. 12.40B).
- Ensure that the tape does not complete a full circle to avoid circulatory issues and use two layers for the strongest effect.
- As with the mobilisation technique, avoid compressing the common peroneal nerve.

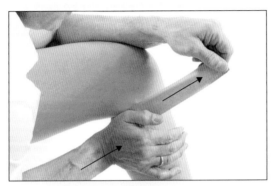

Figure 12.40A
Taping the proximal fibula ventrally

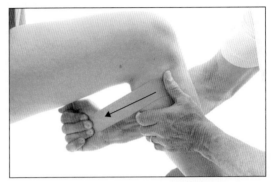

Figure 12.40B
Taping the proximal fibula dorsally

ANNOTATIONS

sup ly R Sup Fib Ant gl MWM Kn F×6
sup ly R Sup Fib Post gl MWM Kn F×6(3)
st R foot on chair R Sup Fib Post gl MWM Kn F×6
st R foot on chair R Sup Fib self Ant gl MWM Kn F×10
R Sup Fib Ant gl tape
R Sup Fib Post gl tape

References

Blond, L., Hansen, L., 1998. Patellofemoral pain syndrome in athletes: a 5.7-year retrospective follow-up study of 250 athletes. Acta Orthop. Belg. 64 (4), 393–400.

Boling, M., Padua, D., Marshall, S., Guskiewicz, K., Pyne, S., Beutler, A., 2010. Gender differences in the incidence and prevalence of patellofemoral pain syndrome. Scand. J. Med. Sci. Sports 20 (5), 725–730.

Dabholkar, A., Kumari, S., Yardi, S., 2014. Comparative study of short term response between Maitland mobilization and Mulligan's mobilization with movement of hip joint in osteoarthritis of knee patients identified as per clinical prediction rule. Ind. J. Physiother. Occup. Ther. 8 (4), 6.

Demirci, S., Kinikli, G.I., Callaghan, M.J., Tunay, V.B., 2017. Comparison of short-term effects of mobilization with movement and kinesiotaping on pain, function and balance in patellofemoral pain. Acta Orthop. Traumatol. Turc. 51 (6), 442–447.

Dillon, C.F., Rasch, E.K., Gu, Q., Hirsch, R., 2006. Prevalence of knee osteoarthritis in the United States: arthritis data from the Third National Health and Nutrition Examination Survey 1991–94. J. Rheumatol. 33 (11), 2271–2279.

Felson, D.T., Naimark, A., Anderson, J., Kazis, L., Castelli, W., Meenan, R.F., 1987. The prevalence of knee osteoarthritis in the elderly. The Framingham Osteoarthritis Study. Arthritis Rheum. 30 (8), 914–918.

12

French, H.P., Brennan, A., White, B., Cusack, T., 2011. Manual therapy for osteoarthritis of the hip or knee – a systematic review. Man. Ther. 16 (2), 109–117.

Jordan, J.M., Helmick, C.G., Renner, J.B., Luta, G., Dragomir, A.D., Woodard, J., et al., 2007. Prevalence of knee symptoms and radiographic and symptomatic knee osteoarthritis in African Americans and Caucasians: the Johnston County Osteoarthritis Project. J. Rheumatol. 34 (1), 172–180.

Katz, J.N., Brophy, R.H., Chaisson, C.E., de Chaves, L., Cole, B.J., Dahm, D.L., et al., 2013. Surgery versus physical therapy for a meniscal tear and osteoarthritis. N. Engl. J. Med. 368 (18), 1675–1684.

Kaya Mutlu, E., Ercin, E., Razak Ozdıncler, A., Ones, N., 2018. A comparison of two manual physical therapy approaches and electrotherapy modalities for patients with knee osteoarthritis: a randomized three arm clinical trial. Physiother. Theory Pract. 34 (8), 600–612.

Kiran, A., Ijaz, M., Qamar, M., Basharat, A., Rasul, A., Ahmed, W., 2018. Comparison of efficacy of Mulligan's mobilization with movement with Maitland mobilization along with conventional therapy in the patients with knee osteoarthritis: a randomized clinical trial. Libyan Int. Med. Univ. J. 3 (1), 26–30.

Nakagawa, T.H., Moriya, E.T., Maciel, C.D., Serrao, F.V., 2012. Trunk, pelvis, hip, and knee kinematics, hip strength, and gluteal muscle activation during a single-leg squat in males and females with and without patellofemoral pain syndrome. J. Orthop. Sports Phys. Ther. 42 (6), 491–501.

Nam, C.W., Park, S.I., Yong, M.S., Kim, Y.M., 2013. Effects of the MWM technique accompanied by trunk stabilization exercises on pain and physical dysfunctions caused by degenerative osteoarthritis. J. Phys. Ther. Sci. 25, 1137–1140.

Page, C.J., Hinman, R.S., Bennell, K.L., 2011. Physiotherapy management of knee osteoarthritis. Int. J. Rheum. Dis. 14 (2), 145–151.

Rao, R.V., Balthillaya, G., Prabhu, A., Kamath, A., 2018. Immediate effects of Maitland mobilization versus Mulligan mobilization with movement in osteoarthritis knee – a randomized crossover trial. J. Bodyw. Mov. Ther. 22 (3), 572–579.

Stathopulu, E., Baildam, E., 2003. Anterior knee pain: a long-term follow-up. Rheumatology 42 (2), 380–382.

Takasaki, H., Hall, T., Jull, G., 2013. Immediate and short-term effects of Mulligan's mobilization with movement on knee pain and disability associated with knee osteoarthritis – a prospective case series. Physiother. Theory Pract. 29 (2), 87–95.

Willy, R.W., Scholz, J.P., Davis, I.S., 2012. Mirror gait retraining for the treatment of patellofemoral pain in female runners. Clin. Biomech. (Bristol, Avon) 27 (10), 1045–1051.

12

Ankle and foot

INTRODUCTION

There are 26 bones in the ankle and foot, which, in combination with the fibula and tibia, form 33 joints. Only the talus, however, articulates with the tibia, as it is gripped bilaterally by the two malleoli, forming the talocrural joint. The talus receives the body weight from the tibia and dissipates it through its articulation with the calcaneus (talocalcaneal joint) and the forefoot through the talocalcaneonavicular joint (Moore et al., 2014). These three joints form the ankle joint complex and allow movement in the sagittal, frontal and transverse planes.

Ankle sprains, usually into inversion with plantarflexion, are common and can become a persistent and recurrent problem for approximately 40% of sufferers (Braun, 1999; Waterman et al., 2010). The mechanism of injury usually involves the ankle joint being somewhat plantarflexed and then superimposed inversion leading to stress at the inferior tibiofibula, talocrural, mid-tarsal and in some cases even the forefoot joints, bones and supporting soft tissue structures. The exact focus of the stress would depend on many factors, including point of foot–ground contact, loads and load vectors experienced within the foot and ankle. The injured joints, bones and their supporting structures might well be localised or distributed. It is reasonably common for plantarflexion–inversion sprains to result in either an injury of the inferior tibiofibular ligament (high ankle sprain), anterior talocrural ligament (the classic ankle sprain) or bifurcate ligament (low ankle sprain). Less commonly the subtalar joint (interosseous ligament) and cuboid metatarsal joints might be involved. Fractures ought to be considered as a differential diagnosis (e.g. talar dome, distal fibula, fifth metatarsal head) (Brukner & Khan, 2012) with key findings including a landing from a height, a mechanism of injury involving dorsiflexion, rapid onset intra-articular effusion and local tenderness over bone prompting follow-up diagnostic examination (e.g. radiographs). Eversion injuries might result in deltoid and spring ligament disruption with signs and symptoms mainly on the medial side of the ankle. Key clinical findings for localised ligamentous and joint injury classically are localised swelling, pain on palpation locally over the injured ligament and joint structures, as well as provocation of pain and/or instability on stress testing. The most appropriate joint to which the MWM should be applied will depend on the clinical examination findings. MWM provides an additional clinical reasoning and assessment tool in that the application of a manual force specifically to a joint can be used to alleviate symptoms – that is, the opposite to the classic symptom provocation approach.

As well as assisting in the assessment of an ankle sprain, MWM is useful in regaining pain-free ROM in a systematic and rapid manner (see Levels of evidence at end of this chapter). A frequent impairment following ankle sprain is a limitation of dorsiflexion (Green et al., 2001). A lack of talocrural dorsiflexion is likely a result of the talus experiencing an anterior positional fault (the talus is drawn forwards in a plantarflexion–inversion injury), which is the opposite to the posterior gliding that occurs at the talocrural joint during dorsiflexion (Denegar et al., 2002). The limited dorsiflexion is usually pain-free and more likely to be stiff/restricted and interfering with such activities as walking down stairs or a slope. A useful technique to improve dorsiflexion is the MWM that employs a relative posterior glide of the talus on the distal leg, in non-weight-bearing dorsiflexion in the early acute stage post-injury and then progressing to weight-bearing dorsiflexion. If there is pain within the joint on dorsiflexion, especially on weight-bearing, the clinician must entertain a high degree of suspicion of the likelihood of a talar dome fracture. This is particularly the case if an MWM cannot be applied in a painless manner.

For some time a number of systems of manual therapy have proposed minor subluxations or positional faults of the ankle joints/bones. Mulligan suggested that when the ankle underwent a plantarflexion–inversion sprain, the anterior talofibular ligament did not rupture but rather it exerted an anterior and caudad force on the fibula (via its attachment thereon) and created a positional fault in that direction (Mulligan, 2010). The fibula was then a more appropriate place to manipulate than the talus and he reported great clinical success with applying a posterior and cephalad glide manually while asking the patient to then repeat a previously symptomatic movement or task (e.g. inversion, plantarflexion or dorsiflexion). Evidence has since emerged showing that in some patients with chronic ankle instability and subacute ankle sprains there is indeed an anteriorly positioned fibula (Hubbard & Hertel, 2008; Hubbard et al., 2006). Minor positional faults probably also occur at other foot joints. For example, a positional fault that has been reported a number of times is the cuboid subluxation syndrome (Matthews & Claus, 2014; Mooney & Maffey-Ward, 1994; Patterson, 2006). It is commonly recommended that a high-velocity low-amplitude thrust is employed to treat this subluxation, but there is no evidence pertaining to its clinical efficacy and some patients might perceive the use of high-velocity thrusts as being too aggressive. MWM offers a gentler way of manually gliding a joint without pain or patient apprehension and, while sustaining that glide, testing the effectiveness of the technique by repeating a previously symptomatic motion (e.g. for a plantar subluxed cuboid, glide it dorsally and then perform the inversion or eversion motion that was previously painful).

13

A clinical utility feature of MWM is that the technique is painless and restores previously limited motion immediately. A positive response to an MWM in this instance helps to confirm the diagnosis and simultaneously directs treatment plans. A failure to improve range and relieve pain (negative response) provides clear indication to stop applying the MWM. This approach could be used at other intertarsal joints.

Structural and functional instabilities are common following injuries of the ankle and foot. Although not a strict contraindication for MWM, structural instabilities require the clinician to apply gentle manual forces to position the joint in its neutral position and to make sure that movements are not excessive. The direction of the applied glide must not be in the direction of the instability and in most cases will be directly opposite the direction of the instability. Most importantly the MWM must not produce apprehension or feelings of giving way or instability either when applied or afterwards.

Apart from managing the sequelae of ankle and foot injuries, MWMs are useful in managing painful limitations of motion in arthritic joints. For example, the great toe is commonly a source of foot pain (Thomas et al., 2011) and is associated with osteoarthritis and hallux valgus deformity. In these cases, first metatarsophalangeal (MTP) extension is often painful during weight-bearing activities, usually in the form of an impingement like pain in the dorsal side of the joint. Applying a transverse glide or rotation prior to performing the extension can provide a substantial amount of relief of this great toe pain.

Levels of evidence

Level 2: six RCTs, three case series, two case reports

Talus posterior glide with dorsiflexion

There is level 2 evidence that an ankle MWM (talus posterior glide with dorsiflexion) produces immediate improvements in dorsiflexion in patients with subacute lateral ankle inversion sprain (standardised mean difference (SMD) 1.18; 95% CI 0.55–1.81) (Bisset et al., 2011). These findings were similar to the effects of the same weight-bearing and non-weight-bearing MWMs in a population of subacute (Collins et al., 2004) and recurrent ankle sprains (Vicenzino et al., 2006). In agreement, a study by Marron-Gomez and colleagues (Marron-Gomez et al., 2015) compared two manual therapy techniques (MWM and high-velocity thrust) and demonstrated an increase in dorsiflexion ROM. Interestingly, Hidalgo and colleagues (Hidalgo et al., 2018) compared the effectiveness of one session of either MWM or osteopathic mobilisation on ankle dorsiflexion ROM and musculoarticular stiffness (MAS) in participants with chronic ankle dorsiflexion rigidity. This group found no significant improvement in ROM or MAS between the two groups. Similarly, Gilbreath and colleagues (Gilbreath et al., 2014), in a within-subjects repeated-measures design, found no significant changes in weight-bearing dorsiflexion ROM or star excursion balance test reach distances after three treatments of MWM in patients with chronic ankle instability. The diverse results presented here clearly indicate the need for further investigation.

Four randomised controlled trials analysed the efficacy of talocrural MWM in ankle ROM and gait parameters in stroke patients (An & Jo, 2017; An & Won, 2016; Kim & Lee, 2016, 2018). The combination of conventional physiotherapy and posterior talar glide and dorsiflexion of the ankle (10(5) daily for 4 weeks) caused greater improvement in weight-bearing lunge test, static balance measures, timed up-and-go and dynamic index than was observed in the control group, which were treated only with conventional physiotherapy and sham MWM (Kim & Lee, 2018). Using the same technique and dosage, Kim and Lee (2016) highlighted the benefits of the inclusion of MWM in a conventional physiotherapy programme in increasing gait functions (i.e. velocity, cadence and single-support time of the affected side) in stroke patients compared with a combined treatment of conventional physiotherapy and exercise (e.g. lunges). Similarly, An and Won (2016) reiterated the superior effects of MWM in improving ROM (passive and active) and gait velocity in stroke patients compared with weight-bearing exercises or traditional physiotherapy.

A repeated-measures case series trial of a set of three treatment sessions with talus posterior glide with dorsiflexion in a cohort of 11 participants with chronic ankle instability (mean number of ankle sprains 3.3, mean number of giving-way episodes in previous 3 months 2.5) did not show any meaningful change in ankle dorsiflexion range or star excursion balance test, but did show a significant moderate to strong effect in the sport subscale of the Foot and Ankle Ability Measure (Gilbreath et al., 2014). This study is level 4 evidence. The finding of self-rated sports performance contrasting with the lack of range and balance effects hints at the likely complex underlying mechanisms of action of MWM. Importantly, a notable difference between this study and the

13

aforementioned two studies is the recurrent ankle sprains and giving way. This study also did not recruit those with limited dorsiflexion on the affected side and so the application of the MWM for dorsiflexion might not have been clinically appropriate. The matter of applying techniques appropriate to the presenting patient's problem is a critical factor in determining outcomes.

Posterocephalad fibula glide

There is some low-level (level 4) evidence of the clinical efficacy of treating both acute and long-term problematic ankle sprains with the posterocephalad fibula glide applied manually, with tape, or both (Hetherington, 1996; O'Brien & Vicenzino, 1998). There are mixed data on the effect of posterocephalad fibula glide tape on balance, with a case series of eight recently sprained ankles showing some beneficial effects (Merlin et al., 2005) but another evaluating 20 patients with chronic ankle instability reporting none (Hopper et al., 2009).

Possibly the most promising and relatively higher-quality evidence (level 3) comes from a pilot study of the injury prevention efficacy of this taping technique. In this study, Moiler and colleagues (Moiler et al., 2006) found only two sprains of a total 11 ankle sprains over the census period occurred in the group allocated to the fibula-taping technique ($n = 125$ basketball players, 433 exposures (224 taped, 209 control), number needed to treat (NNT) 22; 95% CI: 12–312).

TALOCRURAL JOINT

Anteroposterior glide for ankle dorsiflexion in non-weight-bearing

TECHNIQUE AT A GLANCE

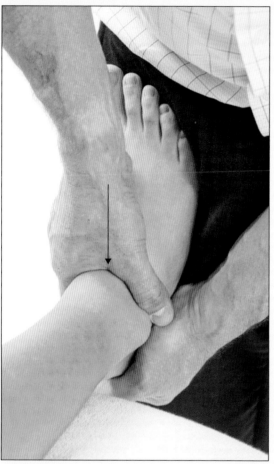

Figure 13.1
Talocrural anteroposterior glide MWM for ankle dorsiflexion: close view hand position

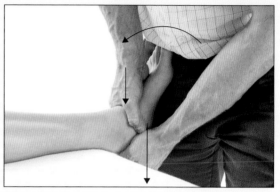

Figure 13.2
Talocrural anteroposterior glide MWM for ankle dorsiflexion: start position

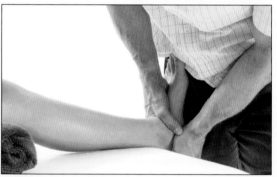

Figure 13.3
Talocrural anteroposterior glide MWM for ankle dorsiflexion: end position

- The patient lies supine with the ankle just over the edge of the treatment table.
- The distal lower leg is supported and the knee slightly bent on a rolled towel.
- One of the therapist's hands holds the calcaneus, while the web-space of the other hand contacts the ventral talus. Both hands contribute to the anteroposterior glide of the talus.
- While maintaining the anteroposterior glide, the patient can perform active dorsiflexion or the therapist can initiate passive dorsiflexion of the ankle.
- See Figs 13.1–13.3.

13

INDICATION

Ankle pain and limitation of ankle dorsiflexion in non-weight-bearing.

POSITIONING

Patient:	The patient lies supine with the foot just over the edge of the plinth.
Treated body part:	Knee slightly flexed, ankle joint close to the limitation of movement or pain onset.
Therapist:	Facing the patient at the end of the treatment table.
Hands/contact points:	One hand grasps the posterior aspect of the calcaneus and the web-space of the other is around the anterior aspect of the talus. The therapist's thigh supports the patient's foot.

APPLICATION GUIDELINES

- Flex the knee slightly to reduce gastrocnemius tension.
- Apply the anteroposterior glide on the talus by pulling the calcaneum towards the floor while applying the anteroposterior pressure on the talus.
- After taking up the slack in the joint, either ask the patient to actively dorsiflex their foot with the assistance of the therapist's pressure from their thigh or the therapist can perform passive dorsiflexion.
- When a new pain-free range is achieved, ask the patient to relax; then the therapist takes up more slack in the joint through the previously described mobilisation.
- This routine is repeated until no more progression can be achieved.
- The number of repetitions will vary upon the progress made, but is typically 6 repetitions in a set, with 3–5 sets per session.
- Additional over-pressure can be given by the patient pulling on a belt wrapped around the foot.

COMMENTS

- Make sure that hand positioning is comfortable, with a broad contact area through the web-space.
- Key to this technique is to avoid squeezing the tendons over the dorsal side of the ankle.
- Use sponge rubber to soften the contact point on the talus.
- If the lower leg moves during the mobilisation, a manual therapy belt can be used to strap the leg to the bed.

13

(continued next page...)

SELF-MANAGEMENT AND TAPING

- Self-management can be achieved with the aid of strapping tape (Fig. 13.4).
- Apply a 1-cm-wide strip of non-stretch sports tape from around the talus to the posterior inferior corner of the calcaneum in a continuous loop.
- Apply two layers for additional strength. Ensure the tape is applied in non-weight-bearing with the ankle in neutral plantar grade position.
- The patient then stands up and performs 5 sets of 10 repetitions of a lunging exercise to increase the range of dorsiflexion, keeping the heel on the floor. Ensure that the tape is removed after completion of the exercise.

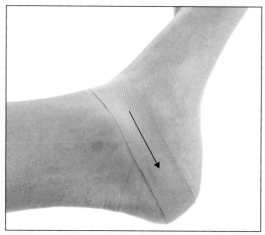

Figure 13.4A
Taping to improve ankle dorsiflexion: application

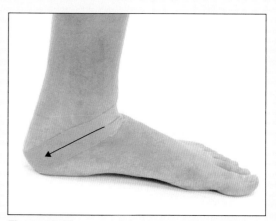

Figure 13.4B
Taping to improve ankle dorsiflexion: in standing

ANNOTATIONS

sup ly R Talus Post gl MWM DF×6
sup ly R Talus Post gl MWM DF +OP(belt)×6
st R Talus tape Post gl MWM Lunge×10(5)

Ankle dorsiflexion MWM in weight-bearing

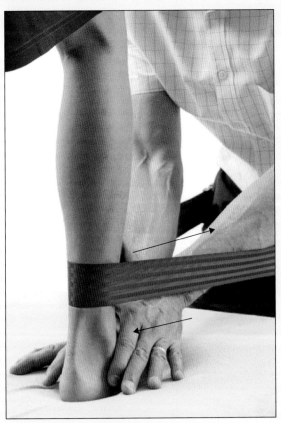

Figure 13.5
Ankle dorsiflexion MWM with belt in weight-bearing: close view hand position

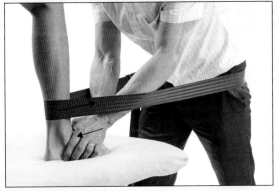

Figure 13.6
Ankle dorsiflexion MWM with belt in weight-bearing: start position

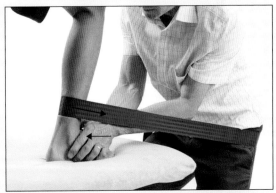

Figure 13.7
Ankle dorsiflexion MWM with belt in weight-bearing: end position

- The patient is standing or kneeling with one foot forwards on a treatment table.
- The treatment belt is looped around the patient's distal lower leg, at a right angle to the lower leg, and around the therapist's hips.
- The therapist fixates the talus and fibula with the web-space of both hands so as to prevent movement of the talus and fibula anteriorly.
- The therapist glides the tibia and fibula anteriorly with the treatment belt. The patient lunges forwards to gain dorsiflexion range.
- See Figs 13.5–13.7.

13

INDICATION

Pain and limitation of range of motion during weight-bearing ankle dorsiflexion.

POSITIONING

Patient:	Step standing or kneeling with involved leg forwards, close to the end of the treatment table.
Treated body part:	Close to the limitation of ankle dorsiflexion.
Therapist:	Facing the patient, in step standing, with knees slightly flexed.
Hands/contact points:	Belt around the hips of the therapist and immediately above the ankle of the patient. The web-spaces of the therapist's hands stabilise the talus and fibula anteriorly.

APPLICATION GUIDELINES

- Provide a support for the patient to lean on to increase stability.
- The therapist glides the tibia and fibula anteriorly with the belt while stabilising the talus with both hands anteriorly.
- Concurrently the patient lunges forwards, to gain pain-free dorsiflexion range.
- Maintain the gliding force through the belt during the movement and ensure that the force is parallel to the treatment plane, which is perpendicular to the lower leg.
- The patient repeatedly moves into dorsiflexion and back to neutral, while the therapist maintains the glide.
- The number of repetitions will vary upon the progress made, but is typically 6 repetitions in a set, with 3–5 sets per session.

COMMENTS

- If an improved range cannot be achieved, try small alterations in the glide direction and/or glide force (e.g. more medial or lateral, or with the knee medially or laterally rotated).
- Note the need for the belt angle to stay in contact with the back of the Achilles tendon. For comfort a foam or towel pad in between the belt and the skin is often required.

13

- One option prior to standing on a table or plinth is to be in a half-kneeling position or alternatively to be in standing with one leg up on a chair (Fig. 13.8).

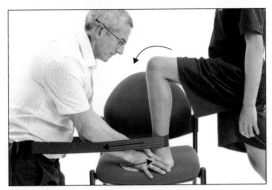

Figure 13.8A
Ankle dorsiflexion MWM in step standing on a chair: start position

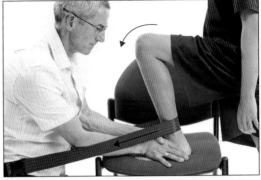

Figure 13.8B
Ankle dorsiflexion MWM in step standing on a chair: end position

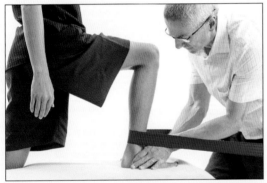

Figure 13.8C
Ankle dorsiflexion MWM in half-kneeling position

SELF-MANAGEMENT AND TAPING

- The patient can replicate this technique as a home exercise using the taping procedure shown in Fig. 13.4.

ANNOTATIONS

R step st on bed R Tib/Fib belt Ant gl MWM DF×10(3)
st R foot on chair R Tib/Fib belt Ant gl MWM Lunge×10(5)
R 1/2 kneel on bed R Tib/Fib belt Ant gl MWM DF×6(3)

13

Plantarflexion MWM in non-weight-bearing

TECHNIQUE AT A GLANCE

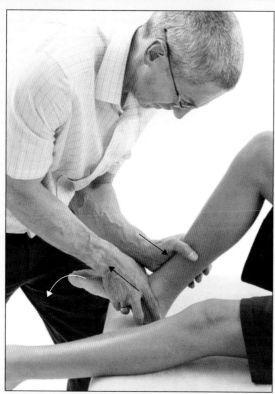

Figure 13.9
Plantarflexion MWM in non-weight-bearing:
positioning of therapist and patient

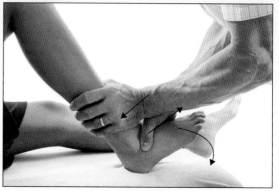

Figure 13.10
Glide of the tibia and fibula – locking ankle into
plantarflexion MWM in non-weight-bearing: start
position

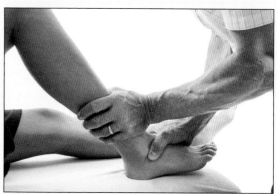

Figure 13.11
Glide and roll of talus forwards with tibia and fibula
locked in plantarflexion MWM in non-weight-bearing:
end position

- The patient lies supine with the knee flexed to 90°, the ankle in neutral plantar grade and the heel on the end of the treatment table.
- The therapist contacts the fibula and tibia distally, applying a posterior force with the ulnar side of the hand.
- The therapist pulls the talus anteriorly and inferiorly with the web-space of the other hand.
- See Figs 13.9–13.11.

13

INDICATION

Pain and limitation of ankle plantarflexion.

POSITIONING

Patient:	Lying supine with the knee flexed to 90° and the heel positioned at the end of the treatment table.
Treated body part:	Ankle in neutral plantar grade.
Therapist:	Standing facing the patient, at the end of the treatment table.
Hands/contact points:	The therapist's stabilising hand contacts the patient's leg (opposite) being treated: the entire palm of the hand should be just proximal to the ankle, over the tibia and fibula, fingers around the leg. The elbow of this hand locks into the therapist's pelvis. Mobilising (talus) contact: web-space grasps around the talus, inferior to the malleoli.

APPLICATION GUIDELINES

- Position the entire palm of the stabilising hand to the ankle being treated over the tibia and fibula, just proximal to the ankle, fingers around the leg, to glide the tibia and fibula posteriorly.
- With the therapist's elbow locked into their pelvis, their body weight can be used to apply the stabilising posterior glide. This effectively locks the ankle so no active talocrural plantarflexion is possible.
- The therapist uses the first web-space of the mobilising hand to grasp the talus and pull it anteriorly. The thumb and fingers should be immediately distal to the malleoli.
- It may be necessary to place more emphasis on the tibia or fibula to achieve more success.
- Without releasing the stabilisation of the lower leg, roll the talus anteriorly and inferiorly to plantarflex the ankle.
- Subtle direction alterations may be useful.
- The number of repetitions will vary upon the progress made, but is typically 6 repetitions in a set, with 3–5 sets per session.

COMMENTS

- It is important that the therapist applies a maximum posterior glide of the tibia and fibula. If slack is successfully taken up, no talocrural plantarflexion will be possible.
- The therapist should avoid using finger flexion to hold the talus and mobilise it as this can create discomfort to the patient. The therapist should use a lumbrical grip to grasp the talus.
- Make sure that hand positioning is comfortable, with a broad contact area through the web-space. Avoid squeezing the tendons over the dorsal side of the ankle. One can use sponge rubber to soften the contact point on the talus, if modifying the hand position at first does not improve comfort.
- Avoid applying pressure with the ulnar side of the mobilising hand on the anterior part of the foot.
- Ensure that the opposite hand to the ankle being treated is used to glide the tibia and fibula (e.g. the therapist's right hand will stabilise the patient's left tibia and fibula). If the wrong hand is used to stabilise, the contact will be only on the tibia.
- This technique is contraindicated in cases that have positive anterior drawer signs of the talocrural joint, which is not uncommon following plantarflexion–inversion ankle sprains.

ANNOTATION

long sit R Talus Ant gl-roll MWM PF×6(3)

INFERIOR TIBIOFIBULAR JOINT – ANKLE SPRAIN

Fibula posterior glide MWM for dorsiflexion / plantarflexion–inversion in non-weight-bearing

TECHNIQUE AT A GLANCE

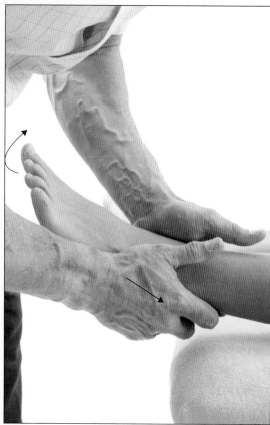

Figure 13.12
Distal fibula posterosuperior glide MWM in non-weight-bearing: start position close view hand position

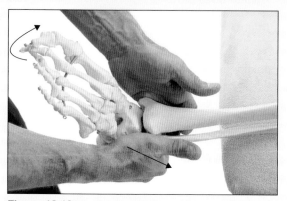

Figure 13.13
Distal fibula posterosuperior glide MWM in non-weight-bearing: model view

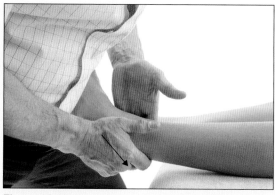

Figure 13.14
Distal fibula posterosuperior glide MWM in non-weight-bearing: plantarflexion–inversion with over-pressure

- The patient lies supine with their foot and ankle off the end of the treatment table.
- A combined posterosuperior glide is applied to the distal end of the fibula.
- The patient moves actively into dorsiflexion or plantarflexion–inversion.
- Over-pressure is applied at the end of range if symptom-free, either by the therapist or by way of a belt.
- See Figs 13.12–13.14.

13

INDICATION

Lateral ankle pain post ankle sprain or limitation in dorsiflexion, plantarflexion or inversion

POSITIONING

Patient/treated body part:	The patient lies supine with affected foot and ankle off the distal edge of the treatment table (see Fig. 13.12).
Therapist:	The therapist stands at the foot end of the treatment table leaning over the patient's foot.
Hands/contact points:	One hand stabilises the patient's tibia posteriorly and medially, while the thenar eminence of the other hand is in contact with the anterior inferior aspect of the lateral malleolus (see Fig. 13.12).

APPLICATION GUIDELINES

- The therapist stabilises the tibia with one hand around the medial malleolus and Achilles tendon.
- The gliding hand moves the fibula posterosuperiorly through a lumbrical action of the first metacarpal and ulnar deviation at the wrist.
- Sponge rubber can be used to maximise comfort.
- While maintaining the fibula glide, move the ankle into the previously restricted or painful direction.
- If full pain-free range can be achieved, apply over-pressure through the therapist's abdomen (Fig. 13.14) or hip, or with the aid of a belt held by the patient (see Fig. 13.15).
- Apply 6–10 repetitions in a set, with 3–5 sets in a treatment session, but only if ROM is pain-free while applying the glide and no latent pain responses occur.
- Return to neutral position before removing the glide force.

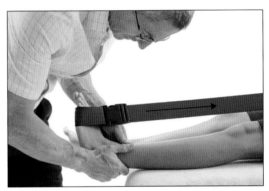

Figure 13.15
Distal fibula posterosuperior glide MWM for dorsiflexion in non-weight-bearing with a belt

COMMENTS

- Ensure that when applying the fibula glide there should be a noticeable movement of the patient's foot into eversion/pronation. If this does not occur the glide is usually being applied in the wrong way or with the wrong hand contact position.
- If pain is not eliminated, adjust by altering the fibula glide direction.
- As the area is usually sensitive to touch, the use of sponge rubber is recommended.
- It is most important to make direct bone contact with the fibula to avoid sensitive soft tissue.
- It is important to distinguish between contact soreness and pain elicited by movement. The latter is important to monitor in terms of the movement being performed (i.e. dorsiflexion, plantarflexion, inversion), but both are important in terms of the overall technique's application.
- This technique should be trialled for any patient presenting following an inversion ankle sprain. If it is found to be ineffective, explore other MWMs to exclude involvement of other possible structures such as the talocrural joint, the calcaneocuboid joint and joints around the base of the fifth metatarsal.
- In the acute phase, combine this MWM with routine management for an acute soft tissue injury and the ankle taping method, which is described next.
- Patients referred with recurrent ankle sprain often benefit from this treatment combined with taping, prior to exercise.
- In patients presenting with functional instability and pain (i.e. not structurally unstable but reporting weakness and giving way), usually of a long-standing nature and recalcitrant to rehabilitation, this manoeuvre seems to be clinically effective in reducing giving way and perception of weakness and lack of confidence in using the ankle, particularly when combined with taping.

(continued next page...)

13

- If the fibula is very sensitive to touch even with sponge rubber, it is possible to apply the glide through a more proximal location.

Fibula posterior MWM for dorsiflexion in weight-bearing

- Progress the technique from non-weight-bearing to partial weight-bearing (foot on a chair; Fig. 13.16A) followed by full weight-bearing (see Fig. 13.16B).
- The patient is step standing with one foot on a chair or standing on a plinth.
- The therapist fixates the tibia with one hand posteriorly and cups the distal end of the fibula (lateral malleolus) with the pisiform/bulk of the hand (making sure not to block the movement of the other hand).
- The therapist glides the fibula in a posterosuperior direction while the patient leans/lunges forwards into dorsiflexion making sure not to overbalance forwards and to maintain equal weight over both feet.
- See Fig. 13.16.

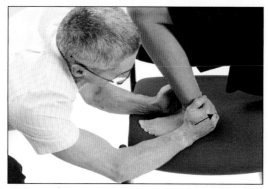

Figure 13.16A
Distal fibula posterior glide MWM: partial weight-bearing end range

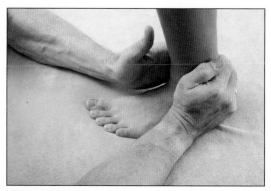

Figure 13.16B
Distal fibula posterior glide MWM: full weight-bearing

Anterior glide of fibula

- If posterior repositioning of the fibula increases pain or if the patient describes the opposite injury mechanism (e.g. eversion sprain) then an anterior fibula glide could be attempted (see Fig. 13.17).

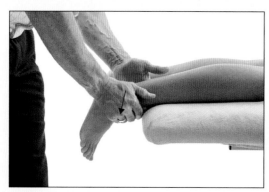

Figure 13.17A
Distal fibula anterior glide MWM for dorsiflexion in non-weight-bearing: start position

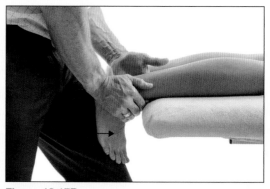

Figure 13.17B
Distal fibula anterior glide MWM for dorsiflexion in non-weight-bearing: end position with over-pressure

13

TAPING

- If sensitivity of the distal fibula will not allow the technique to be applied in a pain-free manner, and trialling a more proximal glide is not effective, then taping the fibula may be more comfortable and achieve a significant improvement in the patient's pain and movement.
- The patient lies supine with their foot supported in neutral ankle position against the therapist's body.
- Use 30–50-mm non-stretch sports tape, depending on the size of the ankle, and apply 5 cm of tape starting 2 cm anterior to the fibula and 1 cm proximally to the tip of the lateral malleolus.
- Start distally with the tape applied to the anterior aspect of the fibula. While applying the fibula glide, spiral the tape obliquely around the lower leg to end the tape on the anterior aspect of the shin (Fig. 13.18).
- Wrinkles in the skin are largely unavoidable, and some think they are important, but in any case minimise them at points of increased tape tension on the skin and over areas of potential compression compromise of underlying tissues and bone (especially over the Achilles tendon).
- Apply two layers of tape in the same location, with equal tension on both layers for maximum effect. To allow circulation to the foot, ensure that there is a gap between the start and end point of the tape.

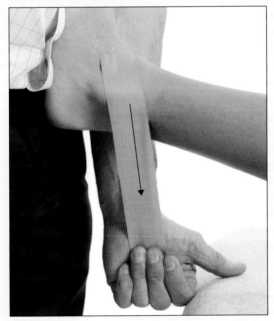

Figure 13.18A
Posterior fibula glide taping technique: start point and direction of the tape

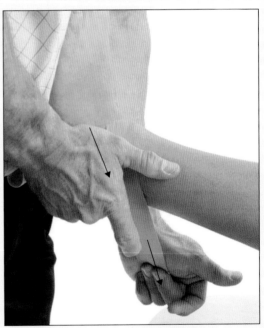

Figure 13.18B
Posterior fibula glide taping technique: spiral application

(continued next page...)

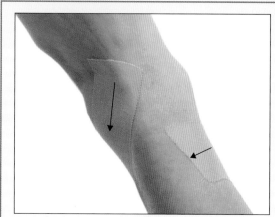

Figure 13.18C
Posterior fibula glide taping technique: completed taping

ANNOTATIONS

long sit L Inf Fib Post-sup gl MWM Inv×6
long sit L Inf Fib Post-sup gl MWM DF +OP(belt)×10(3)
st L Foot on chair L Inf Fib Post-sup gl MWM DF×6(3)
pr R Inf Fib Ant gl MWM DF +OP(therapist)×6
L Inf Fib Post-sup gl tape

13

MID-TARSAL

Medial – cuneiform on navicular

MWM dorsal/plantar glide medial cuneiform on navicular

TECHNIQUE AT A GLANCE

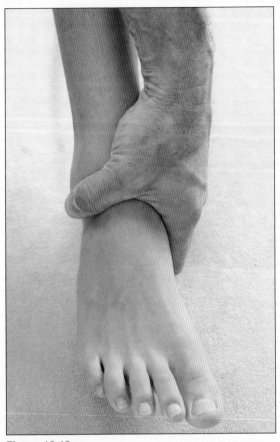

Figure 13.19
Medial cuneiform on navicular MWM: proximal hand

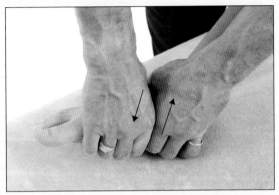

Figure 13.20
Medial cuneiform on navicular MWM: plantar and dorsal glide

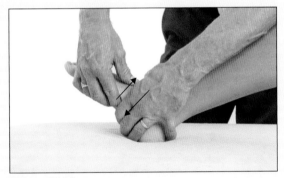

Figure 13.21
Medial cuneiform on navicular MWM: alternative hand placement

- The patient lies supine with the knee extended and foot in neutral position.
- The therapist stabilises the navicular with their proximal hand.
- The therapist glides the cuneiform in a dorsal or plantar direction with the distal hand.
- The pain-free glide is sustained while the patient performs inversion or eversion.
- See Figs 13.19–13.21.

13

INDICATION

Medial foot pain during mid-foot movement (typically inversion or eversion).

POSITIONING

Patient:	Lying supine with leg straight.
Treated body part:	Relaxed neutral foot position.
Therapist:	Standing next to the affected foot.
Hands/contact points:	Stabilising hand: see Fig. 13.19. The entire palm of the proximal hand is used with a focus through the first web-space placed on the navicular tubercle. The index finger is on the plantar aspect of the navicular and the thumb on its dorsal aspect.
	Gliding hand: see Fig. 13.20. The entire palm of the distal hand is used, with a focus through the first web-space placed on the cuneiform and the index finger on its plantar aspect. An alternative is to use the thumb (see Fig. 13.21) on the dorsal side of cuneiform, and the index finger on its plantar side.

APPLICATION GUIDELINES

- Apply a dorsal or plantar glide across the cuneonavicular joint.
- Ensure that both hands are as close as possible, but still have the joint line between them.
- While sustaining the dorsal or ventral glide have the patient repeat the activity that provoked the symptoms.
- If pain is not completely relieved, slightly alter the direction of the glide or the amount of force.
- Apply 6–10 repetitions in a set, with 3–5 sets in a treatment session.

COMMENTS

- Ensure that both hands are as close as possible to have the joint line between them.
- On a weight-bearing position, the patient's position will change from supine to standing. Make sure, before weight-bearing, to have the dorsal glide applied (the hand hold would need to be modified to accommodate weight-bearing).

13

TAPING

- Tape can be applied for both the dorsal and ventral glide techniques (Fig. 13.22A, B). The first tape starts at dorsal aspect of navicular, applied across the plantar fascia, ending on plantar aspect of the foot (Fig. 13.22A).

- The second tape starts at the plantar aspect of the mid foot, adjacent to the medial cuneiform, applied around medial aspect of the mid foot, ending on the dorsal aspect (Fig. 13.22B).

- Reverse the tape procedure for a dorsal glide (Fig. 13.22C).

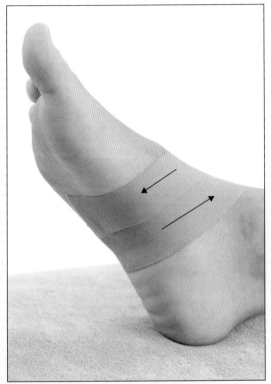

Figure 13.22A
Taping the cuneiform on the navicular

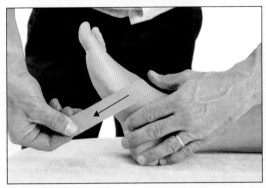

Figure 13.22B
Taping the cuneiform down on the navicular: plantar

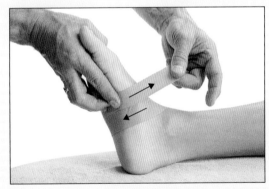

Figure 13.22C
Taping the cuneiform up on the navicular: dorsal

ANNOTATIONS

sup ly R Med Cuneiform on Navicular Plantar gl MWM Inv×3
sup ly R Med Cuneiform on Navicular Dorsal gl MWM Inv×6(3)
sup ly R Med Cuneiform on Navicular Dorsal MWM Inv +OP(belt)×6(3)
sup ly R Med Cuneiform on Navicular Dorsal gl MWM Ev×3
R Med Cuneiform on Navicular Plantar gl tape
R Med Cuneiform on Navicular Dorsal gl tape
R Med Cuneiform Dorsal gl / Navicular Plantar gl tape
R Med Cuneiform Plantar gl / Navicular Dorsal gl tape

13

Lateral – fifth metatarsal on cuboid

MWM dorsal/ventral glide fifth metatarsal on cuboid

TECHNIQUE AT A GLANCE

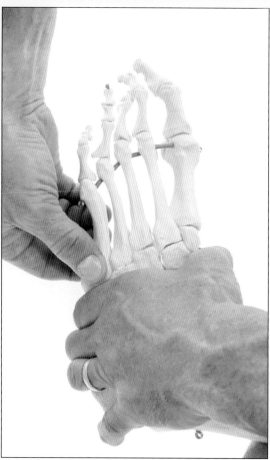

Figure 13.23
Fifth metatarsal on cuboid MWM: model view

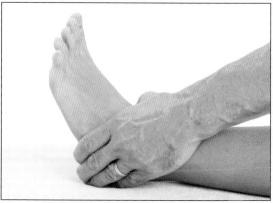

Figure 13.24
Fifth metatarsal on cuboid MWM: proximal fixation

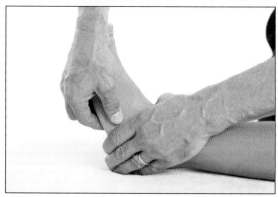

Figure 13.25
Fifth metatarsal on cuboid MWM: hand position

- The patient is in long sitting with the knee extended and foot in relaxed neutral position.
- The therapist stabilises the cuboid with their proximal hand.
- The therapist glides the fifth metatarsal in a dorsal or plantar direction with the distal hand.
- While sustaining the glide, the patient performs mid-foot inversion or eversion.
- See Figs 13.23–13.25.

13

INDICATION

Lateral foot pain during inversion or eversion.

POSITIONING

Patient:	Long sitting with leg straight.
Treated body part:	Relaxed neutral foot position.
Therapist:	Standing on the medial side of the involved foot.
Hands/contact points:	Stabilising hand: the entire palm of the proximal hand, with a focus through the first web-space placed on the dorsal aspect of the foot, the thumb over the navicular tubercule, and the index finger on the plantar aspect of the cuboid (see Fig. 13.24).
	Gliding hand: thumb on dorsal aspect of fifth metatarsal and index finger on ventral aspect of fifth metatarsal (see Fig. 13.25).

APPLICATION GUIDELINES

- The therapist stabilises the cuboid with the proximal hand while the distal hand applies a dorsal or plantar directed glide across the fifth metatarsocuboid joint.
- While sustaining the glide force, have the patient repeat the activity that provoked symptoms. Subtle changes in the glide direction and glide force may be required to render the technique pain-free.
- Apply 6–10 repetitions in a set, with 3–5 sets in a treatment session.
- Ensure that the distance between the stabilisation hand and mobilisation hand is as small as possible and that the therapist's contact does not cross the joint line.

VARIATION

- Try medial or lateral rotation of the fifth metatarsal on the cuboid if pain-free movement cannot be achieved.

13

(continued next page...)

TAPING

- The glide described can then be taped by two complementary pieces of tape that maintain the direction of the inverse glide applied (Fig. 13.26A).

Plantar glide of the fifth metatarsal on the cuboid

- First tape: proximal, on cuboid, start at either the plantar or the dorsal aspect of the cuboid, go around the lateral aspect of the foot and end on the respective aspect of the foot (Fig. 13.26A).

- Second tape: distal, on fifth metatarsal, would inversely either start at the dorsal aspect of fifth metatarsal and either go around lateral aspect of the mid foot, ending on the plantar aspect of the foot (Fig. 13.26B), or start at the plantar aspect of the fifth metatarsal and go around the lateral aspect of the mid foot to end on the dorsal aspect of the foot (Fig. 13.26C).

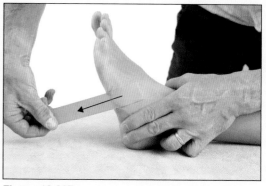

Figure 13.26B
Taping the fifth metatarsal down on the cuboid: plantar

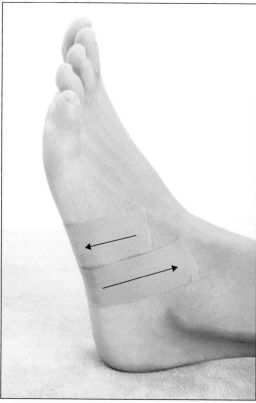

Figure 13.26A
Taping the cuboid on the fifth metatarsal: complete

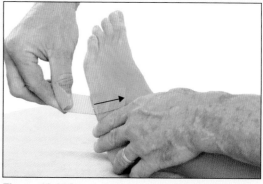

Figure 13.26C
Taping the fifth metatarsal up on the cuboid: dorsal

ANNOTATIONS

long sit R 5th MT on Cuboid Dorsal gl MWM Inv×3
long sit R 5th MT on Cuboid Ventral gl MWM Inv +OP(belt)×6(3)
long sit R 5th MT on Cuboid Dorsal gl MWM Ev×10
long sit R 5th MT on Cuboid Ventral gl MWM Ev +OP(belt)×10(3)
R 5th MT on Cuboid Ventral gl tape
R 5th MT on Cuboid Dorsal gl tape
R 5th MT Plantar gl/Cuboid Dorsal gl tape
R 5th MT Dorsal gl/Cuboid Ventral gl tape

FIRST METATARSOPHALANGEAL JOINT

Lateral glide for flexion and extension

TECHNIQUE AT A GLANCE

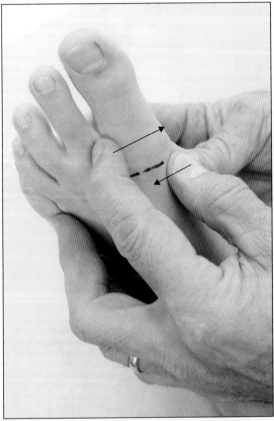

Figure 13.27
First metatarsophalangeal joint lateral glide: overview

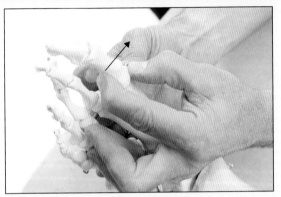

Figure 13.28
First metatarsophalangeal joint lateral glide: model view

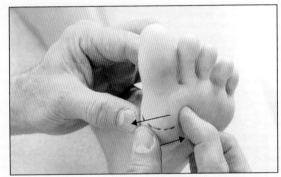

Figure 13.29
First metatarsophalangeal joint lateral glide: great toe extension

- The patient lies supine with their lower limb relaxed.
- The therapist stabilises the distal aspect of the first metatarsal with both thumbs on the medial side, and the index fingers on the proximal aspect of the base of the first phalanx laterally.
- The therapist glides the proximal phalanx laterally.
- While the therapist sustains the glide, the patient actively extends the great toe.
- Apply over-pressure if pain-free.
- See Figs 13.27–13.29.

NB The lateral glide is named from the classical anatomical start position.

13

INDICATION

First metatarsophalangeal joint pain with extension or flexion.

POSITIONING

Patient:	Supine with knee extended and foot in neutral position.
Treated body part:	Neutral metatarsophalangeal joint position.
Therapist:	Standing on the medial side of the affected foot.
Hands/contact points:	Both thumbs contact the lateral aspect of the apex of the first metatarsal. The radial edge of the distal phalanx of each index finger is placed on the proximal aspect of the phalanx medially (see Fig. 13.27).

APPLICATION GUIDELINES

- Glide the proximal phalanx laterally and ask the patient to extend (or flex) the great toe as per their limitation. If painless, apply over-pressure at the end range.

COMMENTS

- The first metatarsophalangeal joint line is more proximal than the first web-space. Ensure that the thumbs and fingers are immediately adjacent to the joint line and that they do not block joint translations.
- Taping may be used if the technique is successful (see taping technique shown in Fig. 13.32).

VARIATIONS

First metatarsophalangeal joint rotation MWM

- A **rotation MWM** can also be applied to the joint as an alternative to a lateral glide.
- The therapist stabilises the first metatarsal with one hand while rotating the proximal phalanx with the other hand using the thumb and the index finger (Fig. 13.30A).
- The therapist sustains the rotation while the patient actively moves their metatarsophalangeal joint into extension (Fig. 13.30B) or flexion (Fig. 13.30C).
- If one direction of rotation is not successful, try the opposite rotation.

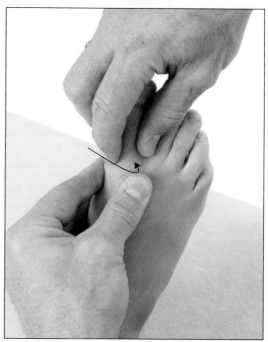

Figure 13.30A
First MTP internal rotation MWM: start point

13

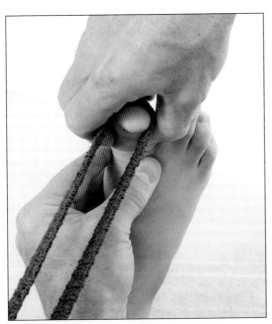

Figure 13.30B
MTP internal rotation MWM for extension with
over-pressure

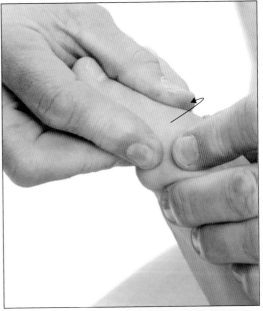

Figure 13.30C
MTP internal rotation MWM with active flexion

Lateral glide MWM extension in weight-bearing

- A lateral glide may need to be progressed into a weight-bearing position (see Fig. 13.31).
- The patient stands on a treatment table with their affected foot forwards.
- The therapist stabilises the distal first metatarsal with a treatment belt, and both thumbs contact the proximal phalanx (Fig. 13.31B)
- The therapist then glides the proximal phalanx laterally with the thumbs.
- The therapist sustains the glide while the patient extends their great toe, raising their heel to increase the ROM (Figs 13.31C).
- Alternatively the therapist can glide the proximal phalanx with one thumb, while holding the patient's heel to guide and stabilise the movement.

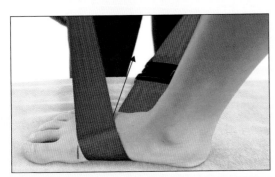

Figure 13.31A
First MTP lateral glide MWM in weight-bearing with
extension: belt fixation

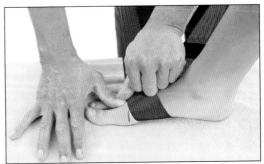

Figure 13.31B
First MTP lateral glide MWM in weight-bearing with
extension: start position

(continued next page...)

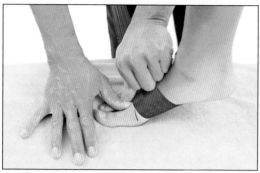

Figure 13.31C
First MTP lateral glide MWM in weight-bearing with extension: end position

TAPING

- The tape is commenced dorsally anchoring it over second metatarsal.
- The tape is spiralled in a lateral distal direction across the proximal lateral aspect of the first phalanx and wrapped around the toe pulling the tape proximally.
- The tape ends at the ventral aspect of the distal first metatarsal.
- Anchoring may be required to hold the tape in place (see Fig. 13.32).

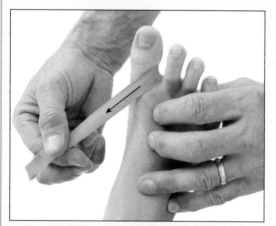

Figure 13.32A
Taping the first metatarsophalangeal joint after MWM: first tape

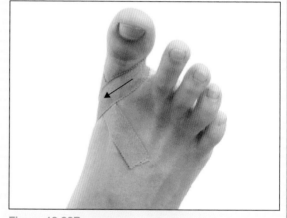

Figure 13.32B
Taping the first metatarsophalangeal joint after MWM: tape completed

ANNOTATIONS

long sit L 1st MTP Lat gl MWM E×6
long sit R 1st MTP IR MWM E +OP(strap)×6(3)
long sit R 1st MTP ER MWM E×10(3)
st R 1st MTP Lat gl MWM E×6(3)
R 1st MTP Lat gl/ER tape

13

References

An, C.M., Jo, S.O., 2017. Effects of talocrural mobilization with movement on ankle strength, mobility, and weight-bearing ability in hemiplegic patients with chronic stroke: a randomized controlled trial. J. Stroke Cerebrovasc. Dis. 26 (1), 169–176.

An, C.M., Won, J., 2016. Effects of ankle joint mobilization with movement and weight-bearing exercise on knee strength, ankle range of motion, and gait velocity in patients with stroke: a pilot study. J. Phys. Ther. Sci. 28 (2), 689–694.

Bisset, L., Hing, W., Vicenzino, B., 2011. A systematic review of the efficacy of MWM. In: Vicenzino, B., Hing, W., Rivett, D., Hall, T. (Eds.), Mobilisation With Movement: The Art and the Science. Churchill Livingstone Australia, Chatswood, NSW, pp. 26–64.

Braun, B.L., 1999. Effects of ankle sprain in a general clinic population 6 to 18 months after medical evaluation. Arch. Fam. Med. 8 (2), 143–148.

Brukner, P., Khan, K., 2012. Brukner & Khan's Clinical Sports Medicine, 4th ed. McGraw-Hill Australia, North Ryde, NSW.

Collins, N., Teys, P., Vicenzino, B., 2004. The initial effects of a Mulligan's mobilization with movement technique on dorsiflexion and pain in subacute ankle sprains. Man. Ther. 9 (2), 77–82.

Denegar, C.R., Hertel, J., Fonseca, J., 2002. The effect of lateral ankle sprain on dorsiflexion range of motion, posterior talar glide, and joint laxity. J. Orthop. Sports Phys. Ther. 32 (4), 166–173.

Gilbreath, J.P., Gaven, S.L., Van Lunen, L., Hoch, M.C., 2014. The effects of mobilization with movement on dorsiflexion range of motion, dynamic balance, and self-reported function in individuals with chronic ankle instability. Man. Ther. 19 (2), 152–157.

Green, T., Refshauge, K., Crosbie, J., Adams, R., 2001. A randomized controlled trial of a passive accessory joint mobilization on acute ankle inversion sprains. Phys. Ther. 81 (4), 984–994.

Hetherington, B., 1996. Lateral ligament strains of the ankle, do they exist? Man. Ther. 1 (5), 274–275.

Hidalgo, B., Hall, T., Berwart, M., Biernaux, E., Detrembleur, C., 2018. The immediate effects of two manual therapy techniques on ankle musculoarticular stiffness and dorsiflexion range of motion in people with chronic ankle rigidity: a randomized clinical trial. J. Back Musculoskelet. Rehabil. 31 (3), 515–524.

Hopper, D., Samsson, K., Hulenik, T., Ng, C., Hall, T., Robinson, K., 2009. The influence of Mulligan ankle taping during balance performance in subjects with unilateral chronic ankle instability. Phys. Ther. Sport 10 (4), 125–130.

Hubbard, T.J., Hertel, J., 2008. Anterior positional fault of the fibula after sub-acute lateral ankle sprains. Man. Ther. 13 (1), 63–67.

Hubbard, T.J., Hertel, J., Sherbondy, P., 2006. Fibular position in individuals with self-reported chronic ankle instability. J. Orthop. Sports Phys. Ther. 36 (1), 3–9.

Kim, S.L., Lee, B.H., 2016. Effect of Mulligan's mobilization with movement technique on gait function in stroke patients. J. Phys. Ther. Sci. 28 (8), 2326–2329.

Kim, S.L., Lee, B.H., 2018. The effects of posterior talar glide and dorsiflexion of the ankle plus mobilization with movement on balance and gait function in patient with chronic stroke: a randomized controlled trial. J. Neurosci. Rural Pract. 9 (1), 61–67.

Marron-Gomez, D., Rodriguez-Fernandez, A.L., Martin-Urrialde, J.A., 2015. The effect of two mobilization techniques on dorsiflexion in people with chronic ankle instability. Phys. Ther. Sport 16 (1), 10–15.

Matthews, M.L.G., Claus, A.P., 2014. Two examples of 'cuboid syndrome' with active bone pathology: why did manual therapy help? Man. Ther. 19 (5), 494–498.

Merlin, D.J., McEwan, I., Thom, J.M., 2005. Mulligan's mobilisation with movement technique for lateral ankle pain and the use of magnetic resonance imaging to evaluate the "positional fault" hypothesis. Paper presented at The Accelerated Rehabilitation of the Injured Athlete, XIV International Congress on Sports Rehabilitation and Traumatology. Isokinetic, Bologna, Italy.

Moiler, K., Hall, T., Robinson, K., 2006. The role of fibular tape in the prevention of ankle injury in basketball: a pilot study. J. Orthop. Sports Phys. Ther. 36 (9), 661–668.

Mooney, M., Maffey-Ward, L., 1994. Cuboid plantar and dorsal subluxations: assessment and treatment. J. Orthop. Sports Phys. Ther. 20 (4), 220–226.

Moore, K.L., Dalley, A.F., Agur, A.M.R., 2014. Clinically Oriented Anatomy, 7th ed. Wolters Kluwer / Lippincott Williams & Wilkins Health, Philadelphia.

Mulligan, B.R., 2010. Manual Therapy: 'NAGs', 'SNAGs', 'MWMs', etc., 6th ed. Orthopedic Physical Therapy Products, Wellington, NZ.

O'Brien, T., Vicenzino, B., 1998. A study of the effects of Mulligan's mobilization with movement treatment of lateral ankle pain using a case study design. Man. Ther. 3 (2), 78–84.

13

Patterson, S.M., 2006. Cuboid syndrome: a review of the literature. J. Sports Sci. Med. 5 (4), 597–606.

Thomas, M.J., Roddy, E., Zhang, W., Menz, H.B., Hannan, M.T., Peat, G.M., 2011. The population prevalence of foot and ankle pain in middle and old age: a systematic review. Pain 152 (12), 2870–2880.

Vicenzino, B., Branjerdporn, M., Teys, P., Jordan, K., 2006. Initial changes in posterior talar glide and dorsiflexion of the ankle after mobilization with movement in individuals with recurrent ankle sprain. J. Orthop. Sports Phys. Ther. 36 (7), 464–471.

Waterman, B.R., Belmont, P.J., Jr., Cameron, K.L., Deberardino, T.M., Owens, B.D., 2010. Epidemiology of ankle sprain at the United States Military Academy. Am. J. Sports Med. 38 (4), 797–803.

13

Pain release phenomenon

TECHNIQUES FOR PAIN RELEASE PHENOMENON

INTRODUCTION

The pain release phenomenon (PRP) procedure is in sharp contrast to the Mulligan Concept of MWM (Mulligan, 2010). The PRP seeks to exert a manual force that is pain provocative at its starting point of application, whereas the manual force applied with an MWM (the first M) does not provoke pain. The analogue to the mobilisation (the second M) in MWM can be a joint compression, joint compression with movement (physiological or accessory), a passive soft tissue stretch or an isometric muscle contraction that provokes the patient's pain.

When a movement of the body is painful, the nervous system will often find ways in which to perform the movement in a different way, most likely in an attempt to avoid further aggravation of pain. Pain avoidance can then lead to mechanical dysfunction. In an acute or a chronic pain situation, it has been established that the second-order neurons can become sensitised (central sensitisation) to the point that even innocuous afferent input can be perceived as painful (Woolf, 1983; Woolf & King, 1987; Woolf & Salter, 2000). Movement of any structure (joint, muscle, tendon, ligament, etc.) results in a cumulative barrage of afferent information into the dorsal horn from multiple segmental levels. This flood of afferent information impedes the ability of the central nervous system to isolate the pain source, perpetuating and sometimes generalising (spreading) the dysfunctional movement and the pain.

A PRP has the unique ability to isolate the structural source of the pain, the specific pain-provoking direction of movement and the amount of force that produces the patient's (familiar) pain. This movement is very specific and may not be a typical movement performed in daily living, such as compression with an accessory glide. This also possibly explains why the pain is often not relieved with more traditional manual therapy. If the familiar pain is reproduced by compression with an accessory glide, it may indicate the nociceptive source is osseous, cartilaginous or capsular. If the painful stimulus is an active muscular contraction, it may indicate a muscular, tendinous or periosteal structural (attachment of muscle and tendon) source to the pain. Reproduction of the familiar pain with a passive end-range stretch of a structure in a very isolated manner may suggest either capsular, ligamentous or musculotendinous involvement.

The amount of manual force that is applied with a PRP must comply with two fundamental rules: (1) the pain must not exceed 4 on an 11-point numerical pain rating scale (NRS, where 0 = no pain and 10 = most severe pain imaginable), and (2) the pain must be 0 on that NRS within 20 seconds of its sustained application. If the pain diminishes to 0 prior to 20 seconds, more force is applied, but the pain must not exceed 4 on the NRS and it still must diminish to 0 within 20 seconds. If the pain does not diminish to 0 within 20 seconds, then less force can be applied in order to achieve this target. The PRP that follows these two fundamental rules is repeated until pain can no longer be elicited. The expectation is that this will occur within a treatment session and might manifest as higher force to provoke pain, earlier abolishment of pain and more difficulty in eliciting the patient's pain at the outset. If a force level cannot be found to comply with these two fundamental rules, then the PRP is not appropriate and should be discontinued.

The success of PRP relies on the patient's understanding that there will be pain up to 4 on an NRS and that they must inform the therapist when the pain is provoked, increased or reduced (including abolished) during the application of the manual force. The patient must inform the therapist if the pain increases once it has been provoked at the outset of the application of the PRP. As for all techniques in this book, the therapist should obtain informed consent from the patient prior to initiating the PRP treatment.

PRP is beneficial in pain states that have been present for at least 6 weeks and there are no clear signs of an acute inflammatory process. The mechanism by which PRP might bring about relief of long-term pain is unknown, but would plausibly involve local receptor hysteresis / creep effects as well as other centrally mediated endogenous inhibitory systems. Some examples of conditions that have responded well to PRP are demonstrated in this chapter.

Thus to effectively employ a PRP, the therapist must be capable of simultaneously reasoning across several categories of decision-making hypotheses, as discussed by Jones and Rivett (2004). Key categories that must be considered in using a PRP include: pathobiological mechanisms (both the stage of tissue healing and the involved pain mechanisms), physical impairments and associated structure / tissue sources for the pain, precautions and contraindications related to treatment, and actual management and treatment decisions (e.g. direction, intensity, dosage). The use of a PRP should therefore be considered only when pain-free MWMs and other less-provocative manual therapy procedures have first been trialled. A PRP should not be used if pain does not subside within the 20-second application period.

14

Levels of evidence

There is only one low-level study on the clinical efficacy of this technique. The randomised controlled trial involving 60 participants compared the effectiveness of the combined treatment of physiotherapy and PRP with physiotherapy alone in the treatment of patella–femoral pain syndrome (Shahid et al., 2016). The group treated with PRP demonstrated greater reduction in pain (VAS) and improved function (in the Functional Index Questionnaire) when compared with the group receiving physiotherapy alone (Shahid et al., 2016). This study, and anecdotal clinical reports of substantial gains made in some cases that were recalcitrant to other treatments, underpins the necessity for clinical trials and case series / studies to be conducted and reported.

14

TRAPEZIUM – FIRST METACARPAL JOINT PRP

TECHNIQUE AT A GLANCE

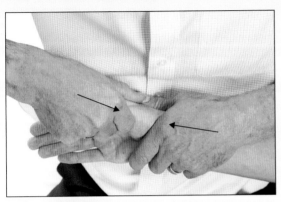

Figure 14.1
Thumb compression PRP: hand placement close
view

- The therapist sits next to patient and stabilises the first metacarpal with the thumb and index finger of one hand and the trapezium with the thumb and index finger of the other hand.
- The therapist reproduces the patient's pain by applying appropriate manual force (compression, or compression with movement).
- The therapist applies a passive compression through the first metacarpal onto the trapezium.
- While the compression is maintained the therapist moves the thumb in a direction that reproduces the patient's pain at a level of no more than 4/10 and diminishes to 0/10 within 20 seconds.
- See Fig. 14.1.

INDICATION

Subacute or chronic pain in the carpometacarpal joint of the thumb that has not responded to other treatment interventions.

POSITIONING

Patient:	Seated, in a chair or on a treatment table.
Treated body part:	The therapist supports the involved hand and thumb.
Therapist:	Seated next to the patient securely supporting the hand and thumb close to their body.
Hands/contact points:	The first metacarpal is stabilised with the thumb and index finger of one hand; the trapezium is stabilised with the thumb and index finger of the other hand.

(continued next page...)

14

APPLICATION GUIDELINES

- The therapist must be able to reproduce the patient's pain (comparable sign) by applying an appropriate compression or compression with movement.
- Apply a passive compression through the first metacarpal onto the trapezium. While the compression is maintained, flex and extend, then abduct and adduct and, if needed, rotate the trapezium until the direction that reproduces the patient's pain is identified.
- When performing these tests avoid end-range movements because you are searching for articular pain (with compression PRP); if the joint is moved to end range the symptoms experienced may be capsular or ligamentous in nature.
- The compression and movement are continued while the patient is questioned about the level of the pain being produced. An appropriate level of pain is in the range of 4/10.
- The compression with movement is continued while the patient's report of pain is closely monitored. The time required to abolish the pain should be less than 20 seconds and will progressively diminish with each application of the technique – that is, 15 seconds, to 10 seconds, to 5 seconds, etc. This procedure is repeated until the pain can no longer be elicited with the PRP technique.
- If the pain abates immediately, the force of the compression with movement should be increased to reach the initial 4/10 appropriate pain report. If, once the pain of 4/10 is reached, the pain increases then the technique should be stopped, the applied force reduced and the PRP technique repeated. If the pain again increases the PRP technique is discontinued.

VARIATIONS

- If the thumb pain cannot be abolished with the PRP technique the therapist might try to position the thumb closer to the midline of the body (or across the midline) and repeat the PRP successfully.
- The underlying mechanism that explains this clinical observation is unknown. It is compelling to speculate that the mechanism by which positioning the thumb nearer the body's midline improves the PRP involves the sensory motor system.

COMMENT

- During performance of the trapezium–first metacarpal PRP there may be a considerable amount of crepitus encountered. This is not unusual at this joint and should not negatively influence the decision to perform a PRP. However, the therapist must adhere to the 4/10 pain and 20-second rules.

SELF-MANAGEMENT

- When a positive treatment effect is achieved in the clinic the therapist may decide to instruct the patient on how to perform the PRP technique as a self-management tool. Precautions on the intensity of the force applied and avoiding exacerbation of the symptoms must be clearly outlined and understood prior to recommending the PRP self-treatment.

ANNOTATIONS

sit L 1st MC/Trapezium Comp PRP×20 sec(3)
sit L 1st MC/Trapezium self Comp PRP×20 sec(3)

14

TENNIS ELBOW PRP WITH A MUSCLE CONTRACTION (LATERAL EPICONDYLALGIA)

TECHNIQUE AT A GLANCE

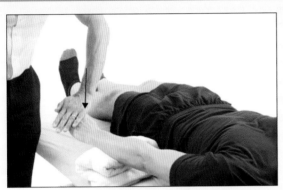

Figure 14.2
Tennis elbow PRP: wrist extension

- The patient is seated or lying on a plinth with their wrist in neutral and their elbow positioned in the most pain-provocative position, which is usually full extension.
- The therapist is next to the patient with one hand on the involved elbow and the other over the dorsum of the involved hand.
- The therapist reproduces the lateral elbow pain (comparable sign) with an isometric contraction (most commonly an isometric wrist extension).
- The patient performs an isometric extension against the therapist producing a pain of 4/10.
- The therapist maintains the same amount of load and the patient contracts to the same effort. Use of a dynamometer would remove any uncertainty about a constant isometric load being maintained.
- The isometric contraction is continued till the patient reports the abolition of pain (approximately 20 seconds).
- This procedure is repeated until the familiar pain can no longer be elicited with the PRP technique.
- See Fig. 14.2.

INDICATION

Subacute or chronic lateral elbow pain that has not responded to other treatment interventions.

POSITIONING

Patient:	Seated, well supported in a chair or lying on a treatment table.
Treated body part:	Wrist is in neutral and the elbow is positioned in the most pain-provocative position, which is usually full extension. However, if the pain cannot be abolished, the elbow will need to be flexed and the procedure repeated.
Therapist:	Seated or standing next to the patient with access to the involved elbow and hand.
Hand contact:	The therapist has one hand on the involved elbow and the other over the dorsum of the involved hand.

(continued next page...)

14

APPLICATION GUIDELINES

- The therapist must be able to reproduce the patient's lateral elbow pain (comparable sign) by asking the patient to actively contract the wrist or finger extensors.
- The patient is instructed to extend the wrist against isometric resistance provided by the therapist and is questioned about the level of pain being produced, which should be no more than 4/10.
- The isometric contraction is continued (at a constant load) while the patient's report of pain is closely monitored. The time required to abolish the pain should be less than 20 seconds and will progressively diminish with each application of the technique – that is, 15 seconds, to 10 seconds, to 5 seconds, etc. This procedure is repeated until the familiar pain can no longer be elicited with the PRP technique.
- If the pain abates immediately, the force of the isometric contraction should be increased to reach the initial 4/10 appropriate pain report. If the pain increases the technique should be stopped, the applied force reduced, and the PRP technique repeated. If the pain again increases the PRP technique is discontinued.

VARIATIONS

- To progress the technique the patient slightly flexes and abducts the shoulder and extends the elbow while resistance is applied to wrist and/or finger extension.
- If muscle contraction PRP is not successful a trial of soft tissue stretching PRP (Fig. 14.3) can be initiated. The therapist must be able to reproduce the patient's lateral elbow pain by applying a soft tissue stretch to the wrist and finger extensors. Follow the same procedure but with the stretch as the provocative movement.
- Initially keeping the patient's arm close to their body may increase the likelihood of a successful outcome. Adding small amounts of pronation or supination of the forearm in addition to the wrist flexion will be helpful in the fine-tuning provocation of the patient's pain.

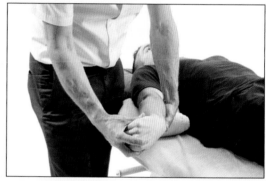

Figure 14.3
Tennis elbow: PRP passive stretch

COMMENT

- In some cases, resisting extension of the third and fourth fingers, versus the wrist, reproduces the patient's pain more specifically and so can be used instead.

SELF-MANAGEMENT

- When a positive treatment effect is achieved in the clinic the therapist may decide to instruct the patient on how to perform the PRP technique as a self-management tool.
- Precautions on the intensity of the force applied and avoiding exacerbation of the symptoms must be clearly outlined and understood prior to recommending the PRP self-treatment.

ANNOTATIONS

sup ly L Elb Contraction PRP Wr E×20 sec
sup ly L Elb Contraction PRP Finger E×20 sec
sup ly L Elb Stretch PRP Wr Extensors×20 sec(3)
sit L Elb self Contraction PRP Wr E×20 sec(3)

14

CHRONIC PAINFUL SHOULDER PRP

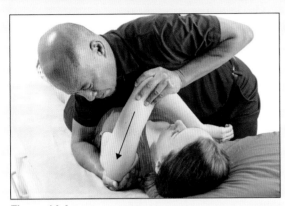

Figure 14.4
Shoulder PRP: hand placement

- The patient lies supine with their involved shoulder in 90° of flexion and a small amount of horizontal adduction and elbow flexed.
- The therapist stands on the uninvolved side of the patient.
- The therapist places one hand over the bent elbow and the other is placed under the scapula.
- The therapist reproduces the patient's shoulder pain by applying a posterior humeral glide, which is most efficiently applied through using the therapist's body weight through the patient's flexed elbow.
- The passive stretch is maintained (i.e. sustain similar load) till the patient reports the abolition of pain (approximately 20 seconds).
- This procedure is repeated until the patient's pain can no longer be elicited with the PRP technique.
- See Fig. 14.4.

14

INDICATION

Subacute or chronic shoulder pain that has not responded to other treatment interventions.

POSITIONING

Patient:	Lying supine.
Treated body part:	Involved shoulder in 90° of flexion and a small amount of horizontal adduction. The elbow is in flexion.
Therapist:	Standing on the uninvolved side of the patient.
Hand contact:	One hand is placed over the posterior aspect of the elbow and the other is placed under the scapula (alternative: a towel can be used under the scapula). The therapist's anterior shoulder and chest is placed on the hand that is covering the elbow.

APPLICATION GUIDELINES

- The therapist must be able to reproduce the patient's shoulder pain (comparable sign) by applying a compression of the glenohumeral joint and associated structures.
- The therapist applies a posterior humeral glide by applying their body weight through the patient's flexed elbow. It may be necessary to add horizontal adduction of the humerus to elicit the patient's precise pain.
- The pressure through the humerus is sustained while the patient's report of pain is closely monitored. The time required to abolish the pain should be less than 20 seconds and will progressively diminish with each application of the technique – that is, 15 seconds, to 10 seconds, to 5 seconds, etc. This procedure is repeated until the patient's pain can no longer be elicited with the PRP technique.
- If the pain abates immediately, the force of the posterior glide should be increased to reach the initial 4/10 appropriate pain report. If the pain increases the technique should be stopped, the applied force reduced and the PRP technique repeated. If the pain again increases the PRP technique is discontinued.

COMMENT

- The addition of the horizontal adduction increases the soft tissue tension on the posterior structures of the shoulder, which may assist in reproducing the patient's pain.

ANNOTATION

 sup ly L Sh Post gl PRP×20 sec(3)

14

HIP PAIN (FABER POSITION) PRP

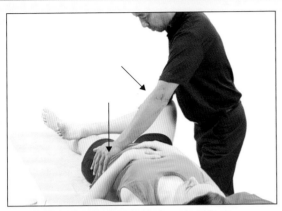

Figure 14.5
FABER PRP: start point

- The patient lies supine on a treatment table with the involved hip placed in a flexed, abducted and externally rotated position (FABER).
- The therapist places one hand on the anterior superior iliac spine (ASIS) on the uninvolved side; the other hand is placed on the medial aspect of the involved side's knee.
- The therapist stabilises the opposite side's ASIS with one hand.
- The hand on the knee applies an anterior to posterior directed force to the medial aspect of the involved side's knee. The force moves the involved hip further into the FABER position.
- The AP force is maintained in this position (i.e. force that is sufficient to obtain a 4/10 pain at the outset) until the patient reports the abolition of pain (approximately 20 seconds).
- This procedure is repeated until the patient's pain can no longer be elicited with the PRP technique.
- See Fig. 14.5.

14

INDICATION

Subacute or chronic hip pain that has not responded to other treatment interventions.

POSITIONING

Patient:	Lying supine on a treatment table.
Treated body part:	The involved hip is placed in a flexed, abducted and externally rotated position.
Therapist:	Stands on the side of the involved hip.
Hands/contact points:	One hand is placed on the ASIS of the uninvolved side; the other hand is placed on the medial aspect of the involved side's knee.

APPLICATION GUIDELINES

- The therapist must be able to reproduce the patient's hip pain (comparable sign) by placing the hip into FABER.
- The therapist stabilises the opposite side's ASIS with one hand (e.g. left hand on left ASIS).
- The other hand applies an anterior to posterior directed force to the medial aspect of the involved side's knee. The force moves the involved hip further into the FABER position.
- The AP force is maintained while the patient's report of pain is closely monitored, which should not exceed 4/10. The time required to abolish the pain should be less than 20 seconds and will progressively diminish with each application of the technique – that is, 15 seconds, to 10 seconds, to 5 seconds, etc. The range of motion into the FABER position may increase as a result of the technique, so on repeating and progressing the PRP the therapist should take up the slack to account for this new range. This procedure is repeated until the patient's pain can no longer be elicited with the PRP technique.
- If the pain abates immediately, the force of the glide should be increased to reach the initial 4/10 appropriate pain report. If the pain increases the technique should be stopped, the applied force reduced, and the PRP technique repeated. If the pain again increases the PRP technique is discontinued.

VARIATIONS

- If the patient's hip pain cannot be elicited with a passive increase in the FABER position then an active increase in FABER through the contraction of the posterior hip muscles can be trialled.
- The therapist's positioning for the muscle contraction technique is the same, with the exception of moving the hand from the medial aspect of the knee to the lateral aspect. The patient is instructed to move their involved side's knee towards the floor while the therapist firmly resists the movement.
- If the contraction reproduces the patient's hip pain, the no more than 4/10 pain level and 20-second rules are followed.

COMMENT

- This technique is described to resolve hip pain but, based on the mechanics of the FABER position, the sacroiliac joint will undergo compression and may be responsible for some of the pain-relieving results.

ANNOTATIONS

sup ly R Hip Contraction PRP FABER×20 sec(3)
sup ly R Hip Stretch PRP FABER×20 sec(3)

14

HIP PAIN (POSTERIOR SHEAR) PRP

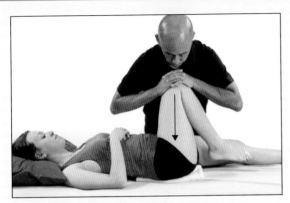

Figure 14.6
Thigh thrust PRP: lateral view

- The patient lies supine on a treatment table with the involved hip flexed to 90° with slight adduction.
- The therapist stands on the opposite side of the involved hip with both hands placed on top of the flexed knee, and against their anterior shoulder and chest.
- The therapist performs a posterior femoral glide by applying their body weight through the patient's flexed knee.
- The posterior glide force through the femur is maintained till the patient reports the abolition of pain (approximately 20 seconds).
- This procedure is repeated until the patient's pain can no longer be elicited with the PRP technique.
- See Fig. 14.6.

14

Subacute or chronic hip pain that has not responded to other treatment interventions.

POSITIONING

Patient:	Lying supine on a treatment table.
Treated body part:	The involved hip is flexed to 90° with slight adduction.
Therapist:	Stands on the opposite side of the involved hip.
Hands/contact points:	Both hands are placed on top of the flexed knee, and against their anterior shoulder and chest.

APPLICATION GUIDELINES

- The therapist must be able to reproduce the patient's hip pain (comparable sign) by applying a posterior glide of the thigh.
- The therapist performs a posterior femoral glide by applying their body weight through the patient's flexed knee. It may be necessary to add horizontal adduction of the femur to elicit the patient's pain.
- The posterior femoral glide is maintained while the patient's report of pain is closely monitored (no more than 4/10). The time required to abolish the pain should be less than 20 seconds and will progressively diminish with each application of the technique – that is, 15 seconds, to 10 seconds, to 5 seconds, etc. This procedure is repeated until the patient's pain can no longer be elicited with the PRP technique.
- If the pain abates immediately, the force of the glide should be increased to reach the initial 4/10 appropriate pain report. If the pain increases the technique should be stopped, the applied force reduced, and the PRP technique repeated. If the pain again increases the PRP technique is discontinued.

COMMENTS

- Like the FABER PRP hip technique, this posterior femoral glide technique applies force to the associated joints (sacroiliac joint and lumbar spine), which may be partially responsible for the pain-relieving results achieved.
- The addition of the horizontal adduction increases the soft tissue tension on the posterior structures of the hip, which may assist in reproducing the patient's pain. This might be more effective than the straight posterior glide for some chronic hip conditions.

ANNOTATION

sup ly R Hip Post gl PRP×20 sec(3)

References

Jones, M.A., Rivett, D.A., 2004. Introduction to clinical reasoning. In: Jones, M.A., Rivett, D.A. (Eds.), Clinical Reasoning for Manual Therapists. Butterworth-Heinemann, Edinburgh, pp. 3–24.

Mulligan, B., 2010. Manual Therapy: 'NAGs', 'SNAGs', 'MWMs', Etc., 6th ed. Orthopedic Physical Therapy Products, Wellington, NZ.

Shahid, S., Ahmed, A., Ahmed, U., 2016. Effectiveness of routine physical therapy with and without pain release phenomenon in patello-femoral pain syndrome. Int. J. Sci. Res. 5 (7), 1891–1919.

Woolf, C.J., 1983. Evidence for a central component of post-injury pain hypersensitivity. Nature 306 (5944), 686–688.

Woolf, C.J., King, A.E., 1987. Physiology and morphology of multireceptive neurons with C-afferent fiber inputs in the deep dorsal horn of the rat lumbar spinal cord. J. Neurophysiol. 58 (3), 460–479.

Woolf, C.J., Salter, M.W., 2000. Neuronal plasticity: increasing the gain in pain. Science 288 (5472), 1765–1769.

14

Index

Page numbers followed by 'f' indicate figures, 't' indicate tables and 'b' indicate boxes.